Handbook of Cardiovascular CT

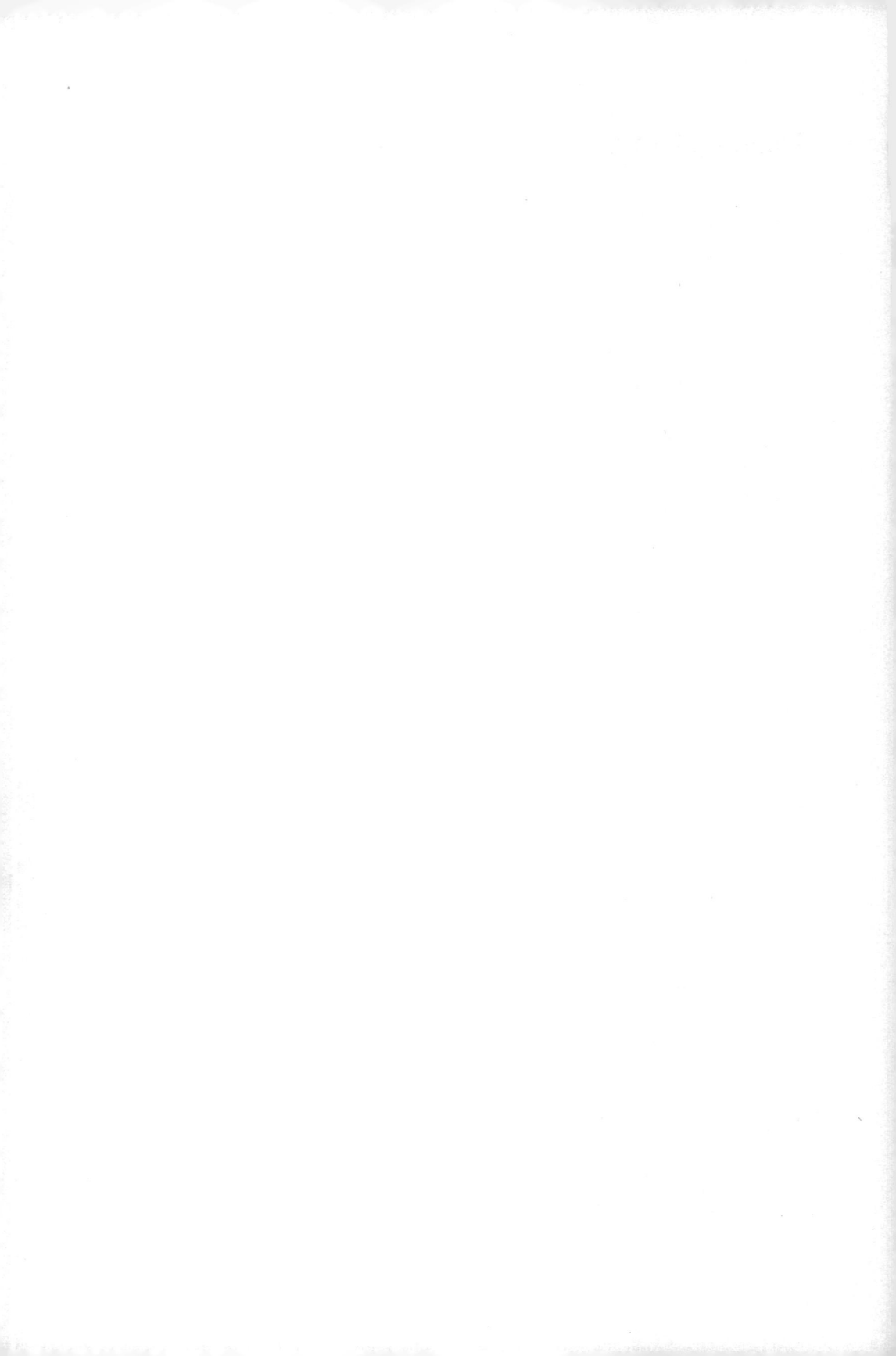

Matthew J. Budoff · Jerold S. Shinbane
Editors

Handbook of Cardiovascular CT

Essentials for Clinical Practice

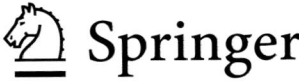 Springer

Editors

Matthew J. Budoff, MD, FACC, FAHA
Los Angeles Biomedical Research Institute at
  Harbor-UCLA Medical Centre
Torrance, CA, USA

Jerold S. Shinbane, MD, FACC
Division of Cardiovascular Medicine
University of Southern California
Keck School of Medicine
Los Angeles, CA, USA

ISBN: 978-1-84800-091-9   e-ISBN: 978-1-84800-092-6
DOI: 10.1007/978-1-84800-092-6

British Library Cataloguing in Publication Data
Handbook of cardiovascular CT : essentials for clinical
    practice
    1. Cardiovascular system - Tomography 2. Cardiovascular
    system - Diseases - Diagnosis
    I. Budoff, Matthew J. II. Shinbane, Jerold S.
    616.1′075722
A catalogue record for this book is available from the British Library

Library of Congress Control Number: 2008931855

Printed on acid-free paper

springer.com

Preface

This book has been created as a primer to help cardiologists, radiologists, and other cardiac-imaging enthusiasts to have a handy reference tool for the answers to important questions related to cardiovascular computed tomography (CCT). CCT has evolved from novel technology to research tool to essential clinical imaging modality at an astounding pace. The technology has great relevance for the multitude of medical and surgical disciplines focused on the treatment of cardiovascular disease. Imaging of anatomy, physiology, and tissue characteristics from large-to-small vessel within seconds, and reconstruction to multimodal 2- and 3-D images within minutes, has facilitated practical clinical applications important to cardiovascular diagnosis, risk stratification, and procedure guidance. The new wave in technology requires education and training of initial generations of readers and users of CCT focused on providing an understanding of the essentials of methodology, technique, and image analysis for clinical application. This text serves as a primer for the practical performance and interpretation of CCT. The breadth and depth of the knowledge of the individual authors have provided concise chapters on essential topics, with additional teaching pearls as well as key images.

Matthew J. Budoff
Torrance, California, USA

Jerold S. Shinbane
Los Angeles, California, USA

Acknowledgments

I would like to thank the authors of the chapters not only for their excellent and concise contributions, but also for their innovations that continue to move this field forward. To my family, especially Vicky, Daniel and Garrett, who put up with my long hours in front of my laptop while creating this book. To Jerold, who did the lion's share of work for this book, for without his encouragement and assistance, this never would have come to be.

Matthew J. Budoff, MD FACC, FAHA

I would like to thank Matthew Budoff, whose dedication, enthusiasm, and intellectual curiosity has continued to move the field of cardiovascular CT forward in innovative directions. I would also like to thank the chapter authors for their ability to instill their significant expertise in cardiovascular CT into clear, concise, and accessible chapters. To my family, especially Rosemary, Anna, and Laura, thank you for your continued encouragement and support.

Jerold S. Shinbane, MD FACC

Contents

Contributors

Antonio Bellasi, MD
Department of Urology, Department of Medicine and Division of Cardiology, Emory University School of Medicine, Atlanta, GA, USA,
e-mail: abellas@emory.edu

Daniel S. Berman, MD
Department of Imaging, Cedars Sinai Medical Centre, Los Angeles, CA 90048, USA, e-mail: bermand@cshs.org

William D. Boswell, MD, FACR
Department of Radiology, Los Angeles, CA, USA, e-mail: wbosw@usc.edu

Matthew J. Budoff, MD, FACC, FAHA
Los Angeles Biomedical Research Institute, Harbor-UCLA Medical Center, Torrance, CA, USA, e-mail: mbudoff@labiomed.org

Tracy Q. Callister, MD
Department of Cardiology, Tennessee Heart and Vascular Institute, Sumner, 353 New Shackle Island Road, Nashville, TN 37075 USA,
e-mail: tracycallister@comcast.net

Patrick M. Colletti, MD
Department of Radiology and Medicine, University of Southern California, Los Angeles, CA, USA, e-mail: colletti@usc.edu

Bjorn P. Flygenring, MD
Cardiovascular Services Division, Minneapolis Heart Institute, Minneapolis, MN, USA, e-mail: bjorn.flygenring@allina.com

John D. Friedman, MD
Department of Imaging, Cedars-Sinai Medical Centre, Los Angeles, CA, USA,
e-mail: John.Friedman@cshs.org

Mario J. García, MD, FACC, FACP
Cardiovascular Institute, Mount Sinai Hospital, New York, NY 10029, USA,
e-mail: garcia@mountsinai.org

Guido Germano, PhD
Artificial Intelligence Programme, Cedars-Sinai Medical Centre, Los Angeles,
CA, USA, e-mail: guido.germano@cshs.org

Ambarish Gopal, MD
Division of Cardiology, Los Angeles Biomedical Research Institute at Harbor-
UCLA Medical Centre, Torrance, CA, USA, e-mail: ambarishgopal@hotmail.com

Ilan Gottlieb, MD
Department of Medicine/Cardiology, John Hopkins University, Baltimore,
MD, USA, e-mail: igottli1@jhmi.edu

Sean W. Hayes, MD
Department of Cardiac Imaging, Cedars-Sinai Medical Centre, Los Angeles,
CA, USA, e-mail: Sean.Hayes@cshs.org

Harvey S. Hecht, MD, FACC
Department of Cardiology, Lenox Hill Heart and Vascular Institute, New York, NY,
USA, e-mail: HHecht@LENOXHILL.NET

Alan T. Hirsch, MD
Vascular Medicine Programme, Minneapolis Heart Institute Foundation and the
University of Minnesota, Minneapolis, MN, USA, e-mail: hirsc005@umn.edu

Udo Hoffmann, MD, MPH
Cardiac MR PET CT Program, Department of Radiology, Massachusetts General
Hospital, Harvard Medical School, Boston, MA, USA,
e-mail: uhoffmann@partners.org

Roland P. Karlsberg, MD
Cardiovascular Medical Group of Southern California, Cedars Sinai Medical
Centre, Los Angeles, CA, USA, e-mail: Karlsberg@CVmg.com

Thomas Knickelbine, MD, FACC, FSCAI
Department of Cardiology, Minneapolis Heart Institute Foundation and the University of Minnesota, Minneapolis, MN, USA, e-mail: thomas.knickelbine@allina.com

Kai H. Lee, PhD
Department of Radiology, Los Angeles County and University of Southern
California Medical Center, Los Angeles, CA, USA, e-mail: kailee@usc.edu

Stamatios Lerakis, MD, PhD
Department of Medicine, Division of Cardiology, Emory University School
of Medicine, Atlanta, GA, USA, e-mail: slerak@emory.edu

John R. Lesser, MD
Department of Cardiology, Minneapolis Heart Institute Foundation and the
University of Minnesota, Minneapolis, MN, USA, e-mail: john.lesser@allina.com

João Lima, MD, MBA
Department of Medicine/Cardiology, John Hopkins University, Baltimore, MD,
USA, e-mail: jlima@jhmi.edu

Terrence F. Longe, MD, FACC
Department of Cardiology, Minneapolis Heart Institute Foundation and the University of Minnesota, Minneapolis, MN, USA, e-mail: Terrence.longe@allina.com

Songshou Mao, MD
Department of Cardiology, Los Angeles Biomedical Research Institute,
Harbor-UCLA Medical Center, Torrance, CA, USA, e-mail: smao@labiomed.org

Khurram Nasir, MD, MPH
Cardiac MR PET CT Programme, Massachusetts General Hospital, Boston,
MA, USA, e-mail: KNASIR@PARTNERS.ORG

Susanna Prat-González, MD
Cardiovascular Institute, Mount Sinai Hospital, New York, NY, USA,
e-mail: susanna.prat@mssm.edu

Paolo Raggi, MD, PhD
Department of Medicine and Division of Cardiology, Emory Cardiac Imaging
Centre, Emory University School of Medicine, Atlanta, GA 30322, USA,
e-mail: praggi@excite.com

Ian S. Rogers, MD, MBA
Cardiac MR PET CT Program, Division of Cardiology and Department of
Radiology, Massachusetts General Hospital, Harvard Medical School, Boston,
MA, USA

Alan Rozanski, MD
Department of Medicine, St Luke's Roosevelt Hospital Centre, Clifton, NJ, USA,
e-mail: Arozonsk@chpnet.org

John A. Rumberger, MD, PhD, FACC
Director of Cardiac Imaging, Cardiovascular Diseases, The Princeton Longevity
Centre, Princeton, NJ, USA; Clinical Professor of Medicine, The Ohio State
University, Columbus, Ohio, e-mail: jrumberger@theplc.net;

Javier Sanz, MD
Cardiovascular Institute, Mount Sinai Hospital, New York, NY, USA, e-mail:
javier.sanz@mssm.edu

Rola Saouaf, MD
Department of Imaging, Cedars Sinai Medical Centre, Los Angeles, CA, USA

Ammar Sarwar, MD
Cardiac MR PET CT Programme, Massachusetts General Hospital, Boston,
MA, USA

Michael D. Shapiro, DO
Cardiac MR PET CT Programme, Massachusetts General Hospital, Boston,
MA, USA, e-mails: mdshapiro@partners.org, shapiromi@gmail.com

David M. Shavelle, MD, FACC, FSCAI
David Geffen School of Medicine at UCLA, Division of Cardiology, Harbor-UCLA
Medical Centre, Torrance, CA, USA, e-mail: dshavelle@hotmail.com

Leslee J. Shaw, PhD
Department of Medicine, Emory University School of Medicine, Atlanta, GA,
USA, e-mail: lshaw3@emory.edu

Jerold S. Shinbane, MD, FACC
Division of Cardiovascular Medicine, USC Keck School of Medicine, Los Angeles,
CA, USA, e-mail: shinbane@usc.edu

Jabi E. Shriki, MD
Department of Radiology, LAC + USC Medical Centre, Los Angeles, CA, USA,
e-mail: jabishriki@gmail.com

Robert S. Schwartz, MD, MS
Minneapolis Heart Institute Institute Foundation and the University of Minnesota,
Minneapolis, MN, USA, e-mail: rss@rsschwartz.com

Piotr J. Slomka, PhD
Department of Imaging, Cedars-Sinai Medical Centre, Los Angeles, CA, USA,
e-mail: Piotr.Slomka@cshs.org

Dr Lance E. Sullenberger, MD
Cardiology Service, Walter Reed Army Medical Center, Washington, DC, USA;
Uniformed Services University of the Health Sciences, Bethesda MD, e-mail:
lancewrame@yahoo.com

Allen J. Taylor, MD
Walter Reed Army Medical Centre, Department of Cardiology, Washington, DC,
USA, e-mail: allen.taylor@na.amedd.army.mil

Louise E.J. Thomson, MBChB
Department of Imaging, Cedars Sinai Medical Centre, Los Angeles, CA, USA;
Uniformed Services University of the Health Sciences, Bethesda MD,
e-mail: Louise.Thomson@cshs.org

Todd C. Villines, MD
Department of Cardiology, Walter Reed Army Medical Centre, Washington,
DC, USA

Wm Guy Weigold, MD
Division of Cardiovascular Disease, Dept. of Medicine, Washington Hospital
Centre, Washington, DC, 20010, USA, e-mail: Guy.Weigold@MedStar.net

Chapter 1
Cardiovascular CT Angiography: Concepts Important to Image Acquisition and Reconstruction

Matthew J. Budoff, Songshou Mao, Patrick M. Colletti,
and Jerold S. Shinbane

Meticulous attention to the methodology of image acquisition and reconstruction is essential to performance and analysis of coronary artery CT angiography. High-quality images must be captured during the most quiescent phase of coronary artery motion while minimizing patient exposure to radiation and intravenous contrast agents. Successful imaging requires an understanding of the temporal interplay of multiple motions including the complexities of cardiac contraction, potential respiratory motion, potential patient movement, table motion, gantry rotation, and timing and movement of the bolus of intravenous contrast through the structures of interest (**Fig. 1.1**). Additional factors relate to the use of x-ray energy to capture adequate images balanced by the limitation of radiation to the lowest level possible.

1.1 Concepts for Image Acquisition

There are many interdependent factors that affect spatial and temporal resolution. The goal of image acquisition is to visualize the target structures in their entirety while limiting the field of view (FOV) to the region of clinical interest. For a given voxel matrix, smaller FOVs yield smaller voxels and greater spatial resolution. Voxel attenuation is measured (on a scale) with the attenuation values of different substances represented by different Hounsfield units (HU) values [1]. Representative HU values include the following: air –1000, fat –50 to –100, water 0, muscle 10–40, contrast 300–500, and calcium 130–1500.

Conceptually, all multidetector computed tomography (MDCT) systems work using similar principles, but vary in regard to specific components and features. A MDCT system has an x-ray tube that is capable of extremely rapid rotation and a collimated array of detectors. The x-ray tube provides radiation energy adjustable through tube current (mAs) and tube voltage (kVP). Multiple rows of detectors are arranged in a variety of arrays with the goal of covering a specified volume during each gantry rotation. Advances in detector number and arrangement have

M.J. Budoff
Los Angeles Biomedical Research Institute, Harbor-UCLA Medical Center, Torrance, CA, USA
e-mail: mbudoff@labiomed.org

M.J. Budoff, J.S. Shinbane (eds.), *Handbook of Cardiovascular CT*,
DOI: 10.1007/978-1-84800-091-9_1, © Springer-Verlag London Limited 2008

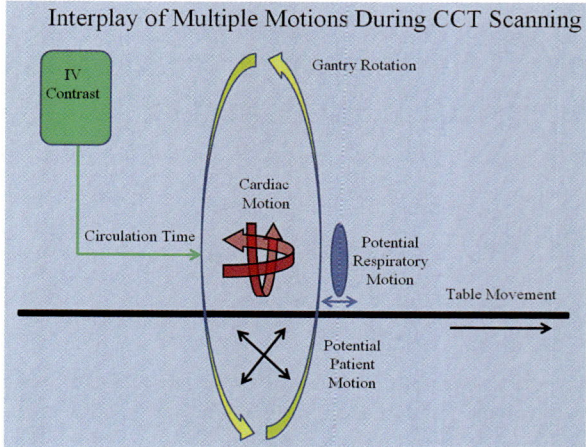

Fig. 1.1 The multiple motions during cardiac CT acquisition. Red signifies the cardiac motion. Yellow represents the gantry movement (rotation of the x-ray tube and detectors around the patient). Black represents the table motion and blue represents potential respiratory motion. An additional consideration is the time from the vein injection to the arrival of contrast in the coronary circulation (green)

lead to increases in the volume of coverage per rotation, with the ultimate goal being imaging the entire heart within one cardiac cycle.

The relationship between table movement, gantry rotation speed, and beam collimation defines the volume coverage per rotation as well as the degree of overlap between rotations. The concept of "pitch" quantifies this relationship. Pitch relates to coverage obtained by the x-ray beam (through beam width and table movement) during one rotation of the gantry and defines the amount of overlap of acquired data. With a pitch value of less than 1, there is overlap between volumes of coverage. Overlapping images allow for oversampling, permitting multisector image reconstruction, at the expense of greater radiation exposure. The definition of pitch has evolved with newer scanner technologies, and various equations have been proposed depending on the specific type of scanner [2]. Newer systems have thinner slice thickness and collimation, allowing for an even lower pitch resulting in more images, thinner reconstruction intervals, and better visualization of the coronary anatomy.

ECG triggering is essential to minimize the effects of cardiac motion on image acquisition. Factors related to motion in the X, Y, and Z directions include coronary artery and cardiac motion during the cardiac cycle related to heart rate and rhythm. In MDCT, images are usually acquired with retrospective ECG gating. With this approach, images are acquired throughout the cardiac cycle, and therefore can be reconstructed at specific points in the cardiac cycle [3]. With image acquisition, an ECG signal is simultaneously recorded with the raw dataset. Given the complexities of coronary motion, the optimal timing for reconstruction can vary by artery or arterial segment. The strength of this approach is that after data acquisition has occurred, images can be reconstructed at the most optimal timing for the coronary arteries. Additionally, acquisition of images throughout the cardiac cycle allows for volumetric assessment of cardiac function. The major drawback of this approach is that radiation exposure is significantly greater than that with a prospective ECG-gated approach. Tube current modulation leads to a significant decrease in radiation by decreasing radiation exposure during the systolic phase of the cardiac cycle [4]. With prospective triggering, images are obtained at a set percentage of the R–R interval. The advantage of this technique is the limitation to radiation exposure [5]. The disadvantage relates to the limited dataset obtained. If the images obtained demonstrate significant motion artifact, there are no other images to reconstruct. Given the variability of heart rate with arrhythmias, prospective gating can be problematic with significant ectopy or atrial fibrillation.

Breath hold is essential to limit motion of structures due to respiration during image acquisition. Breath hold times have decreased significantly with advances in technology and are in the range of 6–10 second. There is some controversy as to the optimal phase of respiration for breath hold. Regardless of the phase chosen in an individual lab, it is important to practice breath hold commands and exercises prior to the scan. As an end-inspiratory breath hold will place structures more caudally than an end-expiratory breath hold, consistent breath hold instructions need to be given for preview images and actual scans.

1.2 Preview Scans

Cardiovascular CT is performed using planar scout images, a non-contrast calcium scan, a timing scan for assessment of the circulation time, and a contrast scan. Planar scout images are obtained in order to define the most cranial and caudal scanning levels (z-axis) of the structures of interest. The scout images are obtained in antero-posterior and lateral views and aligned to the patient by a laser system. The scan volume is selected with the structures of interest placed within the center of the scanning volume. Important landmarks can be identified including the left atrial appendage, which is usually the most cranial structure of the heart, and the ventricular apex, which is the most caudal structure. Although the carina serves as a marker to localize the most cranial aspect of the heart, the distance from carina to left main coronary artery is extremely variable [6]. Additionally, the LAD can course cranial to the left main coronary artery (**Fig. 1.2**). For coronary artery imaging, scanning 10 mm cranial to the left main coronary artery and 10 mm caudal to the apex is subsequently performed with CT angiography. In patients with coronary artery bypass grafts, the starting point is the top of the aortic arch or 10 mm higher than the surgical metal clips. The mid-level of the right pulmonary artery can also be used as the beginning of the scan level, if it can be defined in preview images.

After the scout images, a calcium scan is performed. This is a high-resolution non-contrast cardiac-gated study, which provides important prognostic information regarding future cardiovascular risk. For the calcium scan, the 2-D axial images are analyzed with the identification of calcium using either manual or automated

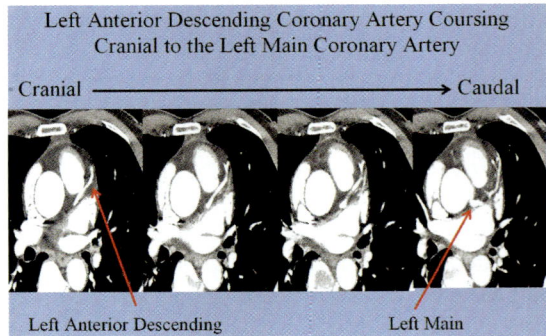

Fig. 1.2 Serial axial slices from cranial (left) to caudal (right) demonstrating a case where the left anterior decending (left panel arrow) is visible above the left main coronary artery (right panel arrow)

methods with quantification of calcium score based on identification of HU units with an attenuation of at least 130 HU in the areas of identified calcium. There are two major methods of quantifying coronary artery calcium: the Agatston score and the volumetric analysis. The Agatston score is based on the summation of plaque area times a coefficient based on the peak HU units in the plaque for all identified plaques [7]. Calcium volume score describes a volumetric analysis of calcium with calculation based on volumetric reconstruction and is more reproducible on serial studies [8]. The calcium score is a marker of plaque burden and is an independent risk factor for CAD beyond traditional risk factors [9, 10].

The calcium scan is useful to the planning, performance, and interpretation of the contrast CT angiogram. Assessment of the images can be used to ensure that there is complete coverage of the coronary anatomy in the image set prior to contrast angiography, as well as to determine the minimum volume to be covered to minimize radiation exposure [11]. Extensive coronary calcification may prohibit the accurate assessment of coronary artery stenoses. The calcium score as well as the calcium distribution should be assessed prior to the performance of the CT angiogram to determine whether the contrast study should be performed. Different imaging centers use various cutoffs for the performance of CT angiography in the setting of a significantly elevated calcium score, with some centers using >500 or >1000. It is important to have an understanding of the specific goal of an individual study, as depending on the question asked and the location of calcium, some studies may still be performed. For example, in cases where the location and patency of coronary artery bypass grafts is the clinical question, calcium in the native coronary arteries may still not necessarily prohibit the study from being performed. In addition to traditional cardiac risk factors, knowledge of the calcium score is helpful in assessing the pretest probability of coronary artery disease when interpreting the contrast angiography images.

After performance of the calcium scan, a contrast angiography study is performed, with the administration of iodinated contrast timed to enhance the structures of interest. This may vary by the type of study, with some studies performed specifically for assessment of coronary artery anatomy, while others performed for additional assessment of thoracic structures, such as in the case of congenital heart disease. Assessment of the circulation time is important for the appropriate timing from contrast injection to the acquisition of images, to assure the optimal enhancement of target structures. The test sequence for this typically consists of repetitively imaging a single slice using a low mAs, low radiation dose technique. For coronary angiography, scans are obtained at the level of the takeoff of the left main coronary artery, to create a time–density curve to assess the time to peak opacification. The measured transit time is then used as the delay time from the start of the contrast injection to the start of the imaging for the CT coronary angiogram. Circulation times vary based on factors including cardiac output and must be individually determined. Patients with low-output states require increased time delays and those with high-output states require decreased time delays. This step can be omitted with the use of bolus-tracking software. These methods track the contrast enhancement within the vessel of interest and automatically trigger image acquisition [12].

After determination of the circulation time, the contrast CT angiogram is performed. The circulation time is useful for determining the time to begin scanning, but the goal is to maintain the same level of vascular enhancement throughout image acquisition. Multiphase contrast injectors with preset volumes and injection velocities are used to maintain uniformity of contrast enhancement throughout the study. The use of a saline bolus after contrast injection moves the residual contrast in the intravenous tubing and arm veins into the heart and coronary vasculature. The timing of the saline bolus is important, as in some studies, clearance of the venous circulation and right heart structures can help in visualization of arterial structures, while in other studies, enhancement of these structures is important for analysis.

1.3 Image Reconstruction and Analysis

Image reconstruction allows creation of a 3-D map of cardiovascular anatomy from larger vessels to smaller vessels. Serial axial 2-D images are reconstructed into a 3-D data cube with subsequent use of software to edit out and analyze cardiovascular structure (**Fig. 1.3**). Interpretation of CT coronary angiography requires reconstruction and analysis of multiple 2-D and 3-D projections so that findings can be confirmed on multiple views and artifacts caused by a particular type of reconstruction can be identified. Improved workstation software has dramatically reduced the time for image editing and reconstruction. Systematic reconstruction, serial automated editing, and analysis of the 3-D data cube allows one to glean information important to characterization of the relationships between structures essential to clinical diagnosis and planning and facilitation of cardiovascular procedures. These reconstructions include the following:

1. Displays of thoracic structures in relation to skeletal structures (an example would be relation of sternum to coronary and vascular structures in a patient undergoing repeat sternotomy after prior coronary artery bypass grafting)

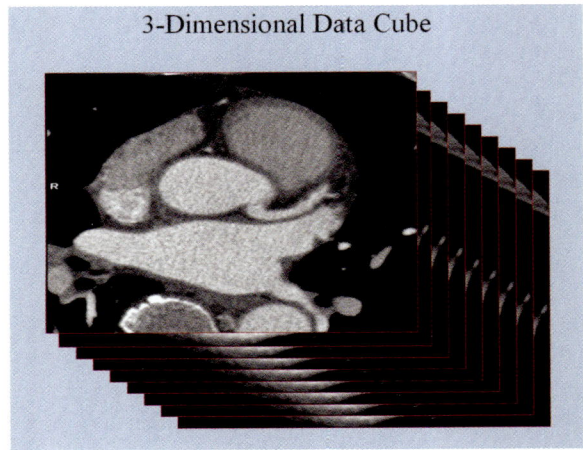

Fig. 1.3 Serial axial slices are taken every 0.5 millimeters (mm) to 0.625 mm (depending on the scanner manufacturer), usually cranial to caudal. The workstation then reconstructs the three-dimensional or curved multiplanar images

2. Relation of large vessel vasculature and structures (relation for surgical approaches, anomalous structures, chest pathology)
3. Cardiac structures and relationships (cardiac chambers, valves, and coronary vasculature)
4. Coronary artery anatomy
5. Global and regional quantification of cardiac function

Image reconstruction is dependent on image acquisition as the reconstructed images are only as good as the acquired data. The raw datasets are imported to workstations with software suitable for the analysis of images in multiple 2-D and 3-D formats. Prior to reconstruction, the 2-D axial dataset must be reviewed to ensure that the structures of interest were scanned in their entirety and that there is uniformity of contrast enhancement throughout the study. For coronary arterial studies assessment, the 2-D images must be analyzed for complete vessel visualization and the degree of contrast uniformity between slices. Decreased contrast in the distal vessels can simulate stenoses. Adequate and uniform enhancement of the distal aorta can be helpful in ensuring that distal coronary arteries have been adequately visualized.

Reconstruction of coronary artery anatomy requires assessment of the correct phase of the cardiac cycle during which an artery or arterial segment is most quiescent. Retrospectively gated axial images can be reconstructed at different diastolic phases of the cardiac cycle and assessed for the most optimal images regarding minimizing cardiac motion. The optimal phase of the cardiac cycle may vary by artery and arterial segment. Once the correct phase or phases have been chosen, 2-D images can be rapidly formatted in axial, sagittal, and coronal planes, as well as along the long and short axes of the heart.

Although the 3-D reconstructed images are both attractive and seemingly intuitive regarding ease of interpretation, it is essential to recognize that the process of reconstruction has limitations. The 2-D views provide an entire dataset, whereas the 3-D views typically use selectively reduced data with potential artifactual information loss. Given the limitations of reconstruction techniques, it is important to continually reference back to the 2-D images and view potential findings using multiple types of reconstructions before making a diagnosis.

Volume-rendering pixels above a chosen threshold are assigned HU depending on their attenuation. Automated editing discards pixels below a certain HU cutoff (lower threshold 80–100 HU). Volume rendering and editing software allow creation of 3-D images with overlying structures removed to adequately visualize structures of interest. There can be loss of data through over-editing of structures with the potential of cutting out portions of the coronary arteries associated with using automated or manual methods, with editing of unenhanced or partially enhanced structures based on certain HU cutoffs. Removal of structures such as the atrial appendage and coronary sinus and great cardiac vein allows for better visualization of the circumflex coronary artery, and removal of the pulmonary trunk allows viewing of the left main coronary artery. Reconstruction of 2-D images can also create artifacts due to motion between slices or volumes, with discontinuous arterial segments that could be misinterpreted if only 3-D image sets of the coronaries are obtained. Volumetric images with differences in cardiac respiratory or patient motion on different slices may result in artifacts that may appear as obstructive lesions. Lack of uniform contrast enhancement on serial slices may result in artifactual appearance of stenoses. Reconstruction may also be limited in structures that course into myocardium such as myocardial bridging.

Reconstruction may be limited by partial volume effects. Isotropic data, where the spatial resolution is equal in the x, y, and z axes, allows for the ability to obtain accurate images with multiplane reconstructions [13]. As CT slice thickness is typically 0.5–0.6 mm, spatial resolution in the z-axis may not be truly isotropic with in-plane resolution of 0.4 mm (e.g., FOV = 200 mm, matrix = 512 × 512 pixels), and some volume averaging of data may occur with reconstruction of longitudinal structures. This can make assessment of the coronary arterial wall challenging for assessment of different tissue components of the plaque wall.

Multiple image display methods are important for comprehensive analysis [14] (**Fig. 1.4**). Maximal intensity projections (MIPs) demonstrate the maximal attenuation point at each point in a 3-D volume. Conceptually, this provides the ability to move through the 3-D data cube with a thick slab focused on the maximum intensity of the images in the slab. MIPs help to demonstrate smaller and more distal vessels. This may be useful for differentiating calcium, contrast enhancement, and metal stents in the coronary arteries. With unedited MIPs, there will be overlap of structures as one moves through the dataset. MIPs may be edited to enhance specific anatomy. Multiplanar reformatting with curved surface reformation allows for longitudinal analysis of an individual vessel [15]. A reconstruction is performed orthogonal to vessel centerline and does not require editing. Vessels can be analyzed in a 360-degree rotation, allowing for assessment of eccentricity of plaque in relation

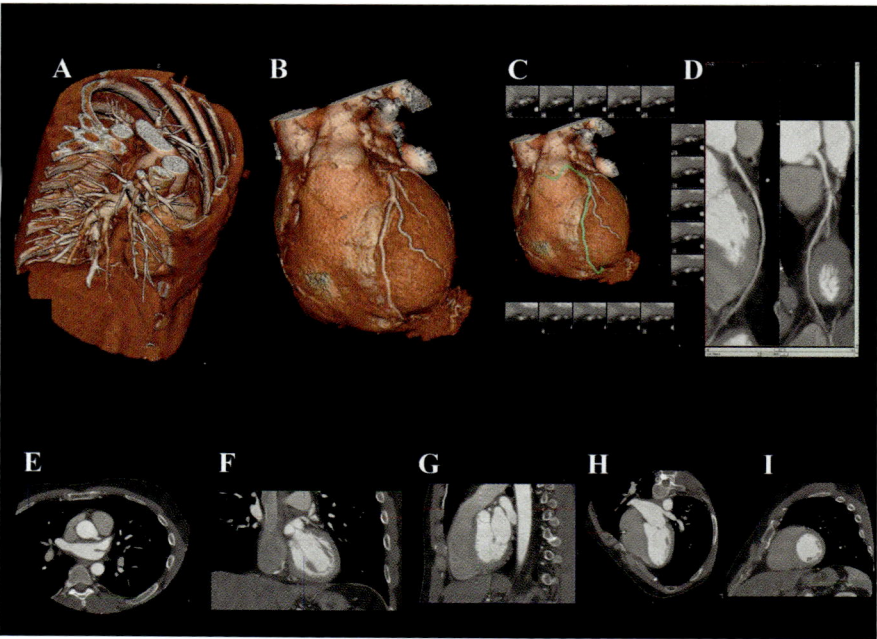

Fig. 1.4 Multiple CT angiography views are demonstrated including: (**A**) 3-D volume-rendered view of thorax, (**B**) 3-D volume-rendered view of the heart and coronary arteries, (**C**) 3-D volume-rendered view with vessel tracking, (**D**) Curved multiplanar reformatted view, (**E**) 2-D axial view, (**F**) 2-D coronal view, (**G**) 2-D sagittal view, (**H**) 2-D four-chamber view, (**I**) 2-D short-axis view

to the vessel lumen. The technique requires accurate vessel tracking and determination of the centerline of the vessel. Interactive display methods may provide greater diagnostic accuracy than pre-rendered images [14]. Virtual endoscopic views that provide a perspective from inside a vessel or chamber have been developed, but are very dependent on filtering, smoothing, and display techniques. Fluoroscopic views are helpful for assessment of metallic structures such as pacemaker leads and prosthetic valves.

Current CT scanners and workstations allow for rapid acquisition and reconstructions of images for the characterization of cardiovascular disease processes. An understanding of the concepts, technology, indication for study, pretest probability of pathology, and strengths and limitations of imaging and analysis of data are essential to the performance and interpretation of cardiovascular CT imaging.

1.4 Clinical Data with Coronary Artery Calcification

Although atherosclerotic vascular disease accounts for more death and disability than all types of cancer, a screening tool to detect subclinical atherosclerosis (such as coronary artery calcium) and target prevention of future cardiovascular events is only now starting to be adopted. In about 50% of individuals, the initial presentation of CAD is a myocardial infarction (MI) or cardiac death. Conventional office-based risk screening methods, such as Framingham risk score (FRS) in the United States or from the *Pro*spective *Car*diovascular *Mü*nster (PROCAM) study in Germany, are among the most common and widely available for estimating multi-factorial absolute risk in clinical practice; however, these prediction models have limitations [16]. In these studies, more than ½ of all cardiovascular events occur in those patients with low or intermediate risk, rather than the high risk cohort. These risk factor assessment tools only predict 60–65% of cardiovascular risk, leaving many individuals to have cardiovascular events in the absence of traditional risk factors for atherosclerosis [17].

1.4.1 Risk Stratification in Asymptomatic Patients

The American Heart Association (AHA), the American College of Cardiology (ACC), and the National Cholesterol Education Program (NCEP) endorse use of the risk prediction algorithm from the Framingham Heart Study, followed by calcium scoring in those persons found to be intermediate risk [18]. Akosah and colleagues highlighted the shortcomings of Framingham assessment in a study of previously asymptomatic younger adults (men <55 and women <65 years of age), who were hospitalized for their first acute myocardial infarction [19]. Of 222 such patients identified in a three year period, 75% would not have been considered for statin therapy according to the NCEP guidelines, suggesting missed opportunities for prevention of CHD. Furthermore, current population-based risk prediction algorithms appear to perform poorly in women [20]. Intermediate risk patients currently do not qualify for the most intensive risk factor interventions, yet they may have risk factors that exceed desirable levels. It is this group that may benefit the most from further risk stratification, as CAC testing is effective at identifying increased risk and in motivating effective behavioral changes.

1.5 Coronary Calcium – Basis and Background

The presence of calcium in coronary arteries is pathognomonic of atherosclerosis [18]. The close correlation between the atherosclerotic plaque burden and the extent of CAC has been confirmed both by histopathology and intravascular ultrasound [18].

Similar to CTA, electrocardiographic gating and breathholding techniques are utilized, however the radiation dose of calcium scoring is only 1 millisievert and studies take less than 5 minutes, with no contrast requirements. While most centers do not employ beta blockade during calcium scoring, it will lead to improved reproducibility and less motion artifacts when quantifying calcium.

1.6 Coronary Artery Calcification and Obstructive Disease

Coronary calcified plaque by cardiac CT has a high sensitivity and negative predictive power for obstructive CAD but limited specificity. CAC can assist the clinician in effectively "ruling out" angiographically significant CAD in symptomatic patients [21]. In a study of 1851 patients undergoing angiography and CAC, a negative score (no calcification) was highly associated with no obstruction on angiography (negative predictive power of 98%). The specificity of CAC for obstructive disease is on the order of 40%. Specificity of CAC for atherosclerosis is almost 100%. Thus, clinicians must understand a positive calcium scan indicates atherosclerosis, but most often, no significant stenosis. The absence of coronary calcium is most often associated with a normal nuclear test and no obstructive disease on angiography. A recent study of 1,195 patients who underwent CAC measurement with CAC and myocardial perfusion SPECT (MPS) assessment demonstrated that CAC was often present in the absence of MPS abnormalities (normal nuclear test), and that <2% of all patients with CAC <100 had positive MPS studies [22]. This is supported by the other published reports and is synthesized in a recent appropriateness guideline from the American Society of Nuclear Cardiology and the American College of Cardiology [23]. The ACC/ASNC appropriateness criteria suggest that a low score precludes the need for MPS assessment, and a high score would warrant further assessment. These criteria suggest nuclear testing may generally be inappropriate in patients with calcium scores < 100, as the probability of obstruction or abnormal scan is very low. A person with an Agatston score >400 may benefit from functional testing to detect occult ischemia.

The vast majority of heart attacks (60–83%) occur at the site of a non-obstructive plaque. Exercise testing or pharmacologic cardiac imaging (nuclear or echo) will only diagnose high grade coronary stenoses. They will fail to identify a vast number of asymptomatic patients at risk because an obstructive coronary plaque (stenosis in the artery of >50% severity) is most often NOT the site of the cardiovascular event (MI or sudden cardiac death). Thus, calcium scoring and functional testing may be synergistic to identify the person with atherosclerosis (CAC) and obstructive disease (functional test).

1.6.1 Prediction of Events in Asymptomatic Persons using Coronary Calcium

The extent of coronary atherosclerosis, rather than the severity of stenosis, is the most important predictor of death due to acute MI or sudden cardiac death [25].The extent of CAC has been shown in many studies to predict cardiac events in asymptomatic individuals [18]. Shaw and colleagues reported the relationship of CAC to all-cause mortality in the largest cohort studied to date, consisting of 10,377 asymptomatic individuals (40% women), followed for an average of 5 ± 3.5 years. In both men and women, CAC was an independent predictor of death (p<0.001), and the risk increased proportionally to the baseline calcium scores (risk factor adjusted relative risk of 1.6, 1.7, 2.5, and 4 for CAC 11–100, 101–400, 401–1000, and greater than 1000 respectively) [26].

The St. Francis Heart Study, a prospective observational study of almost 5000 persons, evaluated coronary calcium scores, risk factors and C-reactive protein, and included these variables in the multivariate model [27]. A calcium score >100 (moderate plaque present) predicted all atherosclerotic cardiovascular disease events and the sum of non-fatal MI and coronary death events with relative risks of 9.5–10.7 at 4.3 years, as compared to patients with scores <100. This prospective study strongly demonstrated the ability to utilize this test to rule out patients who don't need therapy. Thus, a negative scan was associated with a 0.05% per year risk of events. In the St Francis Heart Study with 4,903 asymptomatic persons age 50–70 years, only 8/1504 (0.5%) persons with scores of zero had a coronary event over the next 4.3years; with an annual event rate of only 0.1%, demonstrating a low risk group (zero calcium score) that may be effectively treated with lifestyle changes. EBT was predictive of coronary events, while highly sensitive CRP was not.

The Multi-Ethnic Study of Atherosclerosis (MESA) recently reported assessment of 6,814 adults in diverse ethnic groups including African Americans, Chinese, Hispanics, and Caucasians aged 45–85 who were felt to be free of cardiovascular disease at baseline [28]. According to Detrano et al, after median follow-up of 41 months, the hazard ratios for future hard CHD event (myocardial infarction or MI related death) with CAC >100 vs. CAC = 0 was 10.8 (4.8–24.2, p<0.0001). These risk ratios are very much similar to previous published studies and confirm the pooled summary findings previously reported and lay to rest of any concern regarding the prognostic value of CAC testing. To date, summary data from over 20 prognostic studies have demonstrated that elevated calcium scores are associated with an approximate 10-fold increased risk of cardiovascular events. Therefore, patients with CAC scores >100 should be considered for statin therapy, aspirin and possibly ACE inhibition, given the increased cardiovascular risk associated with this level of coronary atherosclerosis, concurring with the current NCEP Adult Treatment Panel (ATP) III guidelines. This will support the conclusions of the AHA [18] and the National Cholesterol Education Panel that high coronary calcium scores confirm increased risk for future cardiac events: "measurement of coronary calcium is an option for advanced risk assessment in appropriately selected persons. In persons with multiple risk factors, high coronary calcium scores (e.g., >75th percentile for age and sex) denote advanced coronary atherosclerosis and provide a rationale for intensified LDL lowering therapy." By identifying high-risk patients, CAC may help select those patients who would benefit most from additional testing (e.g. non-invasive stress imaging) and intensification of medical therapy. Furthermore, the AHA (American Heart Association) scientific statement states, "A negative test (score = 0) makes the presence of atherosclerotic plaque, including unstable or vulnerable plaque, highly unlikely, and is consistent with a low risk (0.1% per year) of a cardiovascular event in the next 2–5 years" [18]. From the available data, intermediate risk patients benefit most from further risk stratification, as CAC testing is effective at identifying increased risk and in improving adherence to statin therapy [29].

1.7 Clinical Pearls for Coronary Calcium Assessment

- The absence of calcium is associated with normal coronary arteries and low cardiovascular risk.
- The presence of coronary calcium is indicative of atherosclerosis, not necessarily obstructive disease.
- Calcium scores > 100 are associated with a 10 fold increased risk of cardiovascular events.
- Calcium scores >400 in asymptomatic persons may benefit from functional testing to detect occult ischemia.
- The specificity of CAC for obstructive disease is on the order of 40%.
- Specificity of CAC for atherosclerosis is almost 100%.
- Intermediate risk patients (by Framingham assessment) will benefit the most by calcium scanning and restratification.
- The radiation dose is low, approximately 1 milliSeivert per study.

The following chapters will detail the methodology and techniques for the use of cardiovascular CT for the assessment of cardiovascular disease processes.

References

1. Brooks RA. A quantitative theory of the Hounsfield unit and its application to dual energy scanning. J Comput Assist Tomogr 1977, 1(4): 487–93.
2. Silverman PM, Kalender WA, Hazle JD. Common terminology for single and multislice helical CT. AJR Am J Roentgenol 2001, 176(5): 1135–6.
3. Becker CR, Knez A, Ohnesorge B, Schoepf UJ, Reiser MF. Imaging of noncalcified coronary plaques using helical CT with retrospective ECG gating. AJR Am J Roentgenol 2000, 175(2): 423–4.
4. Abada HT, Larchez C, Daoud B, Sigal-Cinqualbre A, Paul JF. MDCT of the coronary arteries: feasibility of low-dose CT with ECG-pulsed tube current modulation to reduce radiation dose. AJR Am J Roentgenol 2006, 186(6 Suppl 2): S387–90.
5. Husmann L, Valenta I, Gaemperli O, Adda O, Treyer V, Wyss CA, et al. Feasibility of low-dose coronary CT angiography: first experience with prospective ECG-gating. Eur Heart J 2008, 29(2): 191–7.
6. Bakhsheshi H, Mao S, Budoff MJ, Bin L, Brundage BH. Preview method for electron-beam CT scanning of the coronary arteries. Acad Radiol 2000, 7(8): 620–6.
7. Agatston AS, Janowitz WR, Hildner FJ, Zusmer NR, Viamonte M, Jr., Detrano R. Quantification of coronary artery calcium using ultrafast computed tomography. J Am Coll Cardiol 1990, 15(4): 827–32.
8. Callister TQ, Cooil B, Raya SP, Lippolis NJ, Russo DJ, Raggi P. Coronary artery disease: improved reproducibility of calcium scoring with an electron-beam CT volumetric method. Radiology 1998, 208(3): 807–14.
9. Greenland P, LaBree L, Azen SP, Doherty TM, Detrano RC. Coronary artery calcium score combined with Framingham score for risk prediction in asymptomatic individuals. Jama 2004, 291(2): 210–5.
10. Greenland P, Bonow RO, Brundage BH, Budoff MJ, Eisenberg MJ, Grundy SM, et al. ACCF/AHA 2007 clinical expert consensus document on coronary artery calcium scoring by computed tomography in global cardiovascular risk assessment and in evaluation of

patients with chest pain: a report of the American College of Cardiology Foundation Clinical Expert Consensus Task Force (ACCF/AHA Writing Committee to Update the 2000 Expert Consensus Document on Electron Beam Computed Tomography) developed in collaboration with the Society of Atherosclerosis Imaging and Prevention and the Society of Cardiovascular Computed Tomography. J Am Coll Cardiol 2007, 49(3): 378–402.

11. Gopal A, Budoff MJ. A new method to reduce radiation exposure during multi-row detector cardiac computed tomographic angiography. Int J Cardiol 2007 [Epub ahead of print].

12. Cademartiri F, Nieman K, van der Lugt A, Raaijmakers RH, Mollet N, Pattynama PM, et al. Intravenous contrast material administration at 16-detector row helical CT coronary angiography: test bolus versus bolus-tracking technique. Radiology 2004, 233(3): 817–23.

13. Tsukagoshi S, Ota T, Fujii M, Kazama M, Okumura M, Johkoh T. Improvement of spatial resolution in the longitudinal direction for isotropic imaging in helical CT. Phys Med Biol 2007, 52(3): 791–801.

14. Ferencik M, Ropers D, Abbara S, Cury RC, Hoffmann U, Nieman K, et al. Diagnostic accuracy of image postprocessing methods for the detection of coronary artery stenoses by using multidetector CT. Radiology 2007, 243(3): 696–702.

15. Achenbach S, Moshage W, Ropers D, Bachmann K. Curved multiplanar reconstructions for the evaluation of contrast-enhanced electron beam CT of the coronary arteries. AJR Am J Roentgenol 1998, 170(4): 895–9.

16. Kannel WB, D'Agostino RB, Sullivan L, et al. Concept and usefulness of cardiovascular risk profiles. Am Heart J 2004, 14: 16–26.

17. Raggi P. Coronary-calcium screening to improve risk stratification in primary prevention. J La State Med Soc 2002, 154: 314–8.

18. Budoff MJ, Achenbach S, Blumenthal RS, et al. Assessment of Coronary Artery Disease by Cardiac Computed Tomography. A Statement from the American Heart Association Committee on Cardiovascular Imaging and Intervention, Council on Cardiovascular Radiology and Intervention, and Committee on Cardiac Imaging, Council on Clinical Cardiology. Circulation 2006, 114(16): 1761–91.

19. Akosah KO, Shaper A, Cogbill C, et al. Preventing myocardial infarction in the young adult in the first place: how do the National Cholesterol Education Panel III guidelines perform? J Am Coll Cardiol 2003, 41: 1475–9.

20. Michos ED, Nasir K, Braunstein JB, et al. Framingham risk equation underestimates subclinical atherosclerosis risk in asymptomatic women. Atherosclerosis 2006, 184: 201–6.

21. Budoff MJ, Raggi P, Berman D, et al. Continuous Probabilistic Prediction of Angiographically Significant Coronary Artery Disease Using Electron Beam Tomography. Circulation 2002, 105: 1791–6.

22. Berman DS, Wong ND, Gransar H, et al. Relationship between stress-induced myocardial ischemia and atherosclerosis measured by coronary calcium tomography. J Am Coll Cardiol 2004, 44(4): 923–30.

23. Brindis RG, Douglas PS, Hendel RC, et al. ACCF/ASNC appropriateness criteria for single-photon emission computed tomography myocardial perfusion imaging (SPECT MPI): a report of the American College of Cardiology Foundation Quality Strategic Directions Committee Appropriateness Criteria Working Group and the American Society of Nuclear Cardiology endorsed by the American Heart Association. J Am Coll Cardiol 2005, 46: 1587–605.

24. Giroud D, Li JM, Urban P, et al. Relation of the site of acute myocardial infarction to the most severe coronary arterial stenosis at prior angiography. Am J Cardiol 1992, 69: 729–32.

25. Schmermund A, Baumgart D, Goerge G, et al. Coronary artery calcium in acute coronary syndromes: a comparative study of electron-beam computed tomography, coronary angiography, and intracoronary ultrasound in survivors of acute myocardial infarction and unstable angina. Circulation 1997, 96: 1461–9.

26. Shaw LJ, Raggi P, Schisterman E et al. Prognostic Value of Cardiac Risk Factors and Coronary Artery Calcium Screening for All-Cause Mortality. Radiology 2003, 28: 826–33.

27. Arad Y, Goodman KJ, Roth M, et al. Coronary calcification, coronary disease risk factors, C-reactive protein, and atherosclerotic cardiovascular disease events: the St. Francis Heart Study. J Am Coll Cardiol 2005, 46: 158–65.
28. Detrano R, Guerci AD, Carr JJ, Bild DE, Burke G, Folsom AR, Liu K, Shea S, Szklo M, Bluemke DA, O'Leary DH, Tracy R, Watson K, Wong ND, Kronmal RA. Coronary calcium as a predictor of coronary events in four racial or ethnic groups. N Engl J Med 2008, 358: 1336–45
29. Kalia NK, Miller LG, Nasir K, et al. Visualizing coronary calcium is associated with improvements in adherence to statin therapy. Atherosclerosis 2006, 185(2): 394–9.

Chapter 2
Cardiovascular CT Imaging: Essentials for Clinical Practice

Patient Selection and Preparation

Tracy Q. Callister

2.1 Patient Selection and Indications for Coronary CTA

The current clinical indications for coronary CTA are in evolution and not firmly established.

Patients who are most likely to benefit from coronary CTA are as follows: (1) intermediate risk patients who have undiagnosed chest symptoms and (2) patients with equivocal results from any other noninvasive test.

Following are the published indications for coronary CTA:

1. Detection of CAD: Symptomatic–Evaluation of Intra-Cardiac Structures
   Evaluation of suspected coronary anomalies.
2. Detection of CAD: Symptomatic–Acute Chest Pain
   Intermediate pre-test probability of CAD with no ECG changes and serial enzymes negative.
3. Detection of CAD with Prior Test Results–Evaluation of Chest Pain Syndrome
   Uninterpretable or equivocal stress test (exercise, perfusion, or stress echo).
4. Structure and Function–Morphology
   Assessment of complex congenital heart disease including anomalies of the coronary, circulation, great vessels, and cardiac chambers and valves.
   Evaluation of coronary arteries in patients with new-onset heart failure to assess etiology.
5. Structure and Function–Evaluation of Intra- and Extra- Cardiac Structures
   Evaluation of suspected cardiac mass (tumor or thrombus).
   Patients with technically limited images from echo, MRI, or TEE.
   Evaluation of pericardial conditions (pericardial mass, constrictive pericarditis, or complications of cardiac surgery.
   Evaluation of pulmonary vein anatomy prior to invasive radiofrequency ablation for atrial fibrillation.

T.Q. Callister
Tennessee Heart and Vascular Institute, Nashville, TN 37075
e-mail: tracycallister@comcast.net

M.J. Budoff, J.S. Shinbane (eds.), *Handbook of Cardiovascular CT*,
DOI: 10.1007/978-1-84800-091-9_2, © Springer-Verlag London Limited 2008

Noninvasive coronary vein mapping prior to placement of biventricular pace-maker.

Noninvasive coronary arterial mapping, including internal mammary artery prior to repeat cardiac revascularization.

6. Structure and Function–Evaluation of Aortic and Pulmonary Disease

Evaluation of suspected aortic dissection or aneurysm.

Evaluation of suspected pulmonary embolism.

Following are the contraindications for coronary CTA:

1. Pregnancy
2. Known contrast allergy
3. Inability to tolerate beta-blockade
4. Creatinine >2.0

2.2 Patient Preparation

Following patient instructions should be given when procedure is scheduled:

1. No food or drink (except clear liquids) for 3–4 h prior to exam.
2. No caffeine products for 12 h prior to exam.
3. Do drink plenty of water prior to exam.
4. No nicotine products for 4 h prior to exam.
5. Take all regular medications the day of exam, especially blood pressure medicines.
6. No Viagra or similar medications for 24 h prior to exam.
7. Diabetic patients should ask their physicians how to adjust their medication for the day of the exam.
8. Metformin (Glucophage) often will be discontinued for 48 h after the scan.

Consent/health history forms should:

1. Include past cardiac surgeries, interventions, risk factors, and current symptoms
2. Include past reactions to contrast agents; other allergic reactions; and issues relating to pregnancy, lung disease, kidney disease, diabetes, or the presence of multiple myeloma.
3. Clearly state that this exam will require an intravenous (IV) injection of contrast material and that the patient may be given cardiac medications for heart rate, rhythm, or vasodilatation as needed [1].
4. Explain any portions of the study that might be used for research and how the patient's privacy will be protected.

Patient preparation includes the following:

Patient preparation should be done by an experienced nurse or nurse practitioner.

All employees should be ACLS or BLS trained.

OSHA standards require that radiation safety policy and Hepatitis B viral vaccination be made available to all employees.

2.3 IV Placement

Use short, 20-gauge IV catheters in normal or younger patients, but use an 18-gauge catheter when necessary for more rapid infusion rates (older and hypertensive patients).

Use antecubital veins if available. Alternate sites include the basilica or median veins of the forearm, the cephalic vein lying lateral (thumb side) of the arm, or the large upper cephalic vein above the antecubital space. If necessary, hand veins may be used, generally with a 20-gauge catheter.

The IV catheter tubing should have pressure rating of 300 psi.

No central lines may be used other than those specifically labeled for power injection.

Connect the IV to an extension tubing.

Secure all connections with Op-Site and tape.

2.4 Hydration Policy

The most effective renal protection from IV contrast is adequate hydration both before and after the scan. Patients with diabetes or renal insufficiency or dehydration are at extra risk for contrast-induced nephropathy (CIN) defined as a rise of >0.5 in serum creatinine [2].

Encourage all patients to drink a liter of water prior to arrival. At discharge give the patient a 500 ml bottle of water to drink and instruct them to drink approximately 1500 ml more by the time they go to bed that evening.

Following are the protocols for patients with elevated creatinine levels:

1. For creatinine level between 1.5 and 1.8: aggressive oral hydration pre- and post-administration of nonionic and low osmolar contrast [3]. Patients *may* be premedicated with four doses of Mucomyst 600 mg.
2. For creatinine level between 1.8 and 2.0: 250 cc NS IV hydration immediately post scan plus aggressive oral hydration pre- and post-administration of nonionic and low osmolar contrast. Patient *must* be premedicated with four doses of Mucomyst 600 mg.

Following are the protocols for single kidney and renal transplant patients:

- Creatinine up to 1.5: use protocol (1) above.
- Creatinine of 1.6–2.0: use protocol (2) above.

Do not scan patients with a creatinine level above 2.0.

2.5 Pre-Procedure Patient Medication

Beta-blockade: Oral or IV metoprolol has become the standard because of demonstrated safety in patients with CHF and significant COPD and because of its low cost and reliability [1].

Oral approach: 50 mg of metoprolol is given 12 h before the scan with another 50 mg at the center, or the total 100 mg can be given as a tablet at the center 1 h prior to scanning. If the heart rate is not < 65, an additional 5 mg IV is given every 5 min to a total of 15 mg. Post-oral beta-blockade requires monitoring for 1 h post-procedure.

IV approach: After the patient is on the cardiac monitor and Blood Pressure (BP) is obtained, 5 mg of IV metoprolol is given as a test bolus with a 1–2 min pause to assess the response. A further 5–50 mg is then given as a slow push of 1 mg per 15 s, carefully monitoring the patients Heart Rate (HR). The average total required dose is 25 mg; however, older patients and smokers often require more dose. BP monitoring continues during the medication delivery, and if it is low (<100 systolic), 30 cc of Normal Saline (NS) is given between each 5 mg of Lopressor delivered. No post-procedure monitoring is required if the patient is stable post-scanning [4].

Nitrates: Sublingual nitroglycerin (400–800 mcgs sublingual = 1–2 tablets or 1–2 sprays), should be given between 3 and 10 min of scan time unless the BP is low [5].

Lidocaine: After beta-blockade if frequent PVCs are noted, 2% Lidocaine can be administered at 5–100 mg IV over 1–2 min.

Reasons to stop Lidocaine administration include marked bradycardia, evidence of heart block, or any neurological changes such as drowsiness or disorientation.

Atropine: If after maximal beta-blockade, significant beat-to-beat variability is noted, or if the HR is < 40, Atropine 0.5–1.0 mg can be given.

Breath-hold training :

1. Always practice breath holding and being still.
2. Have patients hold their breath in maximal inspiration.
3. Oxygen or sedation may help.

Patient observation and instruction after the scan [6]:

1. Have patients stand up slowly.
2. Help them walk to a chair and sit with continued IV hydration and observation for 15 min.
3. If oral beta-blockers were given, let them remain at the center for 1 h.
4. Utilize a teaching sheet to remind patients about post-hydration, when they may eat and when to restart their routine medications (including metformin).

2.6 Contrast Issues

1. Image quality is dependent on the signal-to-noise ratio. Optimal images require intra-arterial densities of 250–350 HU (lying well above the background tissues but not substantially overlapping with calcium deposits) [7].
2. Given injection rates of 4–6 cc/s, this is best obtained with iodine concentrations ≥350 mgl/ml.
3. Patients with high cardiac outputs rapidly dilute out the contrast, resulting in poor image quality. Obese, anemic, hyperthyroid, anxious, and smoking patients will require injection rates of 5–6 cc/s.

4. Total contrast loads should not exceed 100 ccs.
5. Programmable and dual source power injectors that allow smooth transitions to a saline flush optimize contrast delivery [8, 9].
6. A 22-gauge IV delivers 3–4 cc/s, a 20-gauge delivers 4–5 cc/s, and an 18-gauge delivers 5–6 cc/s.
7. Obese and high-output patients will require a full 100 ccs of contrast at 5½–6 cc/s.

Accurately timing the scan to the arrival of the IV contrast in the target structures is a required skill that improves with attention and practice. Timing errors of even 5–10 s can make a substantial difference.

Three strategies are employed to best determine the vein-to-aorta travel time.

1. Fixed "best guess" of 22–25 s.
2. Automatic triggering. A region of interest is selected over the ascending aorta and is sampled every 2 s after the initiation of the contrast bolus. When the density in the aorta rises to preset value (usually 100 HU), the system will automatically tell the patient to take a deep breath and will start scanning.
3. Test bolus with a region of interest placed in the ascending aorta and sampled every 1 s. The contrast travel time can be accurately measured. This strategy offers several advantages: no false starts or delays, identification of contrast dilution problems, checking the quality of the IV, and a chance to observe and practice the patient before the real scan.

Following are the timing bolus protocols:

1. Select the level of the ascending aorta at the bifurcation or the pulmonary artery.
2. Give breath-hold instructions.
3. Inject 20 ml of contrast at 5 ml/s followed by 20 ml of normal saline at 4 ml/s.
4. After images are reconstructed, place a ROI cursor in the aorta.
5. Calculate circulation time from onset to the peak of the aortic curve. Add 8 s to peak aortic time (5 s for the built-in delay in the test injection and 3 s for the time it takes to get contrast into the distal coronary arteries).
6. If the aortic curve peak does not reach 100 HU, consider increasing the flow rate below to 5½ or 6 ml per second.

Injection protocol (for the actual scan) is as follows [10, 11]:

	Flow Rate (ml/s)	Volume (ml)
Pure contrast	5	35
Pure contrast	5	30
Blend 60/40 (contrast to saline)	4	30

Contrast reactions are as follows:

1. Moderate-to-severe itching/flushing/rash: diphenhydramine 12.5–25 mg IV and SoluMedrol 125 mg IV [12].
2. Nausea: Phenergan (promethezine) 12.5 mg IV.
3. Mild respiratory distress such as wheezing: Albuterol inhaler two puffs.
4. Signs of anaphylaxis: call a physician, start aggressive hydration, give diphenhydramine 12.5–25 mg IV, and be ready to administer epinephrine SQ 1 mg of 1:10,000.

Extravasation of contrast [13]:

Initial treatment: Elevate extremity.
Ice pack recommended three times per day and may be alternated with warm soaks.
Notify MD and document the following:

Nonionic contrast extravasation >100 ml
Skin blistering
Altered tissue perfusion
Change in sensation distal to the site of extravasation

Follow up through phone call with the patient next day.
Patient teaching includes the following:

1. Keep arm elevated above your heart for 12 h.
2. Apply ice packs for 15–30 min every 8 h for 1–3 days. Use warm soaks after the first day.
3. For pain, use Tylenol or Motrin as directed.
4. Notify MD of any blistering, redness, skin discoloration, hardness, change in sensation (loss of feeling, numbness, tingling), weakness, or an increase or decrease in temperature in the affected arm.
5. If worsens, go to ER.

2.7 Conclusion

The goal of any imaging center is to obtain the highest quality images with the least risk to and discomfort for the patient.

In general, coronary artery CTA is an elective diagnostic procedure and should be deferred if either the risk to the patient or the chance of an inferior study is increased.

References

1. Le Jemtel TH, Padeletti M, Jelic S. Diagnostic and Therapeutic Challenges in Patients with Coexistent Chronic Obstructive Pulmonary Disease and Chronic Heart Failure. J Am Coll Cardiol 2007, 49: 171–182

2. Hoffman U, et al. Image Quality vs. Heart Rate. Radiology 2005, 234: 86–97
3. Barrett BJ, Katzberg RW, Thomsen HS, et al. The IMPACT Study. Invest Radiol 2006, 41: 815–821.
4. Hoffmann U, Ferencik M, Cury RC, Pena AJ. Coronary CT Angiography. J Nuclear Medicine 2006, 47(5): 797–800.
5. Staffey KS, van Beek EJR, Jagasia D. Clinical performance and considerations in coronary CTA. Suppl Appl Radiol 2007: 33–39.
6. King BF, Hartman GW, Williamson B Jr, LeRoy AJ, Hattery RR. Low-osmolality contrast media: a current perespective. Mayo Clin Proc. 1989, 64: 976–85.
7. Stern EJ, et al. High-Resolution CT of the Chest. 2001 by Lippincott Williams & Wilkins 2001: 1–5.
8. Hopper KD, Mosher TJ, Kasales CJ, et al. Thoracic spiral CT: delivery of contrast material pushed with injectable saline solution in a power injector. Radiology 1997, 205: 269–271
9. Haage P, Schmitz-Rode T, Hubner D, et al. Reduction of contrast material dose and artifacts by a saline flush using a double power injector in helical CT of the thorax. Am J Roentgenol 2000, 174: 1049–1053
10. Fleischmann D, Rubin GD, Bankier AA, Hittmair K. Improved uniformity of aortic enhancement with customized contrast medium injection protocols at CT angiography. Radiology 2000, 214: 363–71
11. Bae KT, Tran HQ, Heiken JP. Multiphasic injection method for uniform prolonged vascular enhancement at CT angiography: pharmacokinetic analysis and experimental porcine model. Radiology 2000, 216: 872–880
12. Schoenhagen P, Stillman AE, Halliburton SS, White RD. *Cardiac CT Made Easy*. Taylor & Francis 2006: 117–118
13. de Feyter PJ, Krestin GP. *Computer Tomography of the Coronary Arteries*. Taylor & Francis 2005, 19: 179–186

Chapter 3
Cardiovascular Calcium: Assessment and Impact of Interventions

Stamatios Lerakis, Antonio Bellasi, and Paolo Raggi

The presence of coronary artery calcium (CAC) is 100% specific for atheromatous plaque in patients with normal renal function. In patients with chronic kidney disease, however, calcification may also occur in the media of the vessel wall, and it is not related to atherosclerotic wall changes [1].

During the past few decades, it has become apparent that the accumulation of calcium within the atherosclerotic plaque is dependent on an active process of hydroxyapatite accumulation similar in many aspects to bone remodeling [1]. In fact, several enzymes and mediators of bone remodeling can be found in the context of the growing atherosclerotic plaque. Furthermore, vascular smooth muscle cells cultured in a variety of different media can transform in osteoblast-like cells capable of laying crystals of hydroxyapaptite in the interstitium [1]. This induced several investigators to study the effect of various treatments for atherosclerosis to reduce the progression of vascular calcification. Indeed, early animal experiments suggested that inducing atherosclerosis regression with aggressive lipid lowering, with either diet or statin treatment, may arrest progression of vascular calcification [2, 3]. The ability to carefully quantify CAC with cardiac computed tomography (CT) raised an interest in assessing two important issues linked with atherosclerosis progression: (1) Can sequential CT imaging be employed to assess effectiveness of therapy? (2) Does progressive accumulation of CAC pose a threat to the patient, or is it a sign of ongoing plaque healing?

Recent imaging protocol refinements have reduced the inter-test variability of a cardiac CT performed to assess CAC to 10% or less with a standard deviation of 10–20% [4]. In contrast, annual CAC progression rates typically exceed 20–30%, therefore allowing the implementation of CT imaging to follow progression of CAC. The accuracy of sequential CAC measurements is greater in patients with intermediate-to-high CAC scores. Therefore, CAC score changes are typically assessed in patients with a minimum absolute score of 20–30. Besides improving the reproducibility of the absolute score, this minimizes the effect of a small

P. Raggi
Department of Medicine and Division of Cardiology, Emory University School of Medicine, Atlanta, GA, USA
e-mail: praggi@excite.com

M.J. Budoff, J.S. Shinbane (eds.), *Handbook of Cardiovascular CT*,
DOI: 10.1007/978-1-84800-091-9_3, © Springer-Verlag London Limited 2008

absolute increase that would translate into a large relative score increase as a percent change from baseline (10 points increase over 10 baseline CAC score is a 100% increase). Although the volume score was introduced to improve the reproducibility of the Agatston score [5], the latter is still the most frequently used and reported in the literature, and it appears to have comparable reproducibility [6]. However, with multidetector CT (MDCT), the volume score is recommended.

Present data indicate that CAC progression is most strongly related to the baseline CAC score, with only a limited relationship to standard cardiovascular risk factors. In this light, few if any current medical regimen might delay CAC progression, although a few have been attempted with variable results.

The effect of statins on slowing progression of CAC was initially reported in two observational studies [7, 8] and one small cross-over prospective study [9]. In all of the three studies, the authors concluded that the addition of statin therapy to the medical regimen slowed the progression of CAC from 30–50% per year to 10–15% per year (**Fig. 3.1**). In limited cases, patients treated aggressively showed a small regression of CAC over time, although this might have been a reflection of the interscan error rather than an actual inversion of direction.

In another observational study, Raggi et al. [10] showed that CAC progression is faster in diabetic patients, even when treated with statins, than in non-diabetic

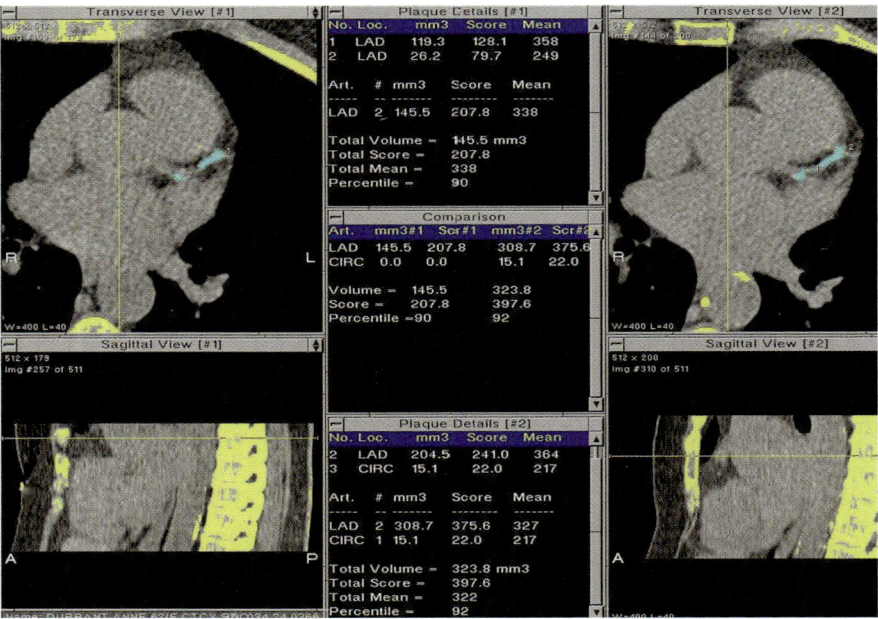

Fig. 3.1 The left upper quadrant shows an axial image of the heart at baseline in a patient not treated with statins. The initial Agatston score (central insert) was 207.8 (volume score: 145.5), and it increased to 397.6 (volume score: 323.8) after 1 year of follow-up. The blue color coding of the calcified plaque seen along the left anterior descending coronary artery indicates a high calcium density

subjects. However, the fact that statin therapy may slow the progression of CAC was disproved in three prospective randomized trials. In two of these trials [11, 12], CAC progression was compared in patients treated with moderate versus intensive statin therapy, while in the third study the effect of atorvastatin was compared to placebo [13]. In each one of the trials, there was no difference in CAC progression between treatment groups. In the Women's Health Initiative (WHI), menopausal women between the ages of 50 and 59 years were randomized to treatment with conjugated estrogens or placebo [14]. In a sub-study of the WHI, 1,064 women were submitted to CAC screening after 8.7 years from trial initiation. The women receiving estrogens showed a lower CAC score compared with those receiving placebo (83.1 vs. 123.1, $P = 0.02$).

While sequential CT imaging may not be helpful in assessing the effect of lipid-lowering therapy on CAC progression in the general population, this approach proved very useful in assessing effectiveness of medical therapy in patients with end-stage renal disease. In fact, in two separate randomized trials, the non-calcium-based phosphate binder sevelamer slowed progression of coronary calcification compared to traditional calcium-based phosphate binders in patients undergoing chronic hemodialysis [15, 16] (**Fig. 3.2**).

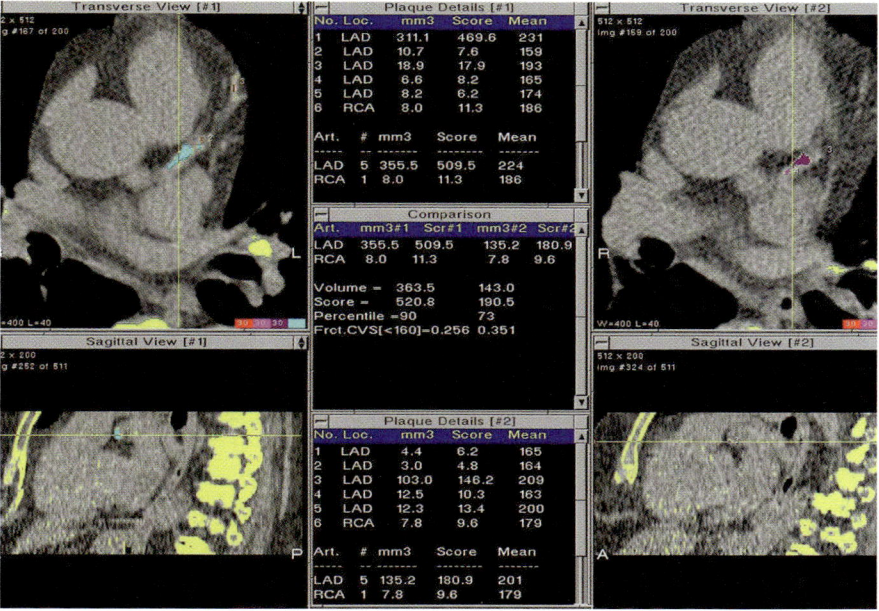

Fig. 3.2 The left upper quadrant shows an axial image of the heart at baseline in a patient undergoing hemodialysis treated with sevelamer (see text). The initial Agatston score (central insert) was 520.8 (volume score: 363.5), and it decreased to 190.5 (volume score: 143.0) after 2 years of treatment. The color coding of the plaque seen along the left anterior descending coronary artery changed from *blue* to *purple* indicating a lower calcium density over time

More importantly, progression of CAC has been shown to be associated with an unfavorable prognosis both in the general population [17] as well as in patients undergoing dialysis [18]. In a randomized trial, hemodialysis patients treated with calcium-based binders had a 2.2-fold greater risk of death after 4.5-year of follow-up compared to those treated with sevelamer [18]. Subjects from the general population with normal renal function and a CAC progression greater than 15% per year had an 11-fold greater risk of death and myocardial infarction than patients showing no progression [17].

Of note, in the clinical studies so far published, patients with no visible CAC on a screening CT remained free of it during a maximum follow-up of 2.5 years even in the presence of renal failure. It would appear, therefore, that rescanning in these subjects might be safely postponed to a minimum of 3 years from screening.

Several other imaging modalities have been used to assess progression of atherosclerosis, some invasive (quantitative angiography and intravascular ultrasound) and others non-invasive (carotid intima media thickness). While all modalities have demonstrated that progression of atherosclerosis is affected by medical management, regression or non-progression on quantitative invasive angiography is the only methodology that has been conclusively linked with a significant reduction in morbidity and mortality. Hence, progression of CAC on cardiac CT, a non-invasive imaging modality that provides a low radiation dose, may prove very useful in assessing future risk of events if the initial experience is confirmed in further studies.

3.1 Imaging Pearls

- Sequential scans should *"preferably"* be performed on the same CT equipment to reduce inter–CT scan variability.
- Scanning parameters should be identical in sequential scans on the same patient. Keep slice thickness, pixel size, and field of view constant.
- The CT scanner should be calibrated often (ideally weekly) to prevent image drifting.
- Using MDCT technology for sequential CAC imaging; it is advisable to use the calcium volume score rather than the Agatston score that was devised for the electron beam tomography scanner with substantially different scanning characteristics. Although mass scores are likely the most reproducible CAC measures on MDCT, they require the use of calibration phantoms, which may not be readily available.
- When performing analyses of repeat CT scans, always compare the new scan with the old one; verify that the same anatomical areas have been covered and that you have interpreted them consistently each time (for example, you have not attributed a calcific lesion to the circumflex coronary artery the first time and to the mitral valve ring the next time).
- Assess your intra-observer variability (*"know your limit"*), and compare yourself to one or two of your colleagues to establish the inter-observer variability. This is

important to set your threshold for change: if your variability is ∼10%, a calcium score increase of 20% could be safely considered a true change.

References

1. Raggi P, Giachelli C, Bellasi A. Interaction of vascular and bone disease in patients with normal renal function and patients undergoing dialysis. Nat Clin Pract Cardiovasc Med 4: 26–33, 2007.
2. Stary HC. Natural history of calcium deposits in atherosclerosis progression and regression. Z Kardiol 89 (suppl 2): 28–35, 2000.
3. Williams JK, Sukhova GK, Herrington DM, Libby P. Pravastatin has cholesterol-lowering independent effects on the artery wall of atherosclerotic monkeys. J Am Coll Cardiol 31: 684–91, 1998.
4. Achenbach S, Ropers D, Mohlenkamp S, Schmermund A, Muschiol G, Groth J, Kusus M, Regenfus M, Daniel WG, Erbel R, Moshage W. Variability of repeated coronary artery calcium measurements by electron beam tomography. Am J Cardiol 87: 210–213, A218, 2001.
5. Callister TQ, Cooil B, Raya SP, Lippolis NJ, Russo DJ, Raggi P. Coronary artery disease: improved reproducibility of calcium scoring with an electron-beam CT volumetric method. Radiology 208: 807–814, 1998.
6. Rumberger JA, Kaufman L. A rosetta stone for coronary calcium risk stratification: agatston, volume, and mass scores in 11,490 individuals. AJR Am J Roentgenol 181: 743–748, 2003.
7. Callister TQ, Raggi P, Cooil B, Lippolis NJ, Russo DJ. Effect of HMG-CoA reductase inhibitors on coronary artery disease as assessed by electron-beam computed tomography. N Engl J Med 339: 1972–1978, 1998.
8. Budoff MJ, Lane KL, Bakhsheshi H, Mao S, Grassmann BO, Friedman BC, Brundage BH. Rates of progression of coronary calcium by electron beam tomography. Am J Cardiol 86, 8–11, 2000.
9. Achenbach S, Ropers D, Pohle K, Leber A, Thilo C, Knez A, Menendez T, Maeffert R, Kusus M, Regenfus M, Bickel A, Haberl R, Steinbeck G, Moshage W, Daniel WG. Influence of lipid-lowering therapy on the progression of coronary artery calcification: a prospective evaluation. Circulation 106: 1077–1082, 2002.
10. Raggi P, Cooil B, Ratti C, Callister TQ, Budoff M. Progression of coronary artery calcium and occurrence of myocardial infarction in patients with and without diabetes mellitus. Hypertension 46: 238–243, 2005.
11. Raggi P, Davidson M, Callister TQ, Welty FK, Bachmann GA, Hecht H, Rumberger JA. Aggressive versus moderate lipid-lowering therapy in hypercholesterolemic postmenopausal women: Beyond Endorsed Lipid Lowering with EBT Scanning (BELLES). Circulation 112: 563–571, 2005.
12. Schmermund A, Achenbach S, Budde T, Buziashvili Y, Forster A, Friedrich G, Henein M, Kerkhoff G, Knollmann F, Kukharchuk V, Lahiri A, Leischik R, Moshage W, Schartl M, Siffert W, Steinhagen-Thiessen E, Sinitsyn V, Vogt A, Wiedeking B, Erbel R. Effect of intensive versus standard lipid-lowering treatment with atorvastatin on the progression of calcified coronary atherosclerosis over 12 months: a multicenter, randomized, double-blind trial. Circulation 113: 427–437, 2006.
13. Arad Y, Spadaro LA, Roth M, Newstein D, Guerci AD. Treatment of asymptomatic adults with elevated coronary calcium scores with atorvastatin, vitamin C, and vitamin E: the St. Francis Heart Study randomized clinical trial. J Am Coll Cardiol 46: 166–172, 2005.
14. Manson JE, Allison MA, Rossouw JE, Carr JJ, Langer RD, Hsia J, Kuller LH, Cochrane BB, Hunt JR, Ludlam SE, Pettinger MB, Gass M, Margolis KL, Nathan L, Ockene JK,

Prentice RL, Robbins J, Stefanick ML. WHI and WHI-CACS Investigators. N Engl J Med 356: 2591–602, 2007.

15. Chertow GM, Burke SK, Raggi P. Sevelamer attenuates the progression of coronary and aortic calcification in hemodialysis patients. Kidney Int 62: 245–252, 2002.

16. Block GA, Spiegel DM, Ehrlich J, Mehta R, Lindbergh J, Dreisbach A, Raggi P. Effects of sevelamer and calcium on coronary artery calcification in patients new to hemodialysis. Kidney Int 68: 1815–1824, 2005.

17. Raggi P, Callister T, Budoff M, Shaw L. Progression of coronary artery calcium and risk of first myocardial infarction in patients receiving cholesterol-lowering therapy. Arterioscler Thromb Vasc Biol 24: 1272–1277, 2004.

18. Block GA, Raggi P, Bellasi A, Kooienga L, Spiegel DM. Mortality effect of coronary calcification and phosphate binder choice in incident hemodialysis patients. Kidney Int 71: 438–41, 2007.

Chapter 4
Assessment of Cardiac Function

John A. Rumberger

4.1 Introduction

Contrast ventriculography has long been the standard to assess cardiac performance including ejection fraction, absolute ventricular volumes, and location and extent of regional wall motion abnormalities. However, non-invasive cardiac imaging has emerged as an alternative that, in many circumstances, has obviated and replaced traditional invasive contrast ventriculography. Today, x-ray computed tomography (CT) imaging of the heart, the coronary arteries, and other vascular structures can be performed using both scanning electron beam tomography (EBT) and validated multi-detector CT (MDCT). The rapid development of computer-assisted image reconstruction with 3-D registration and 4-D rendering of the cardiac, myocardial, and coronary surfaces provides a robust method of non-invasively examining the heart to complement and likely extend the boundaries of all prior and current non-invasive cardiac imaging methodologies. This chapter is intended to discuss the use of state-of-the-art 64+-slice MDCT for clinical quantitation of global and regional cardiac chamber size and systolic function.

4.2 Nomenclature

Nuclear cardiology, echocardiography, cardiac MRI, positron emission tomography (PET), conventional coronary angiography, and cardiac CT have all been used to define cardiac chamber sizes, muscle mass, wall thicknesses, and cardiac chamber function. Although imaging methodologies differ, the major objective in communicating information to colleagues and referring physicians is consistency and standardization of reporting nomenclature as it relates to left ventricular assessment.

Digital cross-sectional or tomographic imaging of the chest and its organs by CT has traditionally oriented and displayed the body using planes parallel to (transaxial) or at 90-degree angles to (sagittal and coronal) the long axis of the body.

J.A. Rumberger
The Princeton Longevity Center, Princeton Forrestal Village, Princeton, NJ 08540
e-mail: jrumberger@theplc.net

M.J. Budoff, J.S. Shinbane (eds.), *Handbook of Cardiovascular CT*,
DOI: 10.1007/978-1-84800-091-9_4, © Springer-Verlag London Limited 2008

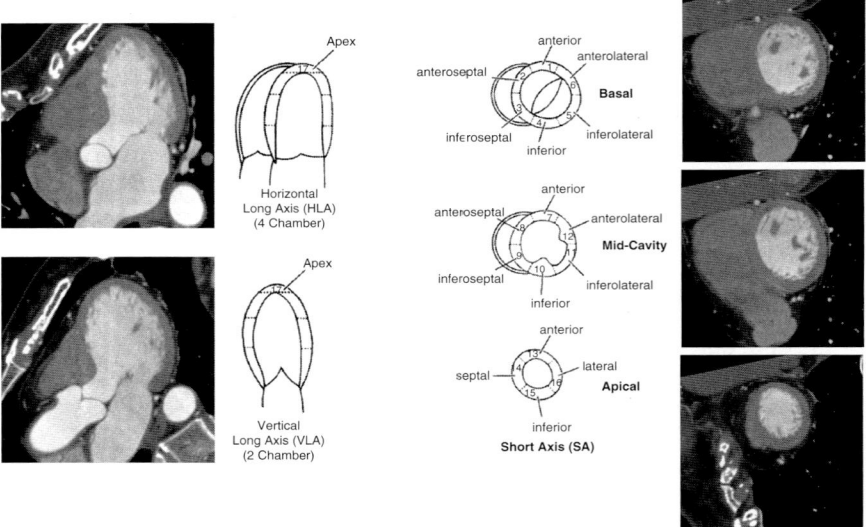

Fig. 4.1 Recommended nomenclature and scanning axis for presentation of CT of the left ventricle. Superimposed are representative images from MDCT in the suggested reference planes. Adapted from reference [2]

However, cardiac displays generated using orthogonal views based on the long axis of the body do not satisfy current standards of cardiac imaging as they do not cleanly transect the ventricles, atria, or myocardial regions as supplied by the major coronary arteries. Rees et al. proposed as early as 1986 that CT adopts standardized "short" and "long" axis cardiac image presentations [1].

The American Heart Association in 2002 [2] published a set of standards of myocardial segmentation and nomenclature for tomographic presentation of the heart regardless of the cardiac imaging modality. Whenever possible, it is recommended that these standards be followed for cardiac function analysis and review using MDCT. This method of image display maintains the integrity of the cardiac chambers as they relate to the distribution of coronary arterial blood flow. For these reasons, it has been agreed that this approach is optimal for use in clinical patient management involving tomographic assessment of cardiac size and function.

The presentation nomenclature employed is as follows: the short axis, the vertical long axis, and the horizontal long axis, as shown in **Fig. 4.1**. For those familiar with 2-D echocardiography, these correspond to the short axis and, roughly, to the apical two-chamber and apical four-chamber views, respectively. These planes are oriented at 90-degree angles relative to each other and optimize viewing of each section of the ventricular myocardium in at least two orthogonal views.

4.3 Methods

For current cardiac functional imaging using 64-slice MDCT, images are acquired generally over a series of 6–10 heartbeats and then "retrospectively" reconstructed at specific "phases" of the cardiac cycle. As greater numbers of "slices" are added

(128, 256, and likely beyond), the actual number of heartbeats required may reduce to a single time event. The methods of actually performing cardiac CT using MDCT are found elsewhere in this volume. Although images are reconstructed so as to display 2-D and 3-D data, analysis of cardiac function employs a 4-D display and analysis (the fourth dimension being the time during the cardiac cycle). There is no "standard" as to how many phases should be reconstructed in order to provide quantitative cardiac functional evaluation, but commonly at least 10 phases (representing consecutive 10% segments of the R–R interval) are retrospectively reconstructed from the raw CT image data. Generally, a display for analysis shows either or both 2-D images using maximum intensity projections (MIP) of variable "thicknesses" (generally 5–15 mm) or a 3-D volume rendering technique (VRT). For ejection fraction and ventricular volume measures, only two sets of images are actually required, end-diastole and end-systole, but for a more qualitative review of regional wall motion, my preference is to view a 10-phase "cine-angiogram" (4-D display) using either a thick MIP or a VRT—this gives an impression more consistent with what is normally utilized in practice using equilibrium nuclear methods, invasive catheterization, or 2-D echocardiography.

4.4 Ventricular Anatomy and Function

CT (EBT and MDCT) has been validated to provide quantitative assessment of the cardiac chambers in patients with no absolute contraindication to the use of iodinated contrast medium. The majority of these validation studies were performed in the 1980s and 1990s using EBT and have been adapted and validated in many instances more recently using MDCT. Since the number of cardiac cycles imaged per scan is generally limited to 5–10, quantitation may be limited to those patients with normal sinus rhythm, although it is possible in patients with significant dysrhythmias, such as atrial fibrillation. **Table 4.1** shows validated norms for left ventricular chamber size, wall thicknesses, ejection fraction, and ventricular volumes using cardiac CT. These were established during the 1980s using EBT [3] but also mimic standards established using 2-D echocardiography [4].

CT imaging using thin sections allows post-processing of images into end-diastolic and end-systolic "short" and "long" axis images to facilitate identification of structures and salient features of the ventricular anatomy (**Fig. 4.1**). Using short- and long-axis imaging also allows for identification of infarct locations and, as noted above, infarct size (**Fig. 4.2**); demonstration of this latter example is a common CT finding in contrast-enhanced images from patients with remote myocardial infarction. The "negative" contrast noted in **Fig. 4.2** is actually due to lack of contrast opacification in the infarcted region causing "contrast rarefaction" (representing a transmural infarction). Long-axis (both vertical and horizontal) imaging of the left ventricle also allows for definition of apical thrombi (**Fig. 4.3**), apical infarcts, and pseudo- and true apical aneurysms (**Fig. 4.4**). 2-D and 3-D reconstruction methods can create nearly an infinite number of imaging planes. The right ventricle can also

Table 4.1 Reference values for left ventricular size, function, and muscle mass for cardiac CT in adult women and men (adapted from data presented in references [3, 4])

Measurement	Women				Men			
	Reference range	Mildly abnormal	Moderately abnormal	Severely abnormal	Reference range	Mildly abnormal	Moderately abnormal	Severely abnormal
Septal wall thickness (mm)*	6–9	10–12	13–15	≥16	6–10	11–13	14–16	≥17
Posterior wall thickness (mm)*	6–9	10–12	13–15	≥16	6–10	11–13	14–16	≥17
LV muscle mass (gm)	66–155	156–176	177–187	>190	96–200	201–227	228–254	>260
LV diameter (mm)*	39–53	54–57	58–61	≥62	42–59	60–63	64–68	≥69
LV global EDV (ml)	60–110	111–122	123–136	>140	70–160	161–190	191–210	≥210
LV global ESV (ml)	20–50	51–60	61–70	≥71	25–60	61–70	71–85	≥86
LV global EF (%)	≥55	45–54	30–44	<30	≥55	45–54	30–44	<30

*end-diastole, mid–left ventricle; EDV = end-diastolic volume; ESV = end-systolic volume; EF = ejection fraction; LV = left ventricular

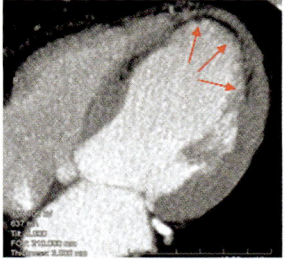 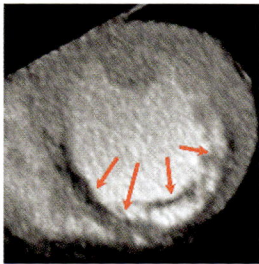

Fig. 4.2 Horizontal long-axis (*left*) and mid-ventricular short-axis (*right*) images from an individual with a remote transmural myocardial infarction of the left ventricular apex and surrounding myocardium. See text for details

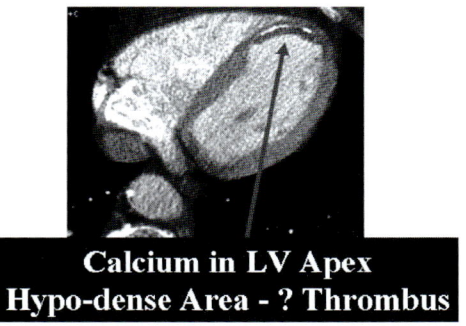 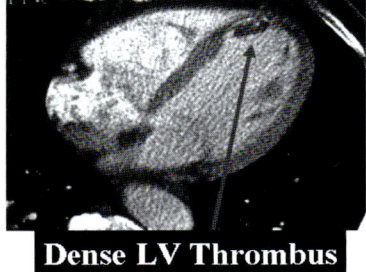

Fig. 4.3 Vertical long-axis tomograms at two different left ventricular tomographic levels. This patient had a 2-D echocardiogram that resulted in incomplete imaging of the ventricular apex and a question of a thrombus. The image on the *left* shows calcification from a remote mural hemorrhage, and the image on the *right* shows the clear delineated ventricular thrombus

be imaged. **Figure 4.5** shows a dilated right ventricle in a patient with arrhythmogenic right ventricular cardiomyopathy; CT can often be an alternative or a confirmatory method to MRI in the evaluation of such patients.

4.5 Chamber Measurements

3-D calipers available on all CT workstations allow for quantitative 2-D and 3-D measures of ventricular size in any axis (**Fig. 4.6**). Additionally, measures of ventricular muscle thicknesses can be performed for all myocardial walls (**Fig. 4.7**). Measures of all myocardial walls as well as the adjacent chambers (**Fig. 4.8**) can also be helpful and augment data on global ventricular volumes, muscle mass, and function by CT.

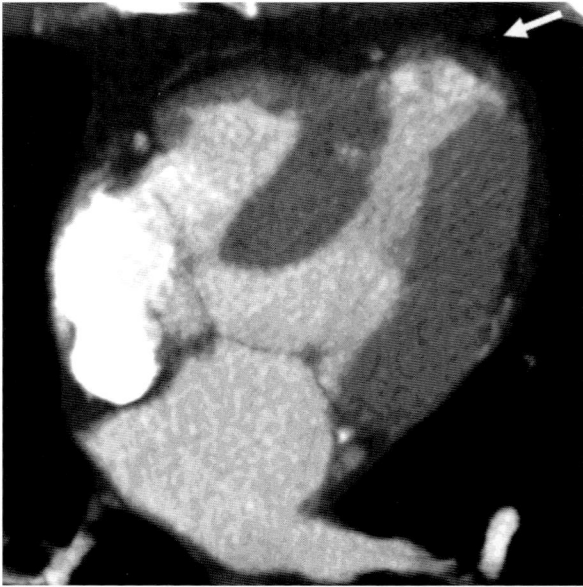

Fig. 4.4 Vertical long-axis image. This shows a distinct apical left ventricular aneurysm with thrombus

4.6 Indications/Appropriateness

Contrast-enhanced cardiac CT using MDCT should include assessment of the cardiac chambers and especially left ventricular function in all instances (if technically possible). Using MDCT and retrospective gating, this information is readily available without administering additional contrast to the patient. Often dose modulation may be applied to reduce the global radiation dose to an individual patient—this is more commonly applied in those with lower heart rates and may not be as practical if the heart rate during acquisition is above 65 beats per minute. Dose modulation can alter the image quality accordingly.

The mandate for a complete cardiac CT angiogram (CTA) in routine clinical practice is to include quantitative left ventricular size, shape, and functional analysis as part of each evaluation performed for assessment of coronary plaque and lumen anatomy.

4.7 Conclusions

There have been historically extensive validations using cardiac CT (EBT and MDCT) for virtually all cardiac size, shape, and functional measures, and these were actually published and established long before such measures were attempted

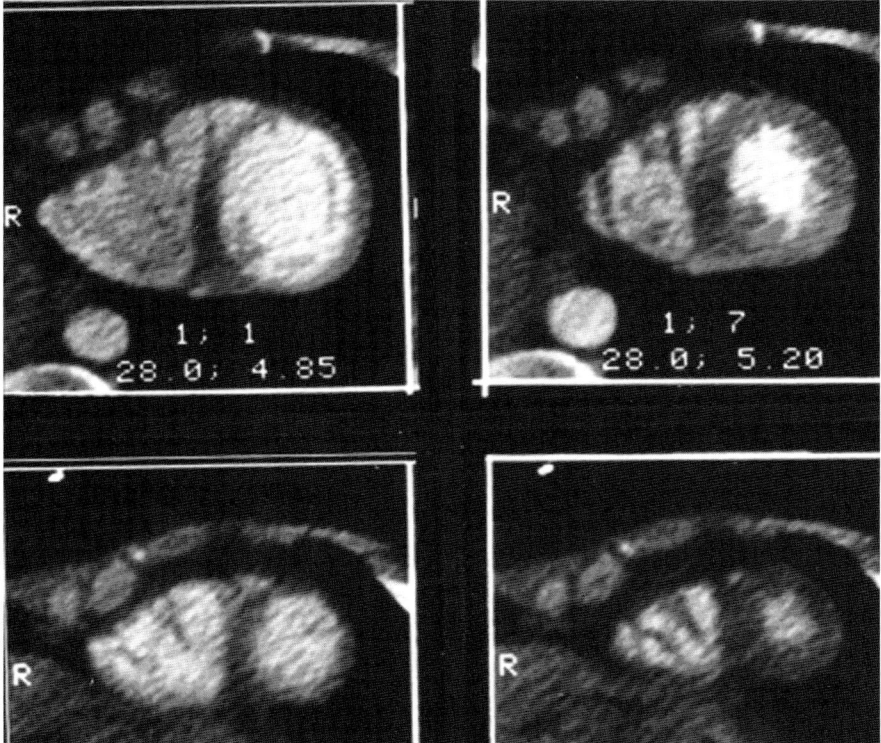

Fig. 4.5 Four short-axis images at four different ventricular levels showing the left ventricle (*right* side of images) and the right ventricle (*left* side of the images); note that the right ventricle is significantly dilated compared to the left ventricle. Furthermore, the right ventricle has deep trabeculations. Both of these characteristics are common in patients with arrhythmogenic right ventricular cardiomyopathy

by MRI. Recent improvements in spiral/helical CT have also accorded this validity to MDCT. CT then becomes a primary method to define the heart and its detailed anatomy in health and in disease. Furthermore, these types of measures can be accomplished during post-processing of images intended to define coronary artery anatomy generally without the need for additional imaging. The disadvantages are that additional sets of cardiac data are required at various portions of the cardiac cycle (nominally at end-diastole and end-systole) and this then obligates concomitant increases in radiation exposure to the patient. That said, CT is a very robust technique that can function as both a primary method and a complementary method (e.g., echocardiography, contrast ventriculography, radionuclide angiography, and MRI) to quantitate details of cardiac anatomy and function.

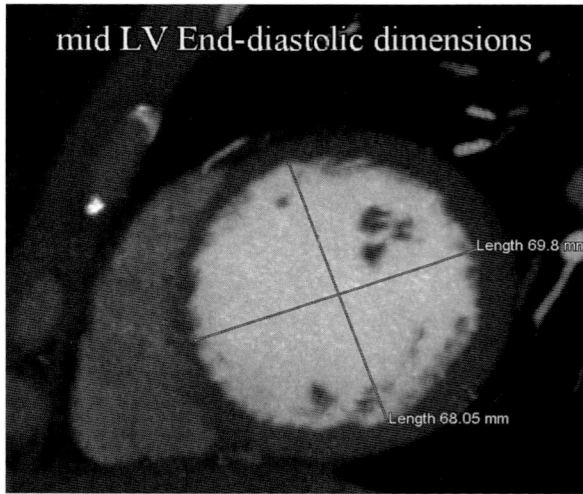

Fig. 4.6 Short axis, mid–left ventricular level showing nominal left ventricular end-diastolic dimensions. This is a 36 year old man with a bundle branch block and recent shortness of breath. The image is consistent with an idiopathic dilated cardiomyopathy

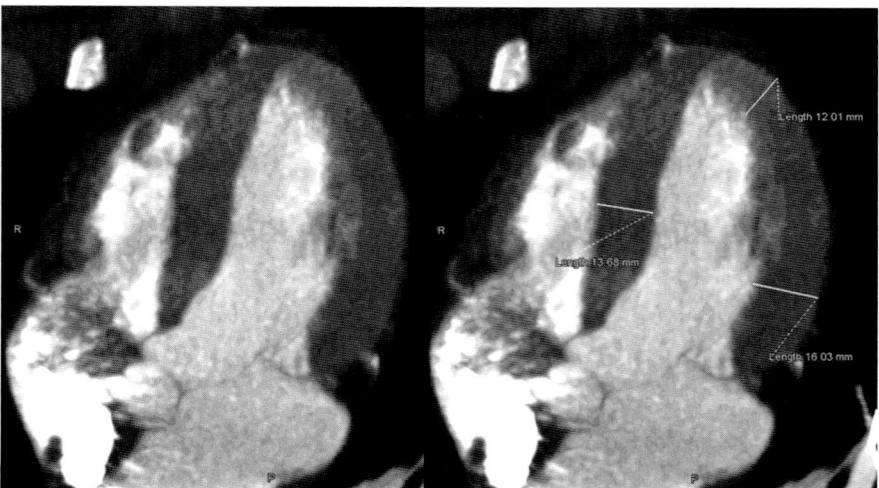

Fig. 4.7 3-D caliber measurements of the left ventricular myocardium; the image on the *left* is without labels and the image on the *right* has the nominal dimensions noted

4.8 Imaging Pearls

- Be consistent in how you approach your analysis—there is no right or wrong way, but you want to have a thorough evaluation of all myocardial segments.

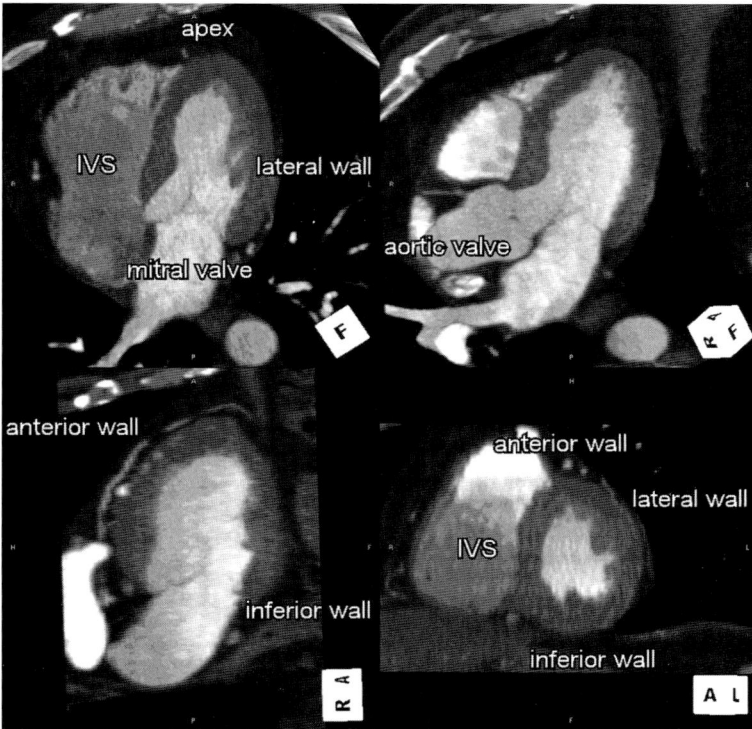

Fig. 4.8 Maximum intensity projection (MIP) of left ventricular chamber in the common display axes—using echocardiographic nomenclature; these are the apical four-chamber view (*upper left*); apical five-chamber view (*upper right*); apical two-chamber view (*lower left*); and mid–left ventricular short axis (*lower right*)

- Start with the left ventricular chamber in the horizontal long-axis view in a dynamic "cine" mode displaying as "apex up"; review the general size of all four cardiac chambers and the motion of the mitral valve and aortic valve; note the thicknesses of the interventricular septum and the lateral (free) wall. View the apex for possible thrombosis/regional wall motion abnormalities. Direct measurements of wall thicknesses and/or left ventricular chamber dimensions can be made in this view (see **Table 4.1** for reference values).
- Rotate the dynamic horizontal long-axis image 90 degrees to your right and you are viewing the vertical long axis; note the thicknesses of the anterior wall and the inferior wall. Again, review the apex for possible wall motion abnormalities. Direct measurements of wall thicknesses and/or left ventricular chamber dimensions can be made in this view (see **Table 4.1** for reference values).
- Rotate the dynamic vertical long-axis image 90 degrees to your left to return to the horizontal long axis and then rotate that image 90 degrees inferiorly to project a roughly short axis (anterior lateral) view. From this view you can visualize

all myocardial walls. Validation of regional wall motion abnormalities requires that these be visualized in two orthogonal views. Direct measurements of wall thicknesses and or left ventricular chamber dimensions can be made in this view (see **Table 4.1** for reference values).

- All MDCT vendors and several independent distributors offer proprietary computer workstations to perform "time volume" analysis of global ventricular function as well as global left ventricular volumes and ejection fraction. Some offer polar displays of regional left ventricular function.

References

1. Rees MJ, Feiring AJ, Rumberger JA, MacMillan RM, Clark DL. Heart Evaluation by Cine CT: Use of Two New Oblique Views. Radiology 1986, 159: 804
2. Cerqueira MD, Weissman NJ, Dilsizian V, Jacobs AK, Kaul S, Laskey WK, Pennell DJ, Rumberger JA, Ryan TJ, Verani MS. Standardized Myocardial Segmentation and Nomenclature or Tomographic Imaging of the Heart – A Statement for Healthcare Professionals from the Cardiac Imaging Committee of the Council on Clinical Cardiology of the American Heart Association. Circulation 2002, 105: 539–542
3. Rumberger JA, Sheedy PF, Breen JF. Use of ultrafast (cine) x-ray computed tomography in cardiac and cardiovascular imaging. IN - Mayo Clinic Practice of Cardiology; Eds: ER Giuliani, BJ Gersh, MD McGoon, DL Hayes, HF Schaff (3rd Edition), Mosby, St. Louis, 1996, Chapter 8, pp. 303–324
4. Lang RM, et al. Recommendations for Chamber Quantification: A Report from the American Society of Echocardiography's Guidelines and Standards Committee and the Chamber Quantification Writing Group, Developed in Conjunction with the European Association of Echocardiography, a Branch of the Europena Society of Cardiology. J Am Soc Echocardiography 2005, 18: 1440–1463
5. Hendel RC, et al. ACCF/ACF/SCCT/SCMR/ASNC/NASCI/SCAI/SIR Appropriateness Criteria for Cardiac Computed Tomography and Cardiac Magnetic Resonance Imaging. JACC 2006, 48: 1475–1497

Chapter 5
CTA as an IVUS Equivalent: Plaque Characterization and Percutaneous Coronary Intervention

Harvey S. Hecht

The excellent negative predictive value of computerized tomographic angiography (CTA) has lead to an emphasis on its ability to exclude significant obstructive disease. Recently, there has been an increasing interest in the ability of CTA to provide a wealth of data about the presence of disease through tomographic intravascular analysis (TIVA), in particular, the stenosis quantitation and plaque characterization potential inherent in its similarity to intravascular ultrasound (IVUS) [1].

5.1 Quantitative CTA

"Eyeballing" the degree of stenosis is, unfortunately, the rule rather than the exception in the catheterization laboratory, resulting in overestimation compared to quantitative coronary angiography (QCA). Even when QCA is performed, the minimum luminal diameter (MLD) correlates poorly with the MLD obtained from IVUS. Nonetheless, MLD and its derived parameter, percent stenosis, is the angiographic standard, and CTA needs to be couched in the same frame of reference. However, rather than repeating the "eyeballing" estimation errors of invasive angiography, QCA analysis of the CTA data is preferable. It is readily applied to the curved MPR image in the angle that demonstrates the most severe stenosis (**Fig. 5.1**); maximum intensity projection (MIP) images are less well suited since they cannot display the entire artery. This technique offers multiple advantages compared to QCA of invasive angiography:

1. The stenosis can be viewed from an infinite number of angles, compared to the limited number of projections in the catheterization laboratory, typically 5–6 for the left and 2–3 for the right coronary artery. Consequently, the likelihood of capturing the stenosis at its most severe is greater by CTA.
2. The appropriate "normal" reference segment can be easily identified (**Fig. 5.1**) because of the ability of CTA to accurately avoid using positively and negatively

H.S. Hecht
Director of Cardiovascular Computed Tomography, Lenox Hill Heart & Vascular Institute, New York, NY
e-mail: HHecht@LENOXHILL.NET

M.J. Budoff, J.S. Shinbane (eds.), *Handbook of Cardiovascular CT*,
DOI: 10.1007/978-1-84800-091-9_5, © Springer-Verlag London Limited 2008

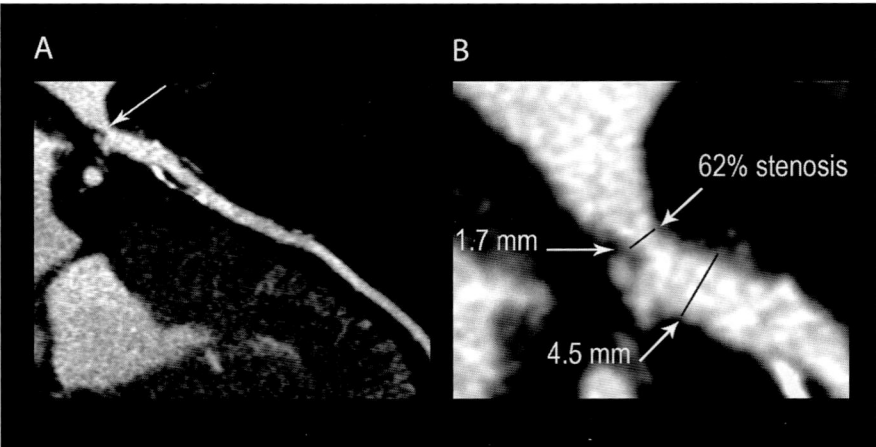

Fig. 5.1 (**a**) Curved MPR of left anterior descending coronary artery demonstrates ostial narrowing in an asymptomatic 58-year-old male. (**b**) Quantitative coronary angiography of ostial lesion; cursors are drawn through the most stenotic and normal reference areas, yielding 62% stenosis. Abbreviation: MPR= multiplanar reformat

    remodeled areas as reference segments, an ability not shared by invasive angiography.

3. A single MLD or percentage stenosis has no physiologic significance except in the rarely occurring perfectly concentric lesion. Rather, the minimum luminal area (MLA) is the best readily available determinant of flow since it incorporates all the possible diameters. It is the cornerstone of IVUS quantitation, and the criteria of <6.0 mm^2 for the left main coronary artery and <4.0 mm^2 for the proximal major vessels have been established to justify percutaneous coronary intervention (PCI) [2]. MLA cannot be measured in the catheterization laboratory without IVUS but is readily calculated from the CTA (**Fig. 5.2**); several studies have supported the correlation between MLA by CTA and IVUS [3, 4].

5.2 Plaque Characterization

Plaque characterization is complex. The simplistic approach would be to assign Hounsfield units (HU; radiologic measure of density) that are applicable in vitro to different plaque components. For instance, lipid would be –150 HU to 0 HU, noncalcified plaque 0 to +130 HU, and calcified plaque >130 HU. However, this method does not work in vivo because HU are affected by the "company they keep." A lipid core adjacent to a calcified plaque may have HU in the >100 range because of the "partial volume effect," whereby sharing voxels with the high-density calcium will elevate the lipid HU and preclude accurate identification as lipid. In addition, calcified plaque cannot be adequately quantified because of the high-density "blooming" that magnifies the true calcified plaque size (**Fig. 5.3**). While this can be partially corrected, there is currently no effective algorithm. A second confounding

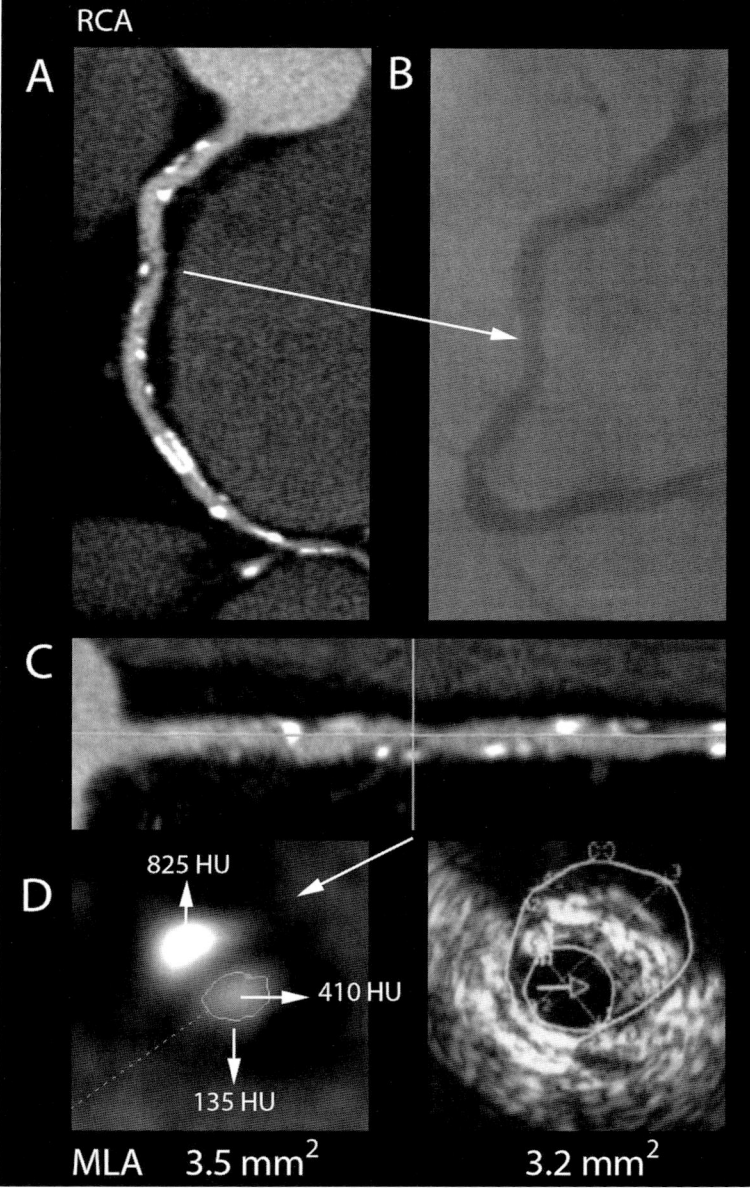

Fig. 5.2 (**a**) Curved MPR of the right coronary artery demonstrates mid-vessel stenosis secondary to combined calcified and noncalcified plaque in a 65-year-old male with new-onset angina. There is proximal plaque and a patent distal stent. (**b**) Corresponding invasive angiogram does not reveal significant narrowing. (**c**) Cross section of the stretched MPR through the stenosis reveals contrast-filled lumen and calcified plaque with a clear noncalcified plaque interface, enabling measurement of the minimum luminal area (3.5 mm²). (**d**) Intravascular ultrasound of the corresponding area confirms the CTA minimum luminal area. Abbbreviation: MPR= multiplanar reformat

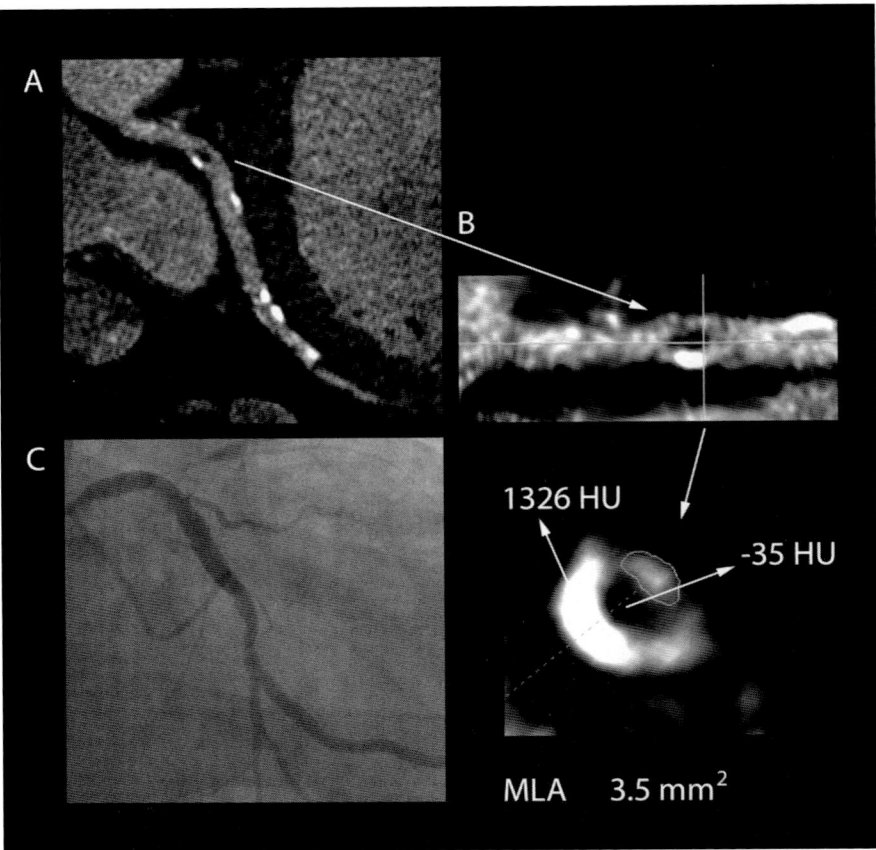

Fig. 5.3 (**a**) Curved MPR of the left circumflex coronary artery reveals a severe ostial lesion secondary to calcified and apparently noncalcified plaque in a 57-year-old female with a prior anteroseptal infarction and atypical chest pain. (**b**) Cross-sectional analysis of the stretched MPR identifies the very low density area with Hounsfield units consistent with lipid, adjacent to densely calcified plaque. Alternatively, the densely calcified plaque is "shadowing" adjacent contrast, mimicking low-density lipid. (**c**) Invasive angiography reveals a normal caliber artery and confirms the "shadowing" etiology. Abbreviation: MPR= multiplanar reformat

factor is "beam hardening" or "shadowing" by very high density calcium of adjacent tissue, which, by decreasing the x-rays reaching this tissue, results in an erroneously low HU (**Fig. 5.3**).

The density gradients between adjacent tissues are much better suited than the absolute numbers for plaque characterization. Gradients in the >150–200 HU range (**Fig. 5.2**) appear to accurately identify different tissue types in an IVUS comparison from our laboratory. There is no absolute gradient criterion that will always suffice; variations in adjacent tissue density, adequacy of coronary filling, and body habitus are always problematic. Nonetheless, accurate MLA measurement is possible even in heavily calcified plaques, provided there is a clear lower density interface between the lumen and the calcified plaque (**Fig. 5.2**).

Plaque quantitation is currently being investigated. The ability to accurately measure plaque burden would provide the basis for the use of serial CTA studies to evaluate the effects of medical therapies, a role currently filled by IVUS. While there is great interest in identifying "vulnerable" plaque, and a lipid core may be readily

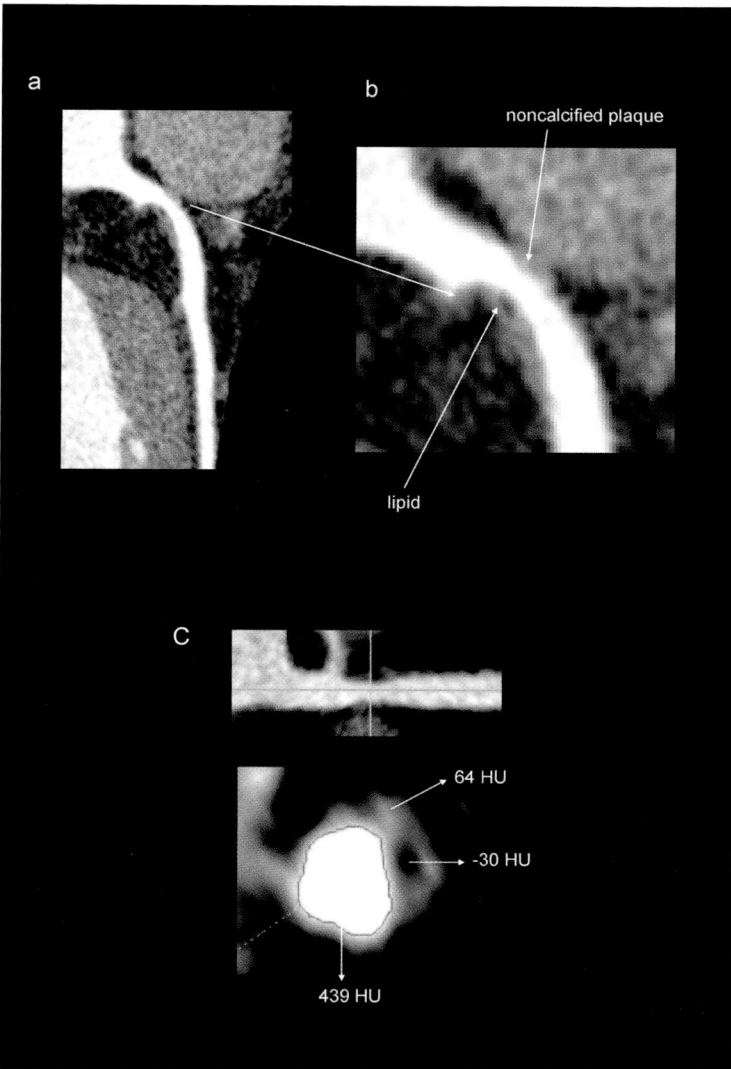

Fig. 5.4 (**a**) 25–50% ostial LAD stenosis in a 43-year-old male who presented to the emergency room with atypical chest pain. The coronary calcium score was 0. (**b**) Magnified view reveals noncalcified plaque of varying density. (**c**) A cross section through the stretched MPR demonstrates exclusively noncalcified plaque, including lipid (–35 HU), representing the CTA equivalent of the thin cap fibroatheroma (TCFA), which is thought to be a strong candidate for plaque rupture and an acute coronary event

identifiable by TIVA (**Fig. 5.4**), if it is not a component of a significantly obstructive plaque, there are no data supporting percutaneous intervention. Nonetheless, identification of such plaques logically mandates very aggressive medical therapy.

5.3 CTA-Guided PCI

5.3.1 Clinical Paradigm

The quantitative and plaque characterization qualities discussed above, by allowing for accurate MLA measurement, provide the basis of CTA-guided PCI [1]. **Figure 5.5** displays the CTA-based paradigm; CTA, rather than stress testing, is the first step in the evaluation of patients for coronary disease. Patients with <50% stenoses are triaged to medical therapy, and those with >75% stenosis are delegated to invasive angiography.

With 50–75% stenoses and MLA <6 mm^2 or 4 mm^2 for the left main and proximal major vessels, respectively, stress testing to determine the functional significance may be appropriate; an abnormal result would indicate a need for PCI, whereas normal perfusion would suggest medical therapy. Since stress testing may be normal in a small but significant number of patients with critical left main or triple vessel disease [5], invasive angiography rather than stress testing may

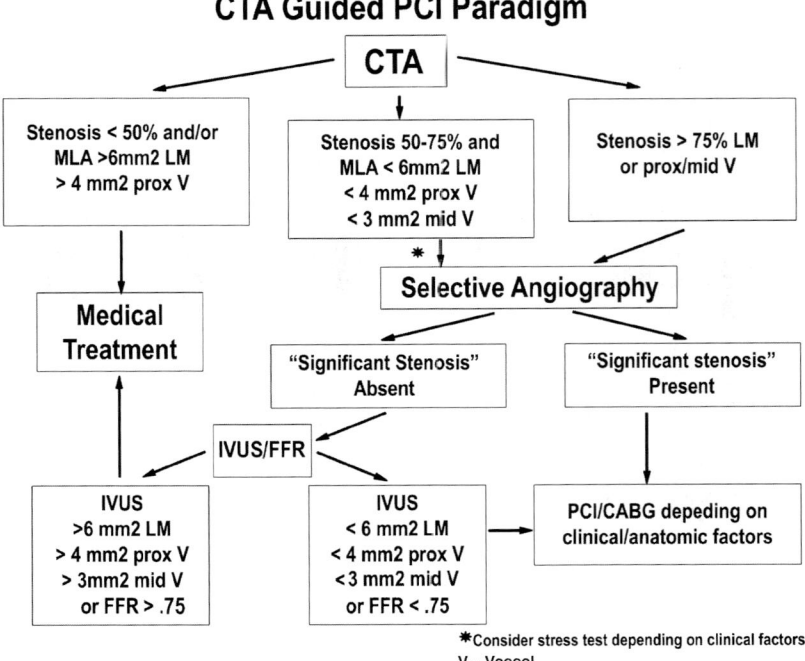

Fig. 5.5 The CTA-guided PCI paradigm (see text)

be preferable. Angiographically apparent significant disease would justify PCI. The absence of angiographically apparent significant disease (**Fig. 5.2**) should be followed by IVUS to confirm the TIVA findings, to be followed by PCI if confirmed and clinically indicated; fractional flow reserve (FFR) may also be utilized as an alternative to IVUS. The decision to perform PCI is not based on the CTA-determined MLA alone; reliance is placed on the CTA-guided IVUS or FFR confirmation rather than on the angiographic appearance. This represents a fundamental change in the traditional paradigm and requires validation of each laboratory's ability to accurately measure MLA, as well as an acceptance of the superiority of IVUS to conventional angiography.

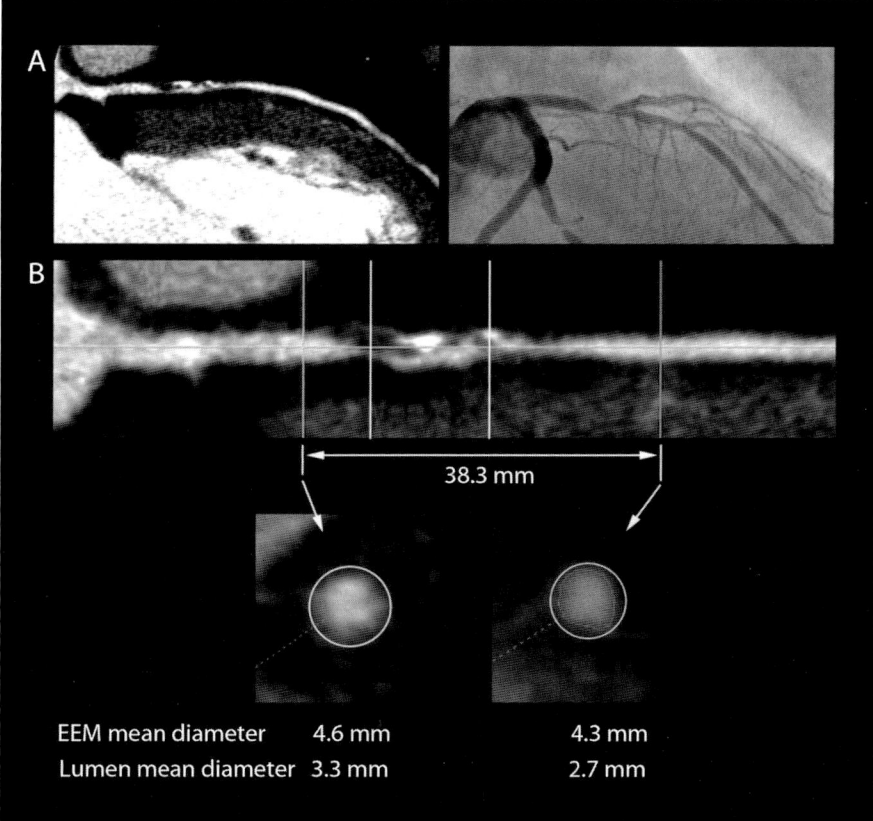

Fig. 5.6 (**a**) A long severely diseased area is seen on the MPR of the left anterior descending coronary artery in a 45-year-old diabetic male with exertional angina (*left*), and on the corresponding invasive angiogram (*right*). The CTA better demonstrates the complexity and extent of the disease. (**b**) Cross-sectional analysis reveals proximal and distal stent-landing zone mean diameters of 3.3 mm and 2.7 mm, respectively, and 38.3 mm of diseased vessel between them, including several critical areas. These data can then be used to size the axial and longitudinal stent dimensions. Abbreviation: MPR= multiplanar reformat

5.4 Optimal Stent Deployment

Stent sizing is readily accomplished (**Fig. 5.6**). By accurately measuring the diameters of the proximal and distal stent landing zones, the axial dimension can be determined. Similarly, the longitudinal stent dimension can be planned, but the decision is dependent on the extent of disease adjacent to the most stenotic area that the operator chooses to cover. For instance, a low-density lipid-laden nonobstructive plaque in the immediate vicinity may be included in the stented area, as well as in the clearly diseased but less obstructive adjacent areas; these cannot be easily appreciated on the conventional coronary angiogram.

The CTA data can be imported directly into the catheterization laboratory and displayed on the monitor next to the invasive angiography (**Fig. 5.7**). The angle of least foreshortening of the stenosis, without vessel overlap, is determined, and the C-arm is automatically rotated to that angle to maximize stent sizing accuracy and to decrease the number of coronary injections. Ultimately, the diagnostic component of the PCI may be shortened to omit the left ventricular angiogram since the CTA

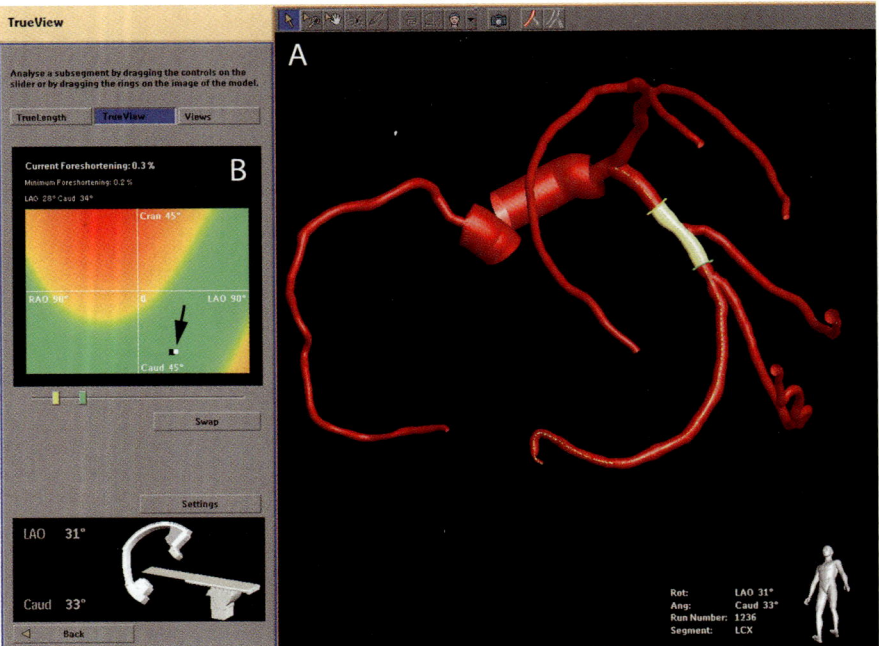

Fig. 5.7 (**a**) A left circumflex stenosis (between the *yellow* and *green* cursors) is delineated on the CTA-generated vessel tree. Computer analysis determines the angles of least foreshortening of the stenotic area and the least overlap (*green* zone). The operator can then rotate the C-arm to move the white dot marking the C-arm position (*arrow*) into the *green* zone; the vessel tree will rotate correspondingly

provides accurate measurement of all but regurgitant parameters, and injection of the non-significantly diseased artery as determined by the CTA.

5.5 Conclusions

The IVUS qualities of CTA have opened the door to an entirely new clinical paradigm in which CTA becomes the triage to the stress testing and catheterization laboratories, and guides the performance of the PCI. Plaque characterization, including identification of the vulnerable plaque, is a work in progress, but can currently be used to direct aggressive medical therapy and choice of areas adjacent to the severe stenosis to be covered by a stent.

5.6 Imaging Pearls

- Curved MPR is superior to MIP for assessment of stenosis severity.
- There are two areas of plaque characterization:

  o Separation of plaque from contrast.
  o Separation of different plaque types.

- Calculation of MLA is dependent on accurate identification of plaque and the ability to separate it from contrast.
- Contrast can never be separated from calcified plaque without an interface of noncalcified plaque between them.
- Tissue characterization cannot be accomplished visually, without quantitation of density by HU measurement.
- Changes in window and center levels, that is, brightness and contrast, will change the visual appearance, and may result in false diagnosis. HU are unaffected by window and center levels.
- Absolute HU may be misleading, since they are affected by the "company they keep"; that is, denser adjacent structures may artificially enhance the density of the tissue in question by a partial volume effect and result in erroneous tissue characterization.
- HU gradients are the key to differentiating between different tissues.
- There are no absolute HU gradient criteria for distinguishing between different tissue types. In general, at least 150–200 HU gradient is required.
- Adjacent structures, if very dense, may have the opposite effect, and may decrease the density of the tissue in question (shadowing), by decreasing the penetration of x-rays through the tissue.
- There are no absolute densities above which there is certainty that adjacent structures will be "shadowed." The most suspicious scenario is the combination of $HU < 0$ adjacent to $HU > 1000$, but exceptions occur.

- There is no clinical gold standard for plaque characterization. Comparison with IVUS, and particularly Virtual Histology, is the only currently available tool and is far from universal acceptance.
- IVUS correlation is essential for each laboratory to have a sense of correctness of their plaque characterization.
- Excellent study quality is essential, including:
  - Uniformity of contrast filling.
  - High signal-to-noise ratio; contrast HU should exceed 300 in proximal vessels.
  - mAs and KV should be adjusted to achieve adequate tissue penetration and must vary with body habitus.
  - Appropriate filtering: smoother filters for larger patients.
  - Minimization of motion and arrhythmias; artifactual alteration of tissue density will result in misdiagnosis of plaque type
- CTA serves as the triage for the cardiac catheterization and stress-testing laboratories.
- CTA identifies arteries that are significantly diseased, and mandates IVUS or FFR even if the stenosis is not angiographically apparent.
- Decision to perform PCI of stenoses that are not angiographically apparent is based on the CTA-guided IVUS and clinical appropriateness.
- CTA guides PCI by providing the least foreshortened angle and accurate stent sizing.
- CTA should be imported directly into the catheterization laboratory.

References

1. Hecht HS, Roubin G. Usefulness of computed tomographic angiography guided percutaneous coronary intervention. Am J Cardiol 2007, 99: 871–5
2. Tobis J, Azarbal B, Slavin L. Assessment of intermediate severity coronary lesions in the catheterization Laboratory. J Am Coll Cardiol 2007, 49: 839–48
3. Moselewski F, Ropers D, Pohle K, Hoffmann U, Ferencik M, Chan RC, Cury RC, Abbara S, Jang IK, Brady TJ, et al. Measurement of cross-sectional coronary atherosclerotic plaque and vessel areas by 16-slice multi-detector CT: comparison to IVUS. Am J Cardiol 2004, 94: 1294–7.
4. Caussin C, Larchez C, Ghostine S, et al. Comparison of coronary minimal lumen area quantification by sixty-four–slice computed tomography versus intravascular ultrasound for intermediate stenosis. Am J Cardiol 2006, 98: 871–6.
5. Lima RSL, Denny D. Watson DD, Goode AR. Incremental value of combined perfusion and function over perfusion alone by gated SPECT myocardial perfusion imaging for detection of severe three-vessel coronary artery disease. J Am Coll Cardiol 2003, 42: 64–70.

Chapter 6
Coronary Angiography of Native Vessels

Matthew J. Budoff

Cardiac computed tomography (CT) is a robust technology for the non-invasive assessment for a spectrum of cardiovascular disease processes. This image modality has been used to provide assessment of atherosclerotic plaque burden and coronary artery disease risk through coronary calcium scoring for 20 years and CT angiography for over 10 years [1].

While electron beam tomography has been used to perform CT angiography (CTA) for well over a decade, this modality has been largely supplanted by multi-detector computed tomography (MDCT) due to higher spatial resolution, improved slice thickness, and greater availability. MDCT scanners with x-ray tubes rotating fast enough to allow coronary artery imaging (500 milliseconds [ms] or less per rotation) became available in the late 1990s. The temporal resolution of MDCT is a little more than half the time it takes for the x-ray gantry to complete a 360° rotation around the patient when using half-scan reconstruction. Thus, typical rotation speeds are 330–420 ms (depending on vendor), so half-scan reconstruction results in rotation speeds of 200–250 ms. The nominal temporal resolution can be improved by a factor of 2–3 (depending on the heart rate) by segmented reconstruction techniques that combine projection data acquired during two or more cardiac cycles into one image. This has been done in two ways. Combining images from consecutive heartbeats is widely available on all current 64-detector systems (multi-segment reconstruction). The Dual Source CT (Siemens, Erlangen, Germany) can also obtain similar temporal resolution by combining images from two detector arrays in the same heartbeat. In this way, current MDCT scanners can acquire up to 64 slices simultaneously with a maximum temporal resolution as low as 100 ms. Because of the high motion velocity of the coronary arteries, CT scanners must have temporal resolution of <50 ms to provide motion-free images of the beating heart. Since that level of temporal resolution is not yet available with current MDCT scanners, use of beta-blockers is routine. Most centers utilize oral beta-blockers prior to patient arrival at the scanning center if possible, and subsequent use of intravenous

M.J. Budoff
Los Angeles Biomedical Research Institute, Harbor-UCLA Medical Center, Torrance, CA, USA
e-mail: mbudoff@labiomed.org

M.J. Budoff, J.S.Shinbane (eds.), *Handbook of Cardiovascular CT*,
DOI: 10.1007/978-1-84800-091-9_6, © Springer-Verlag London Limited 2008

beta-blockers when heart rates exceed 60 beats per minute. If beta-blockers cannot be used due to active asthma or other contraindications, use of diltiazem or vera-pamil is most common.

6.1 Spatial Resolution

The smallest x-ray beam collimation possible with a given CT scanner dictates the minimal thickness of the image slices that can be reconstructed. The slice thickness affects spatial resolution. High spatial resolution allows assessment of small side branches of the coronary arteries, decreases artifacts due to partial-volume effects, and leads to better assessment of calcified coronary artery segments and in-stent stenoses. Spatial resolution has improved with each advance in MDCT technology. "Submillimeter" resolution has been achieved in MDCT scanners ranging from 16 to 256 slices. The spatial resolution of current 64-slice MDCT scanners is approx-imately 0.4 mm [1]. This is an improvement over the 0.7 mm resolution of early 16-slice MDCT scanners, but not as high as catheter-based cine angiography (less than 0.3 mm).

6.2 Coronary CTA for Identification of Native Vessel Coronary Stenoses

The feasibility of coronary CTA was initially demonstrated with EBT and four-slice MDCT [1]. However, image evaluation was impaired in many cases due to limited spatial and temporal resolution. With the introduction of 16-slice MDCT, image quality in coronary CTA has become more consistent. The 16-slice technology with a gantry rotation time below 500 ms and slice collimation of less than 1.0 mm is the minimal technical prerequisite for contrast-enhanced MDCT coronary CTA. Studies that used 16-slice acquisition and rotation times below 400 ms have reported sensi-tivities between 83% and 98% as well as specificities between 96% and 98% [1]. The 64-slice MDCT provides shorter examination times; some scanners also incor-porate improved temporal and spatial resolution compared to early 16-slice MDCT. A recent meta-analysis by Stein et al. [2] reported the diagnostic accuracy by a patient and segmental analysis. These authors noted that the average sensitivity and specificity values were 95% and 84% for four-slice CT and increased to 98–100% for 64-slice CT. Clinicians must weigh the relative advantages of other testing methods such as exercise testing or stress imaging. The choice of testing will be determined by both local expertise in a given hospital as well as the patient's specific clinical history. Functional information demonstrating the physiologic significance of coronary lesions is still paramount for decision making related to revascular-ization. CT has certain advantages over nuclear or functional testing. CT has been shown to be more accurate in determining the presence of obstructive disease [3], providing better prognostic information related to future cardiac events [4], and allowing quantification of plaque burden [1].

In a clinical context, the high negative predictive value is useful to obviate the need for invasive coronary angiography in patients in whom symptoms or an abnormal stress test result requires a clinician to rule out the presence of obstructive CAD. Especially if symptoms, age, and gender suggest a low-to-intermediate probability of hemodynamically relevant stenoses [5], ruling out significant stenoses by CT coronary angiography may be clinically useful and should help avoid invasive angiography. Due to its high negative predictive value, the consensus among most imaging experts is that MDCT can be used as a reliable filter before invasive coronary angiography in the assessment of symptomatic patients with intermediate risk of coronary artery disease and in patients with uninterpretable or equivocal stress tests [6]. Thus, MDCT is often applied as a primary gatekeeper when pretest probability is low, and a secondary gatekeeper in patients with mildly positive SPECT (or equivocal finding) prior to deciding whether to perform conventional coronary angiography in these patients. One major advantage of CT over functional imaging is its ability to determine atherosclerosis burden (targets for lipid lowering and other preventive therapies) as well as the presence of obstructive disease. Currently, "screening" of asymptomatic individuals concerning the presence of coronary artery stenoses is not justified due to radiation and contrast risks.

6.3 Limitations Specific to Coronary CTA

Coronary artery segments with severe calcification may not be evaluable concerning the presence of a hemodynamically relevant stenosis. Coronary CTA requires intravenous injection of iodinated contrast media. Since patients may subsequently require invasive angiography, patients with compromised renal function are generally excluded from coronary CTA. In addition to nephrotoxicity, intravenous administration of iodinated contrast media may also be associated with anaphylactoid reaction [1].

The predominant risk of coronary CTA is radiation exposure. However, newer techniques are now allowing for reduction of radiation doses from 13–18 mSv (64-MDCT, dual source) or higher (256 or 320 MDCT), to doses now averaging only 2–3 mSv with prospective axial gating. This technique will allow for markedly reduced doses of radiation; however, only a small range of images within the cardiac cycle are available. With this new technique, evaluation of ejection fraction and wall motion is not possible, and significant motion artifacts cannot be overcome by evaluating different phases of the cardiac cycle, as is currently done with retrospective triggering with all phases available for analysis.

Careful selection of patients is crucial to increase the diagnostic yield of coronary CTA using MDCT. Relatively fast heart rates (i.e., more than 70 beats per minute after beta-blocker administration), irregular heart rhythm, baseline renal insufficiency, and extensive CAC are three major limitations of MDCT angiography. Newer generation of MDCT technology with even faster gantry rotation may further reduce the motion artifacts of the coronaries, and newer detector arrays may allow for better spatial resolution and blooming artifacts associated with CAC.

6.4 Imaging Pearls

- Use of axial data and selected thin slabs of data can quickly and efficiently allow for evaluation of the coronary tree. A maximum intensity projection (MIP) is a slab of data that can be demonstrated in any plane. The axial plane (the same plane in which images are obtained) is ideal for evaluation of structures that run perpendicular to the long axis of the body ("in-plane" for the axial slices obtained). These include the distal right, posterior descending artery (PDA), and postero-lateral marginal branch (PLMB) by using the axial plane and creating an MIP image (thin but just thick enough to see the distal right coronary artery (RCA), and PDA in one image—**Fig. 6.1**; the left main, proximal, and mid–left anterior descending (LAD) and first and second diagonals, as well as the proximal circumflex are all potentially visible in one axial MIP (**Fig. 6.2**). Axial data is also ideal for evaluation of non-coronary structures, including myocardial enhancement (perfusion).
- Use of a coronal MIP (vertical from head to toe) will allow quick evaluation of the mid-RCA (**Fig. 6.3**) (and RCA grafts if present), as well as visualization of the presence and the magnitude of pericardial effusions and inferior wall infarctions (difficult to assess in axial images).
- Use the sagittal plane (lateral from left to right) images to evaluate the distal LAD (emulates a straight lateral view on invasive catheterization—**Fig. 6.4**), the left internal mammary artery insertion (if present), and the mid-LAD when taking an intra-myocardial course (bridging, **Fig. 6.5**) as well as the entire course of the aorta.

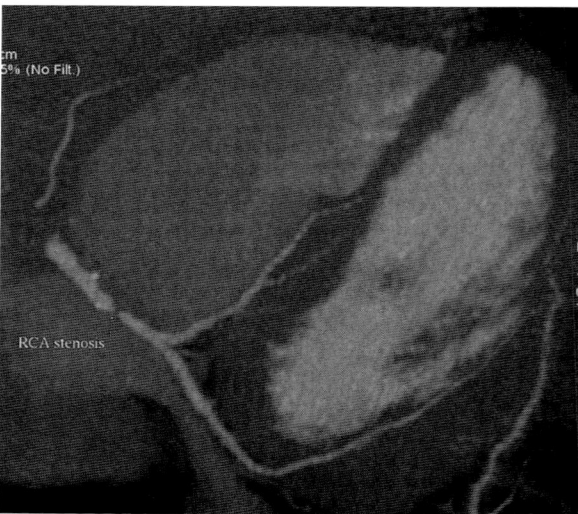

Fig. 6.1 An axial maximum intensity projection (MIP) demonstrating the entire distal right coronary artery distribution (including a high-grade stenosis of the distal right coronary artery)

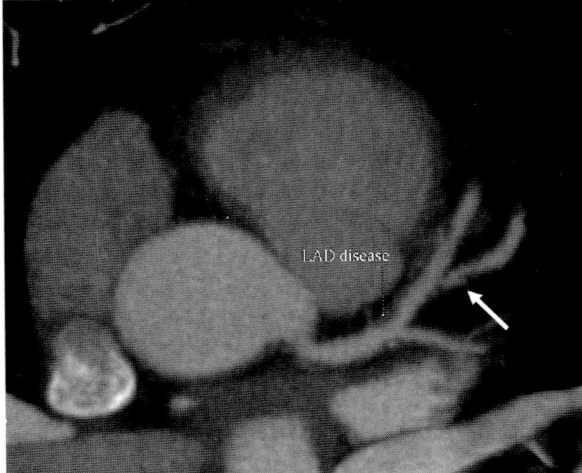

Fig. 6.2 An axial maximum intensity projection (MIP) demonstrating the much of the left anterior coronary artery distribution (including the left main, left anterior descending, diagonal, and proximal circumflex). There is a non-calcific plaque in the left anterior descending and the first diagonal has severe ostial disease (*arrow*)

- Confirm stenoses on the axial data. If it isn't on the axial data but is seen in 3-D reconstructions, it is most likely an artifact.
- Use volume rendering to get an overall 3-D look at the heart. This will help with defining the overall size and distributions of the arteries (which branches are

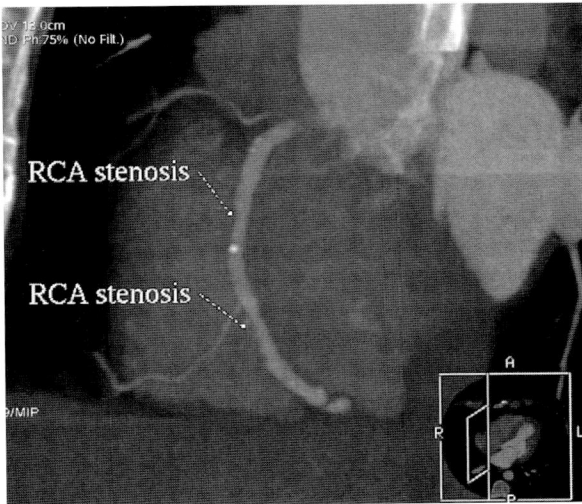

Fig. 6.3 A coronal maximum intensity projection demonstrating the mid-right coronary artery distribution (including mild sequential disease)

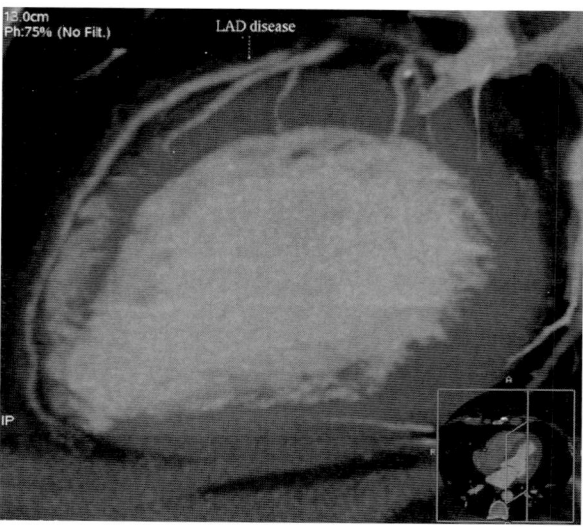

Fig. 6.4 A sagittal maximum intensity projection demonstrating the entire mid- and distal left anterior descending coronary artery (including mild disease of the mid-left anterior descending)

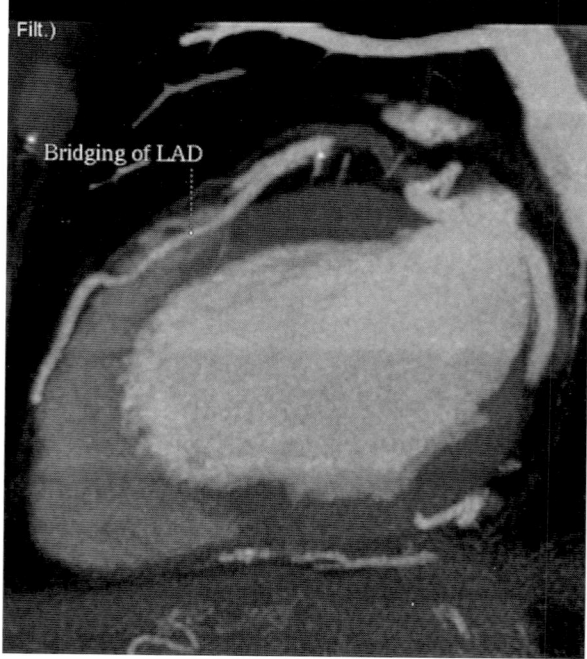

Fig. 6.5 A sagittal maximum intensity projection demonstrating the mid- and distal left anterior descending coronary artery (with the presence of an intramyocardial course or "bridging")

worth further evaluation with CT) and retains a high specificity for obstructive disease (if there is no contrast or calcification in a segment, it is most likely highly diseased).

- After volume rendering, look at selected MIP images or curved multiplanar images of the selected vessels that have concerns.
- Give up after 30 min (once you are facile with the workstation). If interpretation is taking longer than 30 min on a given case, the study is non-diagnostic. Garbage in = garbage out.
- Use different planes to evaluate different walls of the heart: (axial data—apical, septal, and lateral walls; coronal images—inferior wall; sagittal—apical, posterior, and inferior walls).
- When doing two CTA studies, always do the non-cardiac study first. The venous contamination (from prior contrast injection) will make carotids (jugular filling), peripherals (venous filling), or renals (IVC and venous filling) much more difficult. The coronary study always has venous filling due to the low pitch and long injection times, and the software can eliminate the veins.
- The average length required craniocaudally for a cardiac CTA is approximately 12–14 cm (due to the length of the heart). Thus, for every 1 cm of the chest scanned during the CTA, there is a radiation exposure of approximately 1 mSv (male patient). Women typically get up to 50% higher cardiac CTA doses than men, as the breast tissue is radiosensitive. Thus, for younger patients, use prospective triggering and always use dose modulation (except when fast or irregular heart rates are present).

References

1. Budoff MJ, Achenbach S, Blumenthal RS, Carr JJ, Goldin JG, Greenland P, Guerci AD, Lima JAC, Rader DJ, Rubin GD, Shaw LJ, Wiegers SE. Assessment of Coronary Artery Disease by Cardiac Computed Tomography, A Scientific Statement From the American Heart Association Committee on Cardiovascular Imaging and Intervention, Council on Cardiovascular Radiology and Intervention, and Committee on Cardiac Imaging, Council on Clinical Cardiology. Circulation 2006, 114 (16): 1761–91.
2. Stein PD, Beemath A, Kayali F, et al. Multidetector Computed Tomography for the Diagnosis of Coronary Artery Disease: A Systematic Review. Am J Med 2006, 119: 203–16.
3. Budoff MJ, Rasouli ML, Shavelle DM, Gopal A, Gul KM, Mao SS, Liu SH, McKay CR. Cardiac CT Angiography (CTA) and Nuclear Myocardial Perfusion Imaging (MPI)-A Comparison in Detecting Significant Coronary Artery Disease. Acad Radiol 2007 Mar, 14 (3): 252–7.
4. Ramakrishna G, Breen JF, Mulvagh SL, et al. Relationship Between Coronary Artery Calcification Detected by Electron-Beam Computed Tomography and Abnormal Stress Echocardiography Association and Prognostic Implications. J Am Coll Cardiol 2006, 48: 2125–31.
5. Gibbons RJ, Chatterjee K, Daley J, Douglas JS, Fihn SD, Gardin JM, Grunwald MA, Levy D, Lytle BW, O'Rourke RA, Schafer WP, Williams SV. ACC/AHA/ACP-ASIM guidelines for the management of patients with chronic stable angina: executive summary and recommendations. A Report of the American College of Cardiology/American Heart Association Task Force on Practice Guidelines (Committee on Management of Patients with Chronic Stable Angina). Circulation 1999 Jun 1, 99 (21): 2829–48.

6. Hendel RC, Patel MR, Kramer CM, et al. ACCF/ACR/SCCT/SCMR/ASNC/NASCI/SCAI/SIR 2006 appropriateness criteria for cardiac computed tomography and cardiac magnetic resonance imaging: a report of the American College of Cardiology Foundation Quality Strategic Directions Committee Appropriateness Criteria Working Group, American College of Radiology, Society of Cardiovascular Computed Tomography, Society for Cardiovascular Magnetic Resonance, American Society of Nuclear Cardiology, North American Society for Cardiac Imaging, Society for Cardiovascular Angiography and Interventions, and Society of Interventional Radiology. J Am Coll Cardiol 2006, 48: 1475–97.

Chapter 7
Coronary CT Angiography after Percutaneous Coronary Intervention

Wm Guy Weigold

7.1 Introduction

Coronary CT angiography (CTA) is increasingly becoming a more widespread and reliable method of interrogating the coronary vasculature. Its sensitivity makes it an excellent means of detecting coronary artery disease (CAD) in patients with angina and/or abnormal stress test results. It is natural that the technique would be applied to patients who have undergone percutaneous coronary intervention (PCI) for obstructive coronary disease.

As with the imaging of native coronary vessels, general cardiac CT concepts apply: opacify the coronary tree with iodinated contrast material; use helical scanning to acquire the volume data while using ECG gating to "time stamp" that data; and reconstruct the axial dataset using data only from a quiescent time point in the cardiac cycle, thus excluding data acquired during cardiac motion and removing motion artifacts from the images. Performed optimally, the resultant images are motion free and possess exquisite sub-millimeter resolution.

In coronary stent CTA, however, even completely motion-free images will contain, at the least, artifacts that emanate from the stent itself, and may as well confront the reader with coronary calcification, which is more likely to be present in the known CAD patient. "Blooming" artifact from both metal and calcium can obscure visualization of the stent lumen, or create shadows and low-density artifacts that may reduce the specificity of the test. Any degree of motion added to this presents a greater challenge than the same degree of motion in a normal unstented coronary segment. For these reasons, coronary stent CTA is generally considered more challenging, and requires special attention to patient prep, scan protocol, and image reconstruction methods in order to optimize results.

W.G. Weigold
Division of Cardiovascular Disease, Department of Medicine, Washington Hospital Centre, Washington, DC 20010, USA
e-mail: Guy.Weigold@MedStar.net

M.J. Budoff, J.S. Shinbane (eds.), *Handbook of Cardiovascular CT*,
DOI: 10.1007/978-1-84800-091-9_7, © Springer-Verlag London Limited 2008

7.2 Current State of the Literature

Reliably imaging the stented coronary vessel requires at least a 16-row scanner and sub-millimeter collimation. Kruger et al. examined 32 stents in 20 patients using a quad scanner and found that none of the stents were evaluable because volume averaging of the bright, high-density stent struts obscured the lower-density contrast-filled lumens [1]. In this and other reports [2], some authors have proposed defining stent patency by the presence of contrast opacification of the vessel distal to the stent; however, this is not sufficient to establish stent patency, as demonstrated by cases in which the distal vessel remains opacified despite severe in-stent restenosis.

In three 16-slice studies of a combination of 195 patients, the prevalence of non-diagnostic stent images was 17–36% [3, 4, 5]. Determinants of unevaluability included stent size, strut thickness, and stent material. In addition, stents were often unevaluable due to the presence of metal blooming and volume averaging artifact, heavily calcified segments, and motion artifact. In the study by Schuijf et al. [3], 90% of stents >3.0 mm were interpretable, compared with only 72% of stents ≤3.0 mm. In addition, 89% of stents with strut thickness <140 μm were interpretable, compared with only 41% of thicker strutted stents. Similarly, Gilard et al. [4] found that 81% of stents >3.0 mm were evaluable (vs. 50% of stents ≤3.0 mm), and Watanabe et al. [5] reported that unevaluable stents were smaller on average (2.7 mm vs. 3.4 mm).

In the three 16-slice accuracy studies, sensitivity for the detection of ISR ranged from 77% to 83% of evaluable stents, but was as low as 50% when unevaluable stents were included and considered restenosed by default. Specificity for identifying non-obstructed stents was 90–100% for evaluable stents, but 74% when unevaluable stents were included and assigned restenosed status. The prevalence of ISR in these studies was 9–14%; positive predictive value (PPV) ranged from 63% to 100%; and negative predictive value (NPV) ranged from 95% to 96%.

One study using a 40-row scanner examined 111 stents in 65 patients and found 5% of stents unevaluable, and sensitivity and specificity of 74% and 86% for diagnosis or exclusion of ISR [6]. In this group with ISR prevalence of 24%, the PPV of an abnormal reading was only 62%, but the NPV was 91%.

There have been two significant studies of stent imaging using 64-row scanners examining a combined 265 stents in 145 patients, and they report significantly different results. Ehara et al. [7] found that 12% of 163 stents were considered unevaluable, a figure in keeping with most other studies, while Gaspar et al. [8] found that 42% of 102 stents were deemed inadequately visualized for diagnosis. This discrepancy is in part due to the subjective nature of the determination of "evaluability," and likely reflects the stringent criteria applied for considering a stent evaluable.

In the study by Ehara et al. [7], sensitivity and specificity for the diagnosis of ISR were 92% and 81% of stents, and 90% and 79% of patients. Their disease prevalence was 12% of patients, and their PPV and NPV were 58% and 96%. Missed ISR was caused by a technically poor scan or multiple overlapping stents with metal, calcification, and motion artifacts obscuring the stent lumen, while false positive reading was attributed to heavy calcification and motion artifact producing low-attenuation artifacts mistaken for intimal hyperplasia. In the work by Gaspar et al. [8], sensitivity and specificity were only 42% and 50% when unevaluable stents were included. Excluding unevaluable stents, however, sensitivity was 86% and specificity was 98%, and PPV and NPV were 86% and 98%.

Two studies have examined left main stents by CTA. The first examined 162 stents in 70 patients, including 24 patients with complicated left main bifurcation stenting, and used either a 16- or a 64-row scanner [9]. In this study 10 patients had ISR by QCA, and CTA detected ISR in all 10. There were five false positive CTAs, four in patients with left main bifurcation stents, where the excessive and overlapping metal make interpretation of normal more difficult. Still the overall specificity for exclusion of ISR was 92%. In another study, 29 patients were studied by a 16-row scanner and four out of four had their LMCA ISR correctly detected by CTA [10]. Specificity was 88% because of three false positive readings, again predominantly due to metal artifact, calcium, and motion.

In vivo studies of stent artifacts have provided some insights. Maintz et al. [11] looked at 19 stents expanded within contrast-filled tubing to a diameter of 3.0 mm, examined with a four-row scanner, and found significant artificial lumen reductions of 62–94% resulting from metal blooming artifact alone, which varied depending on stent strut material and thickness.

Mahnken [12] performed a similar study using 4- or 16-row scanner and incorporating specialized reconstruction algorithms to enhance edge detection and found artificial lumen reductions from 20% to 100%, again depending on stent material and strut thickness. Maintz et al. [13] re-examined the issue with 64-row scanner, examining 68 stents including stainless steel, cobalt–chromium, cobalt alloy, nitinol, and tantalum, and used four reconstruction algorithms. They found that the "high resolution" reconstruction algorithm permits best lumen visualization, albeit with increased image noise. Stent material was also important, as gold or gold-plated or tantalum stents produced the most metal blooming artifact.

7.3 Strengths and Limitations; Indications and Contraindications

Coronary CTA is a fast, low-risk, noninvasive option for evaluating post-PCI patients. However, in this patient population two new challenges are introduced: (1) imaging a vessel lumen that is surrounded by a jacket of metal and (2) imaging patients with known CAD. As both in vitro and in vivo studies have shown, the stent itself adds new artifacts, and in the known CAD patient, there is an increased likelihood of encountering calcified or diffusely diseased vessels, which make coronary visualization in general more difficult. It is for these reasons, plus the generally low prevalence of ISR in most studies, that the specificity and PPV of coronary CTA for stents has not been higher. Limitations of coronary CTA for the evaluation of stents include spatial resolution that is still less than that of invasive angiography, relatively low temporal resolution that makes the technique vulnerable to image artifacts from cardiac or respiratory motion, and the requirement for strict heart rate modulation and patient compliance. Smaller stents are difficult to adequately visualize, and as such, false positive rates may be high.

Hence, coronary CTA for the evaluation of stents may be described as a mixed bag: the high sensitivity and NPV makes it a useful method of excluding ISR in patients in whom there is sufficient pre-test probability of disease, but on the other hand, its lower specificity makes it less useful as a surveillance modality for follow-up of asymptomatic patients, in whom the false positive rate would likely be unacceptably high and would lead to unnecessary catheterizations. With these ideas in mind, the appropriateness criteria for CT have rated coronary CTA in symptomatic patients as an uncertain (possibly appropriate) indication, pending more data, while its use in the asymptomatic patient after stenting is considered inappropriate [14].

7.4 Comparison to Other Modalities

Assessment of stent patency by coronary magnetic resonance angiography (MRA) has been difficult. Stent lumen visualization by MRA is significantly limited by intraluminal signal void that results from the inability of the radiofrequency signal to penetrate the metal [15]. As is the case with coronary CTA, demonstration of coronary flow distal to the stent, and the assumption that such a finding rules out obstruction within the unvisualized stent lumen, is not sufficient to exclude in-stent restenosis. In addition to the technical difficulties of visualizing the stent lumen, there may also be concern about imaging these metal implants using MRI.

Physiologic studies have performed well in the evaluation of patients after PCI. In one meta-analysis, the overall sensitivity for detection of obstructive disease (either in-stent restenosis or progression of disease) by stress myocardial nuclear perfusion imaging was between 75% and 100% and specificity was between approximately 75% and 80%, while sensitivity of stress echo was slightly lower (63%) but wide ranging (95% confidence interval of 15–100%), and specificity was very good (87%) [16, 17]. Physiologic testing offers the ability to detect ischemia after PCI in general, while coronary CTA can interrogate the stent(s) in particular, and differentiate in-stent restenosis from progression of disease elsewhere in the coronary tree. As restenosis rates decline because of the increased use of drug-eluting stents, indirect assessments of stent patency such as stress nuclear or echocardiographic imaging will suffer from increased false positive rates, while in the low pre-test likelihood patient population, coronary CTA will perform best.

7.5 Future Directions

Improvement in the ability of coronary CTA to evaluate stents will likely come from improvements in the scanners: increased spatial resolution with the use of flat panel detector systems and improvements in detector sensitivity and efficiency, improved temporal resolution with the use of dual-source systems or through increased gantry rotation speed, and improved reconstruction algorithms to better accommodate the stent material and reduce metal blooming artifact. Finally, improvements in stents themselves may contribute to advances in this area, if bioabsorbable stents become robust enough for everyday use, in which case the major limitation of stent imaging by CT will literally disappear.

7.6 Imaging Pearls

7.6.1 Patient Preparation

- Patient preparation is key. The general rules for imaging coronary arteries apply, but are even more critical to high-quality results when imaging stents.
- Modulate the heart rate. The goal should be a heart rate solidly planted within the 55–65 bpm range. Like native coronary vessels, stents are better imaged at lower heart rates.
- Make sure the patient understands the scan instructions, especially the breathing instructions, and is able to comply. Any respiratory motion will degrade the scan and cannot be overcome by the usual reconstruction or post-processing techniques. Having the patient practice a 20-s breath hold before the scan will reduce the chances of respiratory motion during the scan.
- Use nitroglycerin, 400–800 mcgs sublingual, or equivalent, 3–5 min before the CTA. As with native coronary studies, this will help to dilate the vessels and improve contrast opacification and contrast-to-noise ratio of the coronary tree.

7.6.2 Opacification and Scanning

- Use a high flow rate (5 cc/s) and high iodine concentration agent (370–400 mgI/ml) to maximize the contrast-to-noise ratio.
- Tube parameters (voltage [kVp] and current [mA]) are generally the same as for coronary imaging. Just be sure to use adequate tube voltage and current for the patient's particular body habitus.
- Do not use dose modulation if the heart rate and rhythm are not optimal (55–65 bpm in sinus rhythm without ectopy). You may need to reconstruct phases at unusual locations in the cardiac cycle, and will want the entire cardiac cycle available at full resolution.

7.6.3 Image Reconstruction

Figures 1–6: Image reconstruction methods have a dramatic influence on the appearance and diagnostic quality of coronary CTA images. The most important reconstruction parameters for coronary CTA in general, and for stent imaging in particular, are reconstructed slice width, reconstruction kernel, image enhancement, displayed MIP thickness, and window level and width. In this example, the same raw dataset has been reconstructed multiple times, with one factor adjusted for comparison. Other reconstruction parameters are optimized for stent imaging.

- To reduce metal "blooming" artifact, use the thinnest reconstruction slice width possible, with 50% overlap (**Fig. 7.1**). Also use the sharpest reconstruction algorithm (kernel) available, or use a dedicated stent algorithm if available, in order to enhance the stent and vessel edges (**Fig. 7.2**). Together, this will likely increase image noise, so be sure to use adequate tube current.
- To further improve stent and vessel edge definition, use image enhancement either within the reconstruction algorithm and/or in the post-processing (**Fig. 7.3**).

(A) (B)

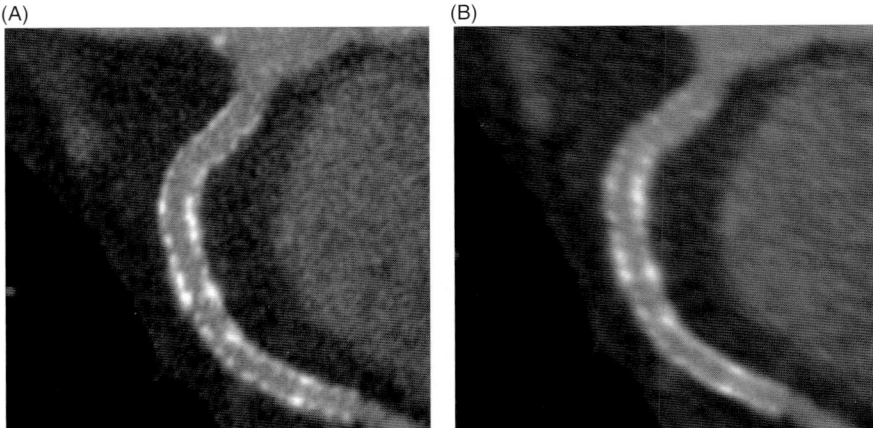

Fig. 7.1 (**A**) The reconstructed slice width is 0.67 mm; the thinner the slice, the better for stents; (**B**) At a slice width of 1.5 mm, volume averaging increases image ambiguity

(A) (B)

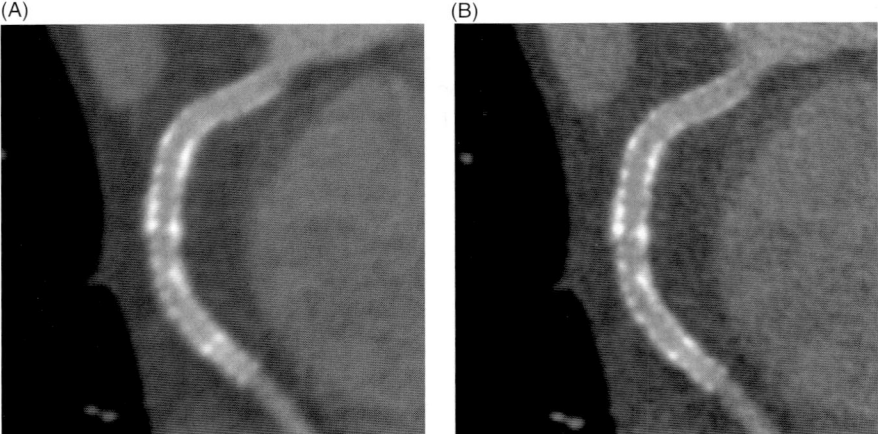

Fig. 7.2 (**A**) A soft reconstruction kernel produces a smoother image, but with less-detailed edges; (**B**) A sharp reconstruction kernel is more appropriate and improves the edge detail and reduces the blooming artifact

(A) (B)

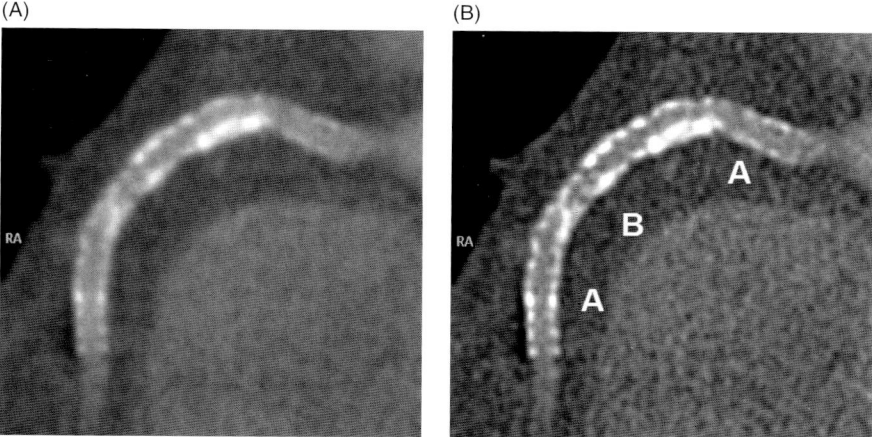

Fig. 7.3 (**A**) Image enhancement is another way to increase edge details and reduce blurring; this image is unenhanced; (**B**) Image enhancement sharpens the image and reduces ambiguity (**A**), but can also introduce new artifacts if the image becomes too grainy (**B**)

(A) (B)

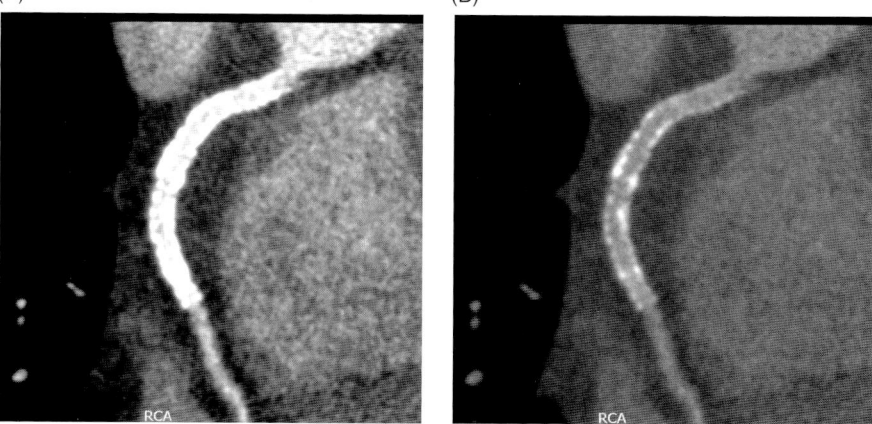

Fig. 7.4 (**A**) A typical CT window level and width increases the metal blooming effect of the stent, and obscures the stent lumen; (**B**) A slightly higher window level, and much wider window width, reduce the blooming and allow visualization of the stent lumen

- Use a wide window width (around 1000–1500 HU) to reduce the appearance of the stent metal and improve visualization of the stent lumen (**Fig. 7.4**).

7.6.4 Interpretation

- Select the most motion-free images. Use multiple phases to evaluate stents for any degree of motion artifact, as this often leads to artifacts that are mistaken for stenosis.

- Use the minimum image thickness for display and analysis—do not use maximum intensity projections (MIPs) (**Fig. 7.5**). The high-density metal of the stent is preferentially displayed by the MIP technique and obscures the lower-density contrast material within the stent lumen (Compare to **Fig. 7.6**).

(A) (B)

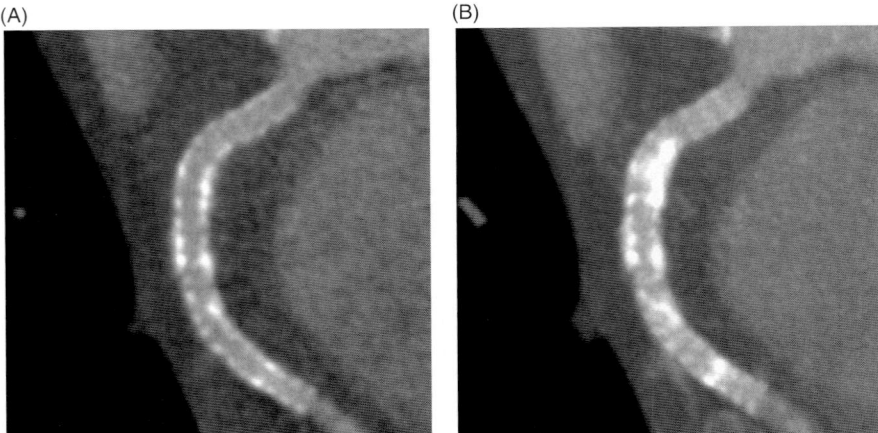

Fig. 7.5 (**A**) When examining stents, the minimum displayed slab thickness should be used; (**B**) Use of the usual 5 mm MIP thickness typically used for non-stented coronary segments will obscure the stent lumen

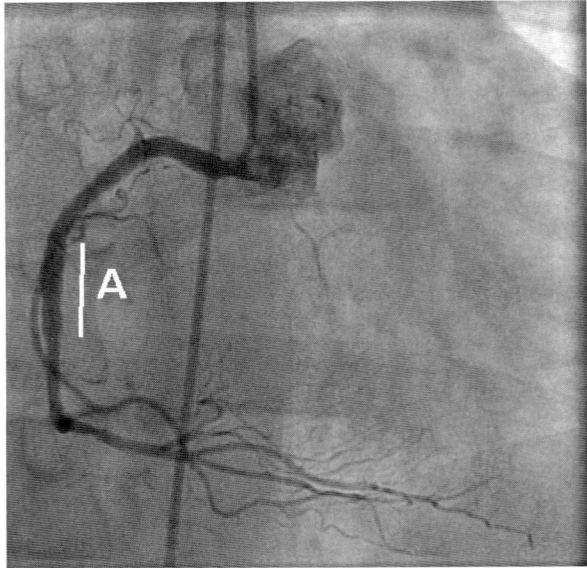

Fig. 7.6 The invasive angiogram of this right coronary artery demonstrates that this is in fact a patent stent (**A**)

- Curved multiplanar reformations (cMPRs) can help to visualize the entire length of a curvilinear stent lumen and facilitate stenosis interpretation.
- Intimal hyperplasia appears as low-density material within or at the edges of the stent. Its appearance is similar to that of non-calcified plaque. Focus on evaluation of the contrast column when trying to differentiate mild intimal hyperplasia from in-stent restenosis (**Figs. 7.7 and 7.8**). Angiographic restenosis by QCA

(A)   (B)

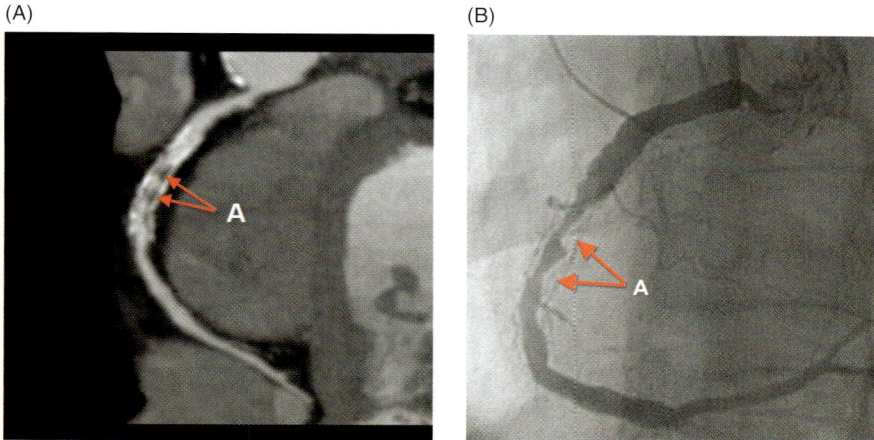

Fig. 7.7 In-stent restenosis demonstrated by coronary CTA (**A**) Significant accumulation of low-density material (intimal hyperplasia) (**A**) within the stent leads to restenosis of the stent lumen. (**B**) Invasive coronary angiogram confirming in-stent restenosis. The contours inside the lumen (**B**) correspond to the low-density material seen in the CT

(A)   (B)

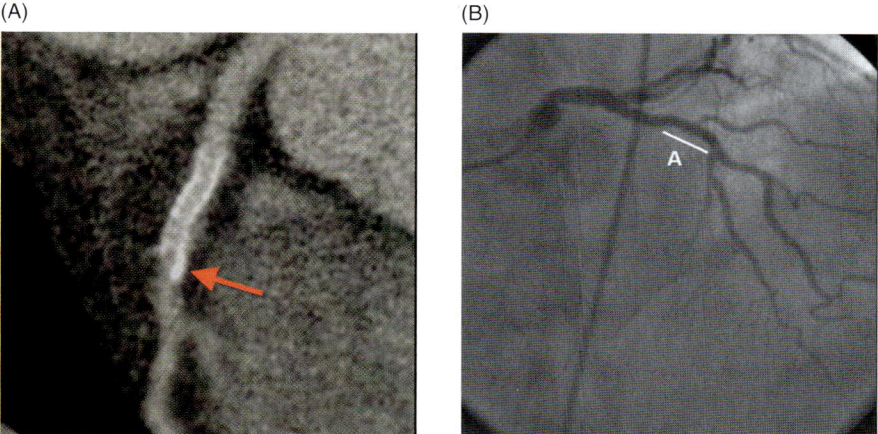

Fig. 7.8 Patent stent (**A**) This stent is patent. The granular appearance of the contrast column represents background image noise, not to be confused with low-density plaque. A small calcification is present at the distal edge of the stent (*arrow*), but does not produce stenosis. (**B**) Invasive coronary angiogram confirming stent (**A**) patency

is usually defined as ≥50% lumen diameter reduction compared to reference diameter.

- Total occlusions are usually fairly obvious. They usually contain very low-density (<50 HU) material throughout all or at least the majority of the stent length. The distal vessel may not be opacified at all, or may be weakly opacified by contrast from collaterals.

(A)   (B)

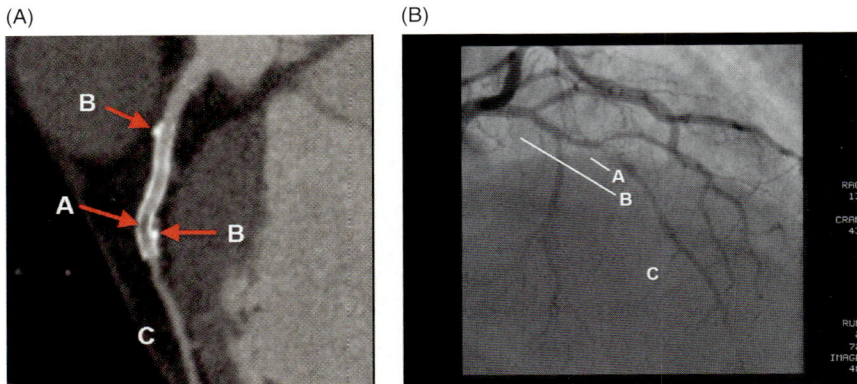

Fig. 7.9 Focal in-stent restenosis (**A**) An accumulation of the same low-density material in this stent (**A**) is more focal, but is still significant because it fills the entire stent diameter. Atherosclerotic plaque and calcification (**B**) that was displaced by the angioplasty is seen behind the stent walls, having been compressed between the stent and the vessel wall. Notice that despite obstructive in-stent restenosis, the distal vessel is opacified (**C**). (**B**) Invasive coronary angiogram confirming in-stent restenosis. The focal, severe stenosis (segment adjacent to line A) is only a fraction of the entire stent length (segment adjacent to line B). Again, distal vessel opacification (**C**) is not a reliable indication of stent patency

(A)   (B)

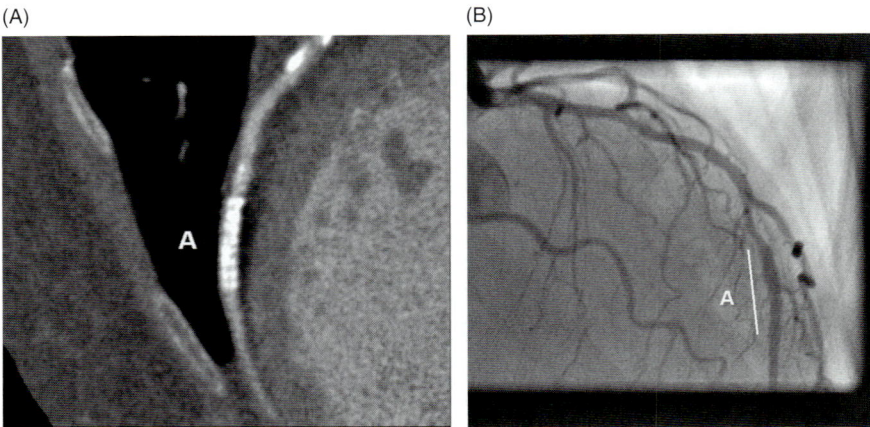

Fig. 7.10 Unevaluable stent (**A**) The lumen of this stent cannot be evaluated, predominantly because of excessive metal blooming artifact, despite image optimization. (**B**) Invasive angiogram reveals that the stent (**A**) is patent

7.6.5 Pitfalls

- Contrast opacification of the vessel distal to the stent does not exclude in-stent restenosis (**Fig. 7.9**). The lumen of the stent itself must be visualized.
- Stents contaminated by motion artifact require extra scrutiny. Metal in motion produces low-density artifacts that may be mistaken for intimal hyperplasia and restenosis. Always examine at least three phases, and create additional reconstructions if necessary.
- Know when you don't know. Some stents just cannot be adequately evaluated using coronary CTA (**Fig. 7.10**).

References

1. Kruger S, Mahnken AH, Sinha AM, et al. Multislice spiral computed tomography for the detection of coronary stent restenosis and patency. Intl J Cardiol 2003, 89: 167–72.
2. Shaohong Z, Yongkang N, Zulong C, et al. Imaging of coronary stent by multislice helical computed tomography. Circulation 2002, 106: 637–38.
3. Schuijf JD, Bax JJ, Jukema JW, et al. Feasibility of assessment of coronary stent patency using 16-slice computed tomography. Am J Cardiol 2004, 94: 427–30.
4. Gilard M, Cornily JC, Pennec PY, et al. Assessment of coronary artery stents by 16 slice computed tomography. Heart 2006, 92: 58–61.
5. Watanabe M, Uemura S, Iwama H, et al. Usefulness of 16-slice multislice spiral computed tomography for follow-up study of coronary stent implantation. Circ J 2006, 70: 691–7
6. Gaspar T, Halon DA, Lewis BS, et al. Diagnosis of coronary in-stent restenosis with multidetector row spiral computed tomography. J Am Coll Cardiol 2005, 46: 1573–9.
7. Ehara M, Kawai M, Surmely JF, et al. Diagnostic accuracy of coronary in-stent restenosis using 64-slice computed tomography: comparison with invasive coronary angiography. J Am Coll Cardiol 2007, 49: 951–9.
8. Gaspar T, Halon DA, Lewis BS, et al. Diagnosis of coronary in-stent restenosis with multidetector row spiral computed tomography. J Am Coll Cardiol 2005, 46: 1573–9.
9. Van Mieghem CA, Cademartiri F, Mollet NR, et al. Multislice spiral computed tomography for the evaluation of stent patency after left main coronary artery stenting: a comparison with conventional coronary angiography and intravascular ultrasound. Circulation 2006, 114: 645–53.
10. Gilard M, Cornily JC, Rioufol G, et al. Noninvasive assessment of left main coronary stent patency with 16-slice computed tomography. Am J Cardiol 2005, 95: 110–12.
11. Maintz D, Juergens KU, Wichter T, et al. Imaging of coronary artery stents using multislice computed tomography: in vitro evaluation. Eur Radiol 2003, 13: 830–5.
12. Mahnken AH, Buecker A, Wildberger JE, et al. Coronary artery stents in multislice computed tomography: in vitro artifact evaluation. Invest Radiol 2004, 39: 27–33.
13. Maintz D, Seifarth H, Raupach R, et al. 64-slice multidetector coronary CT angiography: in vitro evaluation of 68 different stents. Eur Radiol 2006, 16: 818–26
14. Hendel RC, Patel MR, Kramer CM, Poon M. ACCF/ACR/SCCT/SCMR/ASNC/NASCI/SCAI/SIR 2006 appropriateness criteria for cardiac computed tomography and cardiac magnetic resonance imaging. J Am Coll Cardiol 2006, 48: 1475–97
15. Maintz D, Botnar RM, Fischbach R, et al. Coronary magnetic resonance angiography for assessment of the stent lumen: a phantom study. J Cardiovasc Mag Res 2002, 4: 359–67.

16. Georgoulias P, Demakopoulos N, Kontos A, et al. Tc-99m tetrofosmin myocardial perfusion imaging before and six months after percutaneous transluminal coronary angioplasty. Clin Nucl Med 1998, 23: 678–82

17. Garzon PP, Eisenberg MJ. Functional testing for the detection of restenosis after percutaneous transluminal coronary angioplasty: a meta-analysis. Can J Cardiol 2001, 17(1): 41–8.

Chapter 8
Coronary Angiography After Surgical Revascularization

Ian S. Rogers and Udo Hoffmann

Cardiac multidetector computed tomography (MDCT) offers physicians caring for patients who have previously undergone coronary artery bypass grafting surgery (CABG) a highly accurate and non-invasive avenue to evaluate for recurrent cardiac ischemia. In patients presenting with chest discomfort or anginal-equivalent symptoms, stenosis or occlusion of a bypass graft must be considered in addition to ischemia from the patient's native coronary circulation and/or from non-coronary etiologies. The odds of true ischemia are high, as 10% of grafts have been found to occlude during or shortly after surgery, and 59% of venous grafts and 17% of arterial grafts have been found to occlude within 10 years [1]. Fortunately, imaging of venous grafts in particular is easier than imaging of the native coronaries, as the venous grafts are larger and less susceptible to motion than the native vessels.

At our institution, the protocol for the evaluation of patients with CABG is distinct from the standard cardiac MDCT protocol for the evaluation of native coronary arteries in patients without CABG with respect to (1) the field of view, (2) the scanning direction, and (3) the use of volume-rendered images. For bypass graft evaluation, we scan from the level of lung apices to the level of the diaphragm in the caudal–cranial direction. The level of the apices is utilized to ensure complete visualization to the level of the anastomosis of the internal mammary arteries (IMA) with the left subclavian artery. This is critical as recurrent ischemia can result not only from proximal or mid-IMA graft disease, but also from stenosis at the proximal anastomosis and/or in the left subclavian artery itself. In the event that it is known for certain that the patient only has aorta to saphenous vein grafts (i.e., no mammary artery graft), one could choose to scan from the level of the mid-ascending aorta. This decision could carry an element of risk, however, as a smaller field of view could potentially miss saphenous grafts that were implanted unusually high in the ascending aorta.

The decision to scan in the caudal–cranial direction addresses two practical matters relating to scan time: respiratory artifact and contrast opacification. On

U. Hoffmann
Cardiac MR PET CT Program, Division of Cardiology and Department of Radiology, Massachusetts General Hospital, Harvard Medical School, Boston, MA, USA
e-mail: uhoffmann@partners.org

M.J. Budoff, J.S. Shinbane (eds.), *Handbook of Cardiovascular CT*,
DOI: 10.1007/978-1-84800-091-9_8, © Springer-Verlag London Limited 2008

64-slice MDCT scanners, the scan time necessary to image from clavicles to diaphragm with a pitch of 0.2 is typically 20–25 s. As patients with cardiopulmonary disease and/or advanced age may have difficulty maintaining a breath hold for that period of time, the quality of the image is subject to degradation from respiratory artifact, particularly toward the end of the time period. As the native coronary arteries and distal graft anastomoses are more sensitive to motion artifact than the proximal grafts and great vessels, far less damage is done to the scan if respiratory artifact is introduced toward the end of a caudal–cranial scan.

Nieman and colleagues have previously reported that after the start of the breath-hold period, an initial deceleration in heartbeat caused by the Valsalva-induced vagal response takes place, but that this phenomenon fades as the scan approaches 20 s [2]. Hazirolan and colleagues recently demonstrated that this can indeed affect image quality (at least on 16-slice scanners), as the heart rate begins to accelerate at the level of the coronary artery ostia [3]. Moreover, contrast opacification is maximized in the coronary circulation and diluted in the brachiocephalic veins and superior vena cava by the saline chaser, given the length of the exam. This allows improved evaluation of the proximal arterial circulation via the reduction of streak artifact from contrast in these veins.

For the interpretation of the images, we recommend starting with volume-rendered images. These 3-D reconstructions permit the easy identification of the origin, course, and distal anastomosis of the grafts as well as their relation to other cardiac structures (**Fig. 8.1**). This is particularly essential when the operative

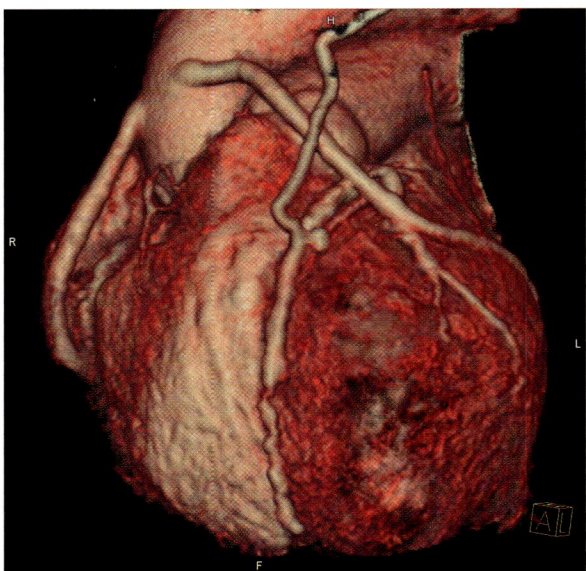

Fig. 8.1 74-year-old woman status-post multi-vessel CABG. Volume-rendered figures suggest patent SVG to LCx and SVG to RCA grafts. Note that the LIMA to LAD also appears patent; however, the run-off (distal LAD) appears occluded

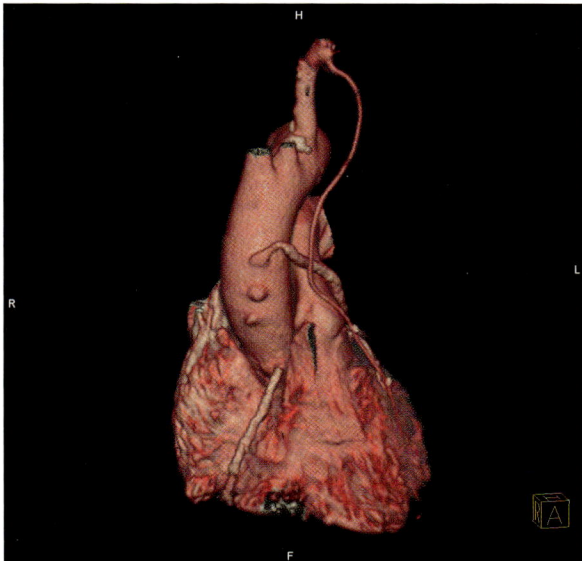

Fig. 8.2 82-year-old woman status-post multi-vessel CABG. Volume-rendered figures reveal two SVG grafts can be clearly identified as proximally occluded

anatomy is unknown. Moreover, proximal graft occlusions are easily identified (**Fig. 8.2**). Care must be taken, however, with the degree of windowing when visualizing grafts in volume-rendered reconstructions, as extreme windows can falsely cause a graft to appear occluded. Also of note, for a patient in whom a CABG revision is being considered, volume-rendered images of the thorax can facilitate localization of the vascular structures in relation to the sternum.

After inspection with volume-rendered reconstructions, the grafts as well as the native coronary arteries should be inspected on axial images for luminal narrowing. It is important to inspect the proximal anastomosis, graft itself, distal anastomosis, and the distal run-off for patency. Maximal intensity projections can be used in non-calcified segments to highlight the vessel course. On axial images, a small diverticulum off the ascending aorta often represents proximal saphenous vein graft occlusion (**Fig. 8.3**).

Evaluation of the anastomosis and distal run-off can be limited by artifact from metallic surgical clips or native coronary artery calcification; however, this can often be mitigated to some extent by the use of multiplanar reconstructions (MPRs), curved MPRs, and inspection at temporal periods within the cardiac cycle (e.g., 65% vs. 75%) (**Fig. 8.4**). The diseased state of the native circulation presents a particular challenge, as these vessels typically are heavily calcified (**Fig. 8.5**). As a result of this calcification, a definite assessment is frequently not possible.

A number of relatively small, single center feasibility studies have reported on the diagnostic accuracy of 64-slice cardiac CT for the detection of graft stenosis. The

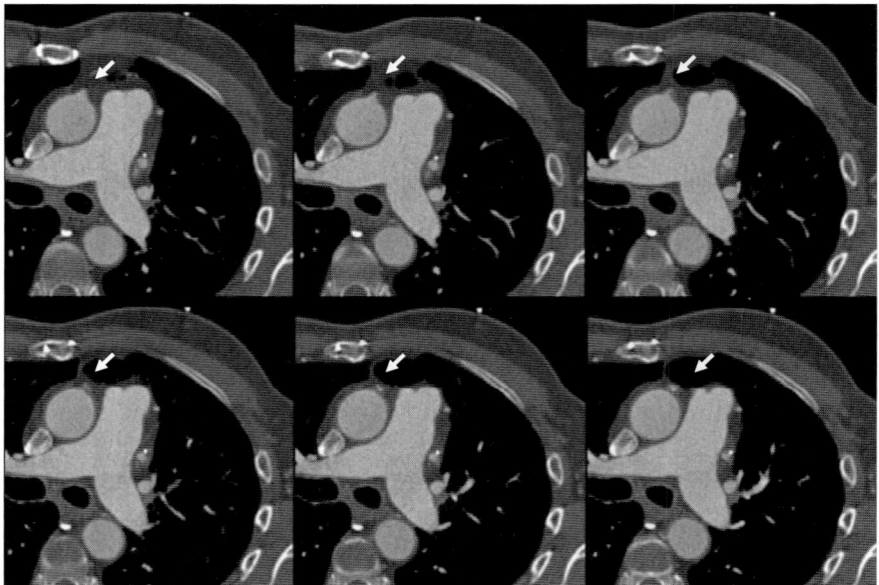

Fig. 8.3 65-year-old man status-post CABG with SVG to LCx graft. Axial figures displayed craniocaudally from *top left* figure to *bottom right* figure. Note patent anastomosis of SVG graft with aorta (*top left* figure); however, a high-grade stenosis is seen in the *top right* and *bottom left* figures. *Bottom right* figure displays reconstitution past the stenosis

patients in the majority of these studies were rather homogenous: mostly in their late 60 s, overwhelmingly male, and with BMIs around 27. Analysis from the studies indicates that most grafts are evaluable, even in unselected patients. Excellent diagnostic test characteristics have been reported for the evaluation of venous grafts, slightly lower sensitivity and specificity for arterial grafts, and a limited ability to assess the native coronary arteries (**Table 8.1**).

The specific aim of a study by Meyer et al. [4] was to evaluate 64-slice MDCT in an unselected patient population. Patients with arrhythmias or elevated heart rates were not excluded. Fifty (36%) of the patients had a heart rate $\geq$65 beats per minute during the scan. In patients with arrhythmias or heart rates $\geq$65 beats per minute, the evaluability decreased significantly from 98% to 95% (arterial grafts) and from 99% to 94% (venous grafts); however, sensitivity, specificity, PPV, and NPV did not suffer in those grafts that were evaluable.

Pache et al. published a similar, but smaller, trial in 2006 [5]. Here also, patients with arrhythmias or elevated heart rates were not excluded. As the study was small and three non-evaluable grafts were not excluded from the statistical analysis (but instead estimated as stenotic by the authors), specificity and PPV suffered in a subanalysis of the arterial grafts. However, overall sensitivity was reported as 97.8%, with specificity 89.3%, PPV 90%, and NPV 97.7%, and the NPV was 92.3% for arterial grafts and 100% for venous grafts. These results are also similar

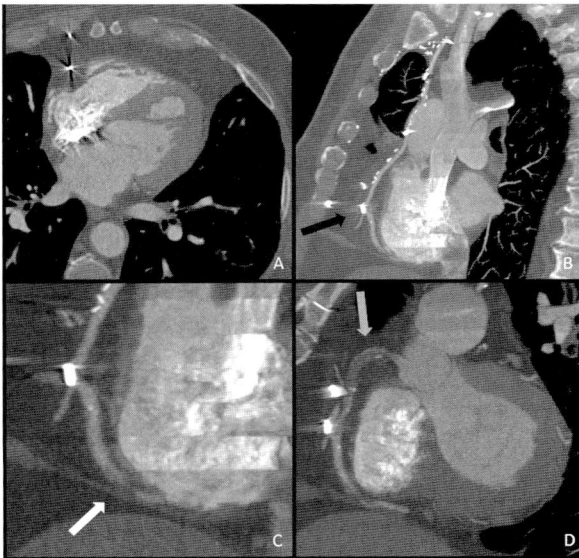

Fig. 8.4 72-year-old man status-post CABG with RIMA—RCA graft presenting with recurrent chest pain. (**A**) Example of metallic clip artifact in mid-RCA territory on axial figure. (**B**) Conclusive evaluation of seemingly patent RIMA graft and anastomosis limited by clip artifact proximally and at the RCA anastomosis (*black arrow*). (**C**) Closer view of clip artifact at anastomosis as well as occlusive disease of the patient's native distal RCA (white arrow). (**D**) Focused sagittal figures demonstrating occlusive native proximal (*grey arrow*) and distal RCA disease

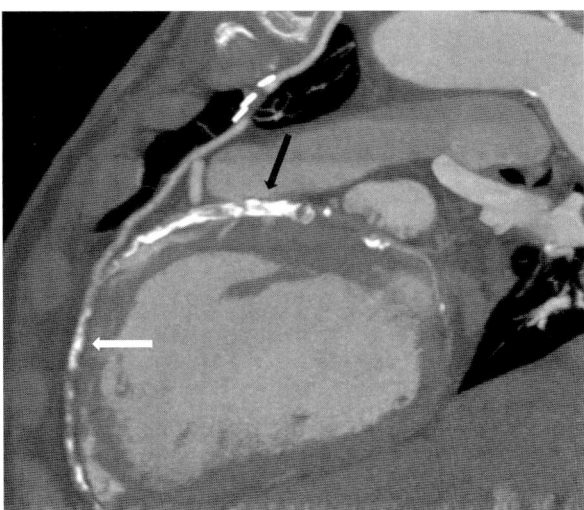

Fig. 8.5 76-year-old man status-post CABG presenting with recurrent chest pain. Sagittal maximal intensity projection (MIP) figure demonstrates a patent LIMA graft and anastomosis. However, the native proximal to mid-LAD (*black arrow*) and the distal run-off LAD (*white arrow*) demonstrate significant disease

Table 8.1 Results of recent studies assessing 64-slice MDCT test characteristics for evaluation of bypass grafts

| | Venous bypass grafts | | | | | | Arterial bypass grafts | | | | | |
	n (grafts)	Evaluable segments	Sensitivity	Specificity	PPV	NPV	n (grafts)	Evaluable segments	Sensitivity	Specificity	PPV	NPV
Meyer (2007)	259	98% (253/259)	99%	98%	96%	99%	147	98% (144/147)	93%	97%	86%	98%
Pache (2006)	72	99% (70/71)*	100%	96.8%*	97.6%**	100%	24	91% (20/22)	83.3%	75%**	55.5%**	92.3%
Malagutti (2006)	64	100% (64/64)	100%	96%	97.5%	100%	45	100% (45/45)	100%	100%	100%	100%
Ropers (2006) †	138	100%	100%	94%	92%	100%						

*Statistics include one non-evaluable graft (estimated as stenotic by the authors). Specificity 100% and PPV 100% when this graft is excluded.
**Statistics include two non-evaluable grafts (estimated as stenotic by the authors). Specificity 85.7% and PPV 71.4% when these grafts are excluded.
† Ropers et al. did not delineate statistics for venous vs. arterial grafts. Data listed in this table reflect all grafts.

to those found by Malagutti and colleagues using 64-slice MDCT in their trial of 52 patients, which did exclude patients with arrhythmia but not elevated heart rates [6]. Assessment of 57 arterial grafts yielded sensitivity, specificity, PPV, and NPV of 100%, and assessment of 64 venous grafts yielded a sensitivity of 100%, specificity of 96%, PPV of 97.5%, and NPV of 100%.

Finally, Ropers et al. also reported the analysis of the native coronary arteries and distal run-off vessels in the studied patients [7]. For the per-segment evaluation of native coronary arteries and distal run-off vessels, sensitivity in evaluable segments was 86% and specificity was 76%; however, 9% of segments were unevaluable. When analyzed on a per-patient basis, MDCT had an overall sensitivity of 97% and specificity of 86% for identifying patients with at least one detected stenosis in a CABG, a distal run-off vessel, or a nongrafted artery or with at least one unevaluable segment.

In summary, the goal of a cardiac MDCT examination in patients who have previously undergone CABG surgery should be to evaluate the bypass grafts, including their proximal and distal anastomoses, the run-off vessels, and whenever possible, the native coronary arteries for patency and the presence of luminal obstruction.

8.1 Imaging Pearls

- The scanning protocol for these patients is specific and deviates from the standard coronary CTA protocol as it should involve scanning to the lung apices and should be in the caudal–cranial direction.
- Otherwise, the standard practice to achieve high image quality applies similar to the assessment of native coronary arteries, including the administration of beta blocker and nitroglycerin.
- 3-D surface volume-rendered images are useful to identify the postoperative anatomy of bypass grafts and their relation to the native coronary arteries and other cardiac structures.
- The assessment of patency and luminal obstruction should be performed on axial and MPR images.
- The most common limitation to evaluability is calcium and metallic clip artifact, which can be mitigated to some extent by the use of MPRs, curved MPRs, and inspection at different temporal periods within the cardiac cycle.
- The accuracy of cardiac MDCT compared to invasive angiography for identification of stenosis is excellent for venous grafts, good for arterial grafts, and limited for native coronary vessels, as derived from small feasibility studies.
- No data from randomized trials are available on the clinical utility, cost, or cost effectiveness.
- Further improvement of CT technology, specifically improvement in temporal and spatial resolution, may help to overcome these limitations.

References

1. Bryan AJ, Angelini GD. The biology of saphenous vein graft occlusion: etiology and strategies for prevention. Curr Opin Cardiol 1994, 9: 641–649.
2. Nieman K, Rensing BJ, van Geuns RJ, et al. Non-invasive coronary angiography with multislice spiral computed tomography: impact of heart rate. Heart 2002, 88: 470–474.
3. Hazirolan T, Turkbey B, Karcaaltincaba M, et al. Impact of Scanning Direction on Heart Rate at Certain Levels of Heart in Electrocardiogram-gated 16-Multidetector Computed Tomography Angiography of Coronary Artery Bypass Grafts. J Comput Assist Tomogr 2007, 31–1: 5–8.
4. Meyer TS, Martinoff S, Hadamitzky M, et al. Improved Noninvasive Assessment of Coronary Artery Bypass Grafts With 64-Slice Computed Tomographic Angiography in an Unselected Patient Population. J Am Coll Cardiol 2007, 49: 946–950.
5. Pache G, Saueressig U, Frydrychowicz A, et al. Initial experience with 64-slice cardiac CT: non-invasive visualization of coronary artery bypass grafts. Eur Heart J 2006, 27: 976–980.
6. Malagutti P, Nieman K, Meijboom W, et al. Use of 64-slice CT in symptomatic patients after coronary bypass surgery: evaluation of grafts and coronary arteries. Eur Heart J 2007, 28: 1879–85.
7. Ropers D, Falk-Karsten P, Kuettner A, et al. Diagnostic Accuracy of Noninvasive Coronary Angiography in Patients After Bypass Surgery Using 64-Slice Spiral Computed Tomography With 330-ms Gantry Rotation. Circulation 2006, 114: 2334–2341.

Chapter 9
Perfusion and Delayed Enhancement Imaging

Joao Lima and Ilan Gottlieb

9.1 Overview

A 54-year-old male with diabetes and a family history of CAD comes to a cardiologist for the first time for atypical chest pain. The patient reports "having to grasp for air" while having chest pain. A rest ECG is done at the office, in which non-specific T-wave changes were the only abnormality. Besides blood tests, the cardiologist orders an echocardiogram that shows reduced left ventricular (LV) function and akinesis of the mid and apical anterior-septal walls and a stress SPECT study that shows a perfusion defect in the same regions, with little reversibility on the rest images. Thinking this is most likely ischemic coronary disease, the cardiologist orders a cardiac MRI for viability evaluation prior to the invasive coronary angiography, which showed an occluded mid-LAD artery with distal filling via collaterals. Given the presence of viability on the MRI scan, the patient successfully undergoes PTCA of the mid-LAD lesion, and 2 months later LV function shows improvement and the patient is asymptomatic.

Cardiologists are familiar with relying on a number of different imaging modalities for a thorough assessment of cardiovascular disorders. Coronary anatomy evaluation is usually performed using invasive catheterization or more recently by non-invasive MDCT scans. Global and regional myocardial function as well as structural abnormalities can be assessed with echo, MRI, and MDCT. Subclinical atherosclerosis is usually assessed via detection of coronary calcium using MDCT or EBCT scanners or via measuring carotid intima-media thickness with ultrasound, while stress tests for ischemia detection and quantification are usually performed with nuclear SPECT or PET, echo stress, or stress MRI imaging. Finally, myocardial fibrosis for viability and prognosis assessment is usually detected and quantified by MRI and nuclear techniques.

From the list above, myocardial fibrosis and perfusion are the only two assessments MDCT does not currently provide, but as will be discussed in this chapter, recent developments have demonstrated initial feasibility for MDCT to be a

J. Lima
Department of Medicine/Cardiology, John Hopkins University, Baltimore, MD, USA
e-mail: jlima@jhmi.edu

M.J. Budoff, J.S. Shinbane (eds.), *Handbook of Cardiovascular CT*,
DOI: 10.1007/978-1-84800-091-9_9, © Springer-Verlag London Limited 2008

complete imaging modality, which in a single scan, could provide a wide array of complementary information. Ideally, using one imaging modality to perform all these assessments during a single scan could have substantial economic implications, may serve to reduce patient anxiety, and may improve workflow.

9.2 MDCT for Detection of Myocardial Fibrosis and Viability

The ability to distinguish dysfunctional, but viable, myocardium from nonviable tissue after acute or chronic ischemia has important implications for the therapeutic management of patients with coronary artery disease [1, 2]. Image-based characterization of myocardial scar morphology can identify those patients with hibernating myocardium who may achieve functional systolic recovery with revascularization [3]. The assessment of myocardial viability and infarct morphology with delayed contrast-enhanced MRI has been well validated over the past several years and is performed routinely by several clinical cardiac MRI centers.

The recent advent of MDCT technology has expanded its potential for a more comprehensive evaluation of cardiovascular diseases. While hypo-attenuation in the non-contrasted scan (due to fatty degeneration of the infarcted area) or during the contrast-enhanced coronary angiography scan has been shown to demonstrate areas of previous myocardial infarction (MI), it is largely underestimated by MDCT [4, 5]. Delayed MDCT myocardial imaging can accurately identify and characterize morphological features of acute and healed myocardial infarction, including infarct size, transmurality, and the presence of microvascular obstruction and collagenous scar (**Fig. 9.1**) [6, 7]. Infarcted myocardial tissue by MDCT is characterized by well-delineated hyper-enhanced regions, whereas regions of microvascular

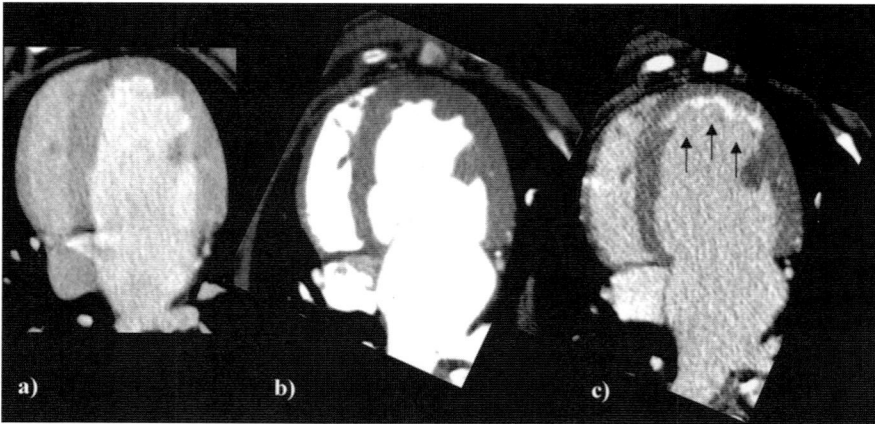

Fig. 9.1 Typical contrast-enhanced myocardial MDCT images showing axial slices (**a**) at baseline (preinfarct) 5 min after contrast, (**b**) postinfarct during first-pass contrast injection, and (**c**) postinfarct 5 min after contrast injection. The infarcted region is represented by the subendocardial anterior hyper-intense region (*arrows*)

obstruction by MDCT are characterized by hypo-enhancement on imaging early after MI [6, 7]. The mechanism of myocardial hyper-enhancement and hypo-enhancement in acutely injured myocardial territories after iodinated contrast administration is similar to that proposed for delayed gadolinium-enhanced MRI [1]. Under conditions of normal myocyte function, sarcolemmal membranes serve to exclude iodine from the intracellular space. After myocyte necrosis, however, membrane dysfunction ensues, and iodine molecules are able to penetrate the cell. Because 75% of the total myocardial volume is intracellular, large increases in the volume of distribution are achieved, which results in marked hyper-enhancement relative to the non-injured myocytes. The mechanism of hyper-enhancement of healed myocardial infarction or collagenous scar is thought to be related to the accumulation of contrast media in the interstitial space between collagen fibers and thus an increased volume of distribution compared with that of tightly packed myocytes. The low signal intensity of microvascular obstruction regions despite restoration of normal flow through the infarct-related artery is explained by the death and subsequent cellular debris blockage of intramyocardial capillaries at the core of the damaged region. These obstructed capillaries do not allow contrast material to flow into the damaged bed, which results in a region of low signal intensity compared with normal myocardium. In minutes to hours, contrast material is able to penetrate this "no reflow" region, and the necrotic myocytes that reside in that myocardial territory then become hyper-enhanced as iodine is internalized by the cell. In weeks the microvascular obstruction area is replaced by collagenous scar tissue, and the former dark area now becomes bright. Since the transmurality of delayed enhancement predicts functional recovery after revascularization [3], the better spatial resolution of MDCT as compared to CMR may influence the accuracy of viability assessment, but no study thus far has tested this hypothesis. For a comprehensive cardiac evaluation, in the future, at least three consecutive scans should be performed: the first one would be a low-dose unenhanced calcium score scan; the second one with contrast injection for the acquisition of coronary angiography, LV function, stress perfusion, and morphology; and a third scan without contrast for the delayed enhancement images. **Figure 9.2** shows a proposed timeline for a comprehensive cardiac evaluation with a 64-detector MDCT scanner. Clearly, radiation dose is a major concern in this scheme, and some evolutions in our scanning machinery and technique may allow us to reduce it to accepted

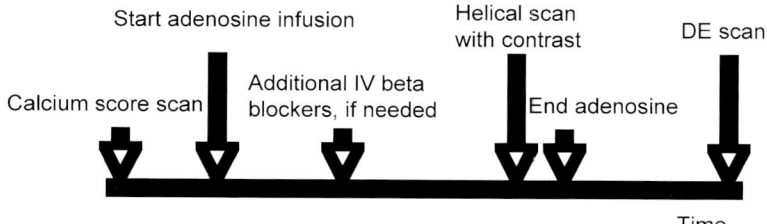

Fig. 9.2 Proposed timeline for a comprehensive MDCT scan. DE: Delayed enhancement

levels. Applying prospective gating to the delayed enhanced scan has been shown to provide similar results, while drastically decreasing radiation dose [8]. With the development of wider detector arrays, complete coverage of the heart will be possible in one gantry rotation, also decreasing the radiation dose in the contrast-enhanced coronary angiography scans, as will be discussed below.

9.3 Ischemia Detection by MDCT

Coronary anatomic information is much more valuable when combined with a functional test, since most decisions regarding treatment are based on the detection of myocardial ischemia [9]. The poor correlation between anatomic modalities such as invasive coronary angiography [10, 11] and MDCT [12] with stress perfusion tests underscores the fact that one cannot substitute for the other. Furthermore, the presence of heavy calcification or stents on the coronary tree generates artifacts that significantly impair analysis [13]. While progress in multi-detector technology has improved our ability to study such patients, greater coverage and improved temporal resolution are unlikely to eliminate the problem of these artifacts. The idea that computed tomography could provide information on myocardial perfusion has been explored in the past by investigators using electron beam computed tomography (EBCT) [14]. However, the combination of a reliable coronary angiogram with stress-induced myocardial perfusion by EBCT is difficult. The recent development of the 64-detector MDCT scanner as well as improvements in temporal and spatial resolutions have enabled the possibility of combining coronary angiograms with measurements of relative differences in myocardial blood flow during stress [15]. Myocardial perfusion measurements by MDCT are derived from the upslope differences in contrast enhancement between the ischemic and remote areas (**Fig. 9.3**).

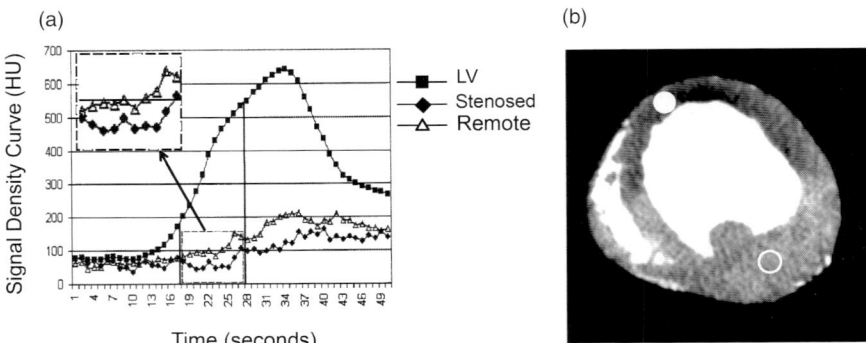

Fig. 9.3 Myocardial enhancement upslope curves for the left ventricular cavity, and remote and ischemic regions (**a**). The usual timing of a coronary CT angiogram is shown as the region between the vertical bars. Following the contrast bolus with an ROI placed at the ischemic (*filled circle*) and remote (*open circle*) areas presents a delta in myocardial enhancement intensity (**b**) that can be measured, as shown inside the *dashed box* (**a**)

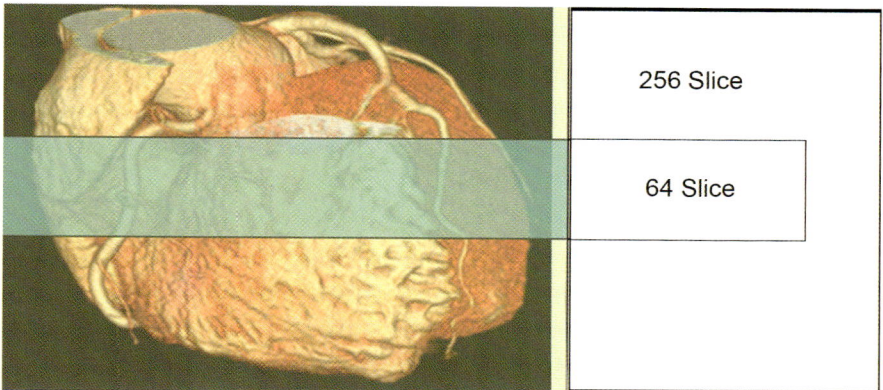

Fig. 9.4 Schematic coverage of a 256-detector as compared to a 64-detector MDCT scanner

Current-generation 64-detector scanners still have limited coverage of the heart, resulting in the base of the heart being scanned earlier in time than the apex, making comparisons in signal intensities between the two areas problematic. In this regard, the development of MDCT technology that would allow the entire heart to be imaged in one gantry rotation (**Fig. 9.4**) combined with the capability of programming such gated image acquisitions to occur only during specific portions of a given cardiac cycle (**Fig. 9.5**) has created a brand new horizon of possibilities to reduce radiation exposure enough to enable the performance of combined angiography and myocardial perfusion assessment during stress, which associated with the angiographic and delayed enhanced images should provide a comprehensive cardiac assessment. Also, with more coverage, scan times will likely decrease, potentially reducing the amount of contrast material per scan. Such techniques would be ideal for the assessment of patients with chest pain who also have calcified coronaries, as well as the follow-up of patients with advanced heart disease post-coronary artery bypass surgery or multiple stent implantations.

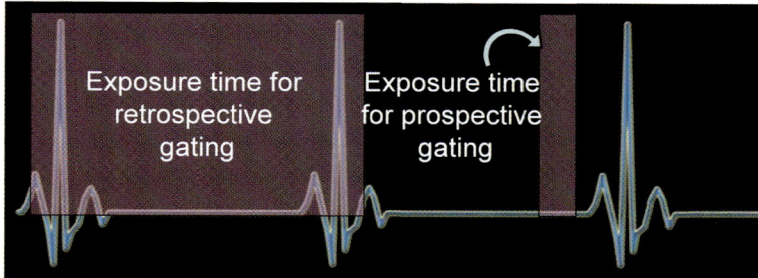

Fig. 9.5 Schematic demonstration of the radiation exposure time differences between retrospective gating (single heart beat) and prospective triggering used in the 256-detectors scanner

At present, clinical quantification of myocardial blood flow is possible only with positron emission tomographic techniques [16]. Using iodine molecules as a tracer, current research has demonstrated that by measuring the concentration in time of the tracer in the myocardium, MDCT can determine absolute blood flow in different regions of the myocardium. Recent attention to patients with chest pain but no obstructive epicardial CAD (syndrome X) has demonstrated that in a substantial proportion of these individuals, microvascular processes can be identified by perfusion reserve measurements in association with traditional CAD risk factors such as hyper-cholesterolemia, hypertension, and smoking as well as with diabetes [17]. The possibility of quantifying epicardial coronary plaque while also assessing microvascular disease during maximal vasodilatation enables coronary MDCTA to characterize macrovascular atherosclerosis as well as microvascular dysfunction secondary to atherosclerosis or other disease processes. The capability of quantifying myocardial blood flow by contrast-enhanced MDCT could represent a "quantum leap" in our ability to assess and characterize the entire process of cardiac atherosclerosis.

9.4 Imaging Pearls: Delayed Enhancement

- The optimal contrast dose to be used for delayed enhancement images is still not defined, but studies in humans [5, 7] showed that the usual amount used for a 16-detector coronary CTA (120–140 ml) provides good enhancement.
- For optimal contrast between the infarcted and the remote regions, the delayed enhanced scan should be done between 5 and 10 min after contrast injection [6].
- Most of the studies done so far reconstructed the images in end-diastole for delayed enhancement analysis.
- The delayed enhancement pattern is important to differentiate between ischemic and non-ischemic etiologies, the former being found as a wave front from the endocardium to the pericardium. Non-ischemic cardiomyopathies can also result in myocardial scar that appears on delayed enhancement images, but those tend to be patchy and do not follow the endocardium-to-epicardium pattern seen in ischemic cardiomyopathy [18].
- Molecular size of the iodinated contrast material may affect the uptake of the tissue by that agent. Two trials used a smaller molecule with high iodine concentration (iomeprol) [5, 7], while another one used a larger molecule with a lower iodine concentration (iodixanol) [6]. It is still unclear which one is the best, if any, or whether other factors (such as ionic polarization) are important.
- Delayed enhancement imaging by MDCT can be obtained both in patients with an acute MI as well as in patients who had infarcts more than 6 months prior to imaging [5, 6, 7].
- Microvascular obstruction can be imaged in the early phase after MI, and it is gradually replaced by fibrous tissue that appears bright on the delayed enhancement images 2–4 weeks after the MI [19].

9.5 Imaging Pearls: Ischemia

- Work on myocardial perfusion is in progress, and most of the published data is experimental.
- Adenosine is the drug most often tested for stress perfusion in MDCT, due to its short onset and offset, safety profile, and proved efficacy in diverging blood from ischemic to non-ischemic territories.
- Since adenosine usually increases heart rate, aggressive beta-blockade should be pursued. Adequate hydration prior to the scan may potentially blunt the reflex increase in heart rate from the adenosine infusion.
- Nitroglycerin should not be given concomitantly to adenosine, since it can reverse the ischemic effects of the latter, as well as decrease blood pressure and increase heart rate even further.
- The visual contouring of the underperfused myocardial areas is the method currently being applied, but as new dedicated software becomes available, this will probably be done semi-automatically. Also, the best threshold for quantitatively discriminating ischemia from remote myocardium is still not defined.
- Balanced ischemia is still a problem with current-generation MDCT scanners, since there are no remote areas to compare to. The 256-detector scanner will potentially solve this problem by allowing absolute quantification of myocardial blood flow.
- Whether stress perfusion scans will be recommended to everyone or just selected patient populations (such as the ones with high calcium scores) is still under investigation.

References

1. Wu KC, Lima JA. Noninvasive imaging of myocardial viability: current techniques and future developments. *Circ Res.* 2003, 93: 1146–1158.
2. Pagley PR, Beller GA, Watson DD, Gimple LW, Ragosta M. Improved outcome after coronary bypass surgery in patients with ischemic cardiomyopathy and residual myocardial viability. *Circulation.* 1997, 96: 793–800.
3. Kim RJ, Wu E, Rafael A, Chen EL, Parker MA, Simonetti O, Klocke FJ, Bonow RO, Judd RM. The use of contrast-enhanced magnetic resonance imaging to identify reversible myocardial dysfunction. *N Engl J Med.* 2000, 343: 1445–1453.
4. Sanz J, Weeks D, Nikolaou K, Sirol M, Rius T, Rajagopalar S, Dellegrottaglie S, Strobeck J, Fuster V, Poon M. Detection of healed myocardial infarction with multidetector-row computed tomography and comparison with cardiac magnetic resonance delayed hyperenhancement. *Am J Cardiol.* 2006, 98: 149–155.
5. Mahnken AH, Koos R, Katoh M, Wildberger JE, Spuentrup E, Buecker A, Gunther RW, Kuhl HP. Assessment of myocardial viability in reperfused acute myocardial infarction using 16-slice computed tomography in comparison to magnetic resonance imaging. *J Am Coll Cardiol.* 2005, 45: 2042–2047.
6. Lardo AC, Cordeiro MA, Silva C, Amado LC, George RT, Saliaris AP, Schuleri KH, Fernandes VR, Zviman M, Nazarian S, Halperin HR, Wu KC, Hare JM, Lima JA. Contrast-enhanced multidetector computed tomography viability imaging after myocardial infarction: characterization of myocyte death, microvascular obstruction, and chronic scar. *Circulation.* 2006, 113: 394–404.

7. Gerber BL, Belge B, Legros GJ, Lim P, Poncelet A, Pasquet A, Gisellu G, Coche E, Vanoverschelde JL. Characterization of acute and chronic myocardial infarcts by multidetector computed tomography: comparison with contrast-enhanced magnetic resonance. *Circulation.* 2006, 113: 823–833.

8. George RT, Schuleri KH, Bluemke DA, Hare JM, Lima JA, Lardo AC. Prospectively ECG-Gated Multidetector Computed Tomography Viability Imaging Accurately Quantifies Infarct Size While Lowering the Radiation Dose by an Order of Magnitude. Circulation 2006, 114:(Supplement) II-818.

9. Smith SC Jr, Feldman TE, Hirshfeld JW Jr, Jacobs AK, Kern MJ, King SB 3rd, Morrison DA, O'Neil WW, Schaff HV, Whitlow PL, Williams DO, Antman EM, Adams CD, Anderson JL, Faxon DP, Fuster V, Halperin JL, Hiratzka LF, Hunt SA, Nishimura R, Ornato JP, Page RL, Riegel B, American College of Cardiology/American Heart Association Task Force on Practice Guidelines, ACC/AHA/SCAI Writing Committee to Update 2001 Guidelines for Percutaneous Coronary Intervention. ACC/AHA/SCAI 2005 guideline update for percutaneous coronary intervention: a report of the American College of Cardiology/American Heart Association Task Force on Practice Guidelines (ACC/AHA/SCAI Writing Committee to Update 2001 Guidelines for Percutaneous Coronary Intervention). *Circulation.* 2006, 113: e166–e286.

10. Rodes-Cabau J, Candell-Riera J, Angel J, de Leon G, Pereztol O, Castell-Conesa J, Soto A, Anivarro I, Aguade S, Vazquez M, Domingo E, Tardif JC, Soler-Soler J. Relation of myocardial perfusion defects and nonsignificant coronary lesions by angiography with insights from intravascular ultrasound and coronary pressure measurements. *Am J Cardiol.* 2005, 96: 1621–1626.

11. Ragosta M, Bishop AH, Lipson LC, Watson DD, Gimple LW, Sarembock IJ, Powers ER. Comparison between angiography and fractional flow reserve versus single-photon emission computed tomographic myocardial perfusion imaging for determining lesion significance in patients with multivessel coronary disease. *Am J Cardiol.* 2007, 99: 896–902.

12. Schuijf JD, Wijns W, Jukema JW, Atsma DE, de Roos A, Lamb HJ, Stokkel MP, Dibbets-Schneider P, Decramer I, De Bondt P, van der Wall EE, Vanhoenacker PK, Bax JJ. Relationship between noninvasive coronary angiography with multi-slice computed tomography and myocardial perfusion imaging. *J Am Coll Cardiol.* 2006, 48: 2508–2514.

13. Gaspar T, Halon DA, Lewis BS, Adawi S, Schliamser JE, Rubinshtein R, Flugelman MY, Peled N. Diagnosis of coronary in-stent restenosis with multidetector row spiral computed tomography. *J Am Coll Cardiol.* 2005, 46: 1573–1579.

14. Budoff MJ, Gillespie R, Georgiou D, Narahara KA, French WJ, Mena I, Brundage BH. Comparison of exercise electron beam computed tomography and sestamibi in the evaluation of coronary artery disease. *Am J Cardiol.* 1998, 81: 682–687.

15. George RT, Jon Resar, Caterina Silva, John Texter, Kathy Citro, David A. Bluemke, Albert C. Lardo, Joao A. Lima. Combined computed tomography coronary angiography and perfusion imaging accurately detects the physiological significance of coronary stenoses in patients with chest pain. *AHA Scientific Sessions 2006.* 2006, Abstract 3264.

16. Lodge MA, Braess H, Mahmoud F, Suh J, Englar N, Geyser-Stoops S, Jenkins J, Bacharach SL, Dilsizian V. Developments in nuclear cardiology: transition from single photon emission computed tomography to positron emission tomography-computed tomography. *J Invasive Cardiol.* 2005, 17: 491–496.

17. Buchthal SD, den Hollander JA, Merz CN, Rogers WJ, Pepine CJ, Reichek N, Sharaf BL, Reis S, Kelsey SF, Pohost GM. Abnormal myocardial phosphorus-31 nuclear magnetic resonance spectroscopy in women with chest pain but normal coronary angiograms. *N Engl J Med.* 2000, 342: 829–835.

18. Gottlieb I, Macedo R, Bluemke DA, Lima JA. Magnetic resonance imaging in the evaluation of non-ischemic cardiomyopathies: current applications and future perspectives. *Heart Fail Rev.* 2006, 11: 313–323.

19. Wu KC, Kim RJ, Bluemke DA, Rochitte CE, Zerhouni EA, Becker LC, Lima JA. Quantification and time course of microvascular obstruction by contrast-enhanced echocardiography and magnetic resonance imaging following acute myocardial infarction and reperfusion. *J Am Coll Cardiol.* 1998, 32: 1756–1764.

Chapter 10
Cardiac SPECT and PET: Complementary Roles with Cardiac CT

Daniel S. Berman, Leslee J. Shaw, Alan Rozanski, John D. Friedman, Sean W. Hayes, Louise E.J. Thomson, Piotr J. Slomka, and Guido Germano

10.1 Introduction

When choosing an imaging test in a cardiovascular patient, different tests are appropriate for different purposes. These purposes can be conceptually divided into imaging for prevention, diagnosis, and intervention.

10.2 Imaging for Prevention

Subclinical coronary atherosclerosis remains a major medical problem, with nearly 50% of patients developing myocardial infarction or sudden death from coronary artery disease (CAD) while having no symptoms or knowledge of disease before the event. Standard clinical risk assessment has proven to be inadequate in identifying these patients. Atherosclerosis imaging with coronary artery calcification (CAC) measurements by computed tomography (CT) has emerged as an effective screening method in asymptomatic patients (**Fig. 10.1**) [1]. In patients found to be at high risk, estimated to be about 10% of patients undergoing CAC testing, further testing for ischemia will be indicated [2]. Stress myocardial perfusion imaging (MPI) with SPECT and positron emission tomography (PET) are widely available modalities that have been well documented to be effective in this setting, allowing accurate selection of the asymptomatic patients at highest risk to undergo invasive coronary angiography and possible coronary intervention [2]. In this regard, a recent report demonstrating the excellent prognosis of a large group of patients with varying amounts of coronary atherosclerosis and normal SPECT MPI is particularly relevant (**Fig. 10.2**) [3]. The findings indicated that the 4-year cardiac event rate in patients without ischemia was equally low in patients with and without extensive coronary atherosclerosis. Given the known adverse prognostic implications of high CAC scores, these findings are somewhat surprising, but imply that in the absence

D.S. Berman
Department of Imaging, Cedars-Sinai Medical Center, Los Angeles, CA 90048, USA
e-mail: bermand@cshs.org

M.J. Budoff, J.S. Shinbane (eds.), *Handbook of Cardiovascular CT*,
DOI: 10.1007/978-1-84800-091-9_10, © Springer-Verlag London Limited 2008

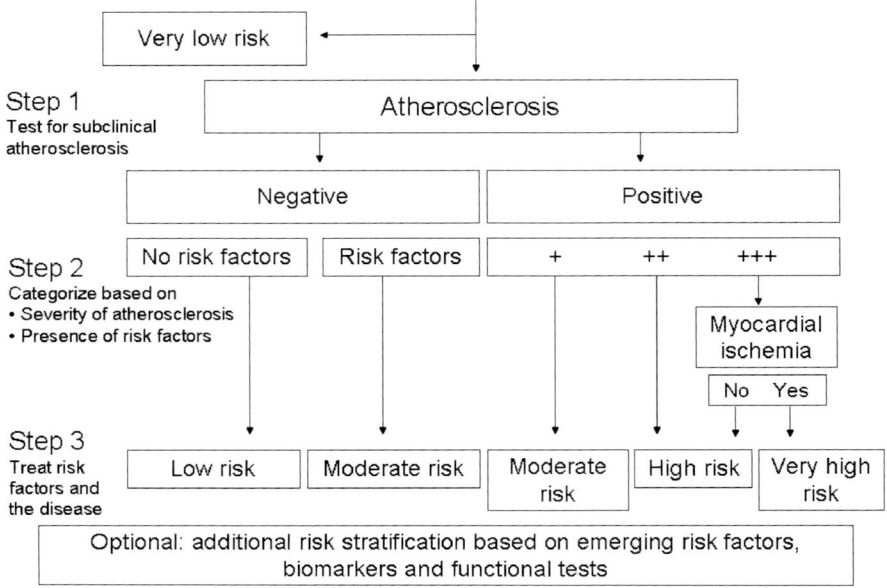

Fig. 10.1 An approach to screening for atherosclerosis advocated by the Association for the Eradication of Heart Attacks (AHEA). y = years. (Adapted with permission from Am J Cardiol [1])

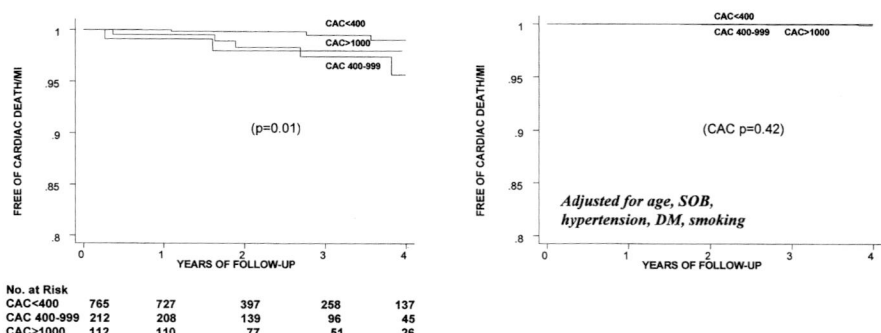

Fig. 10.2 Survival curves for freedom from cardiac death or non-fatal MI (y-axis) among the coronary artery calcium (CAC) patients who had nonischemic exercise myocardial perfusion scintigraphy studies. The *left panel* represents Kaplan Meier survival curve analysis as a function of CAC scores before adjustment for covariates of outcome. The *right panel* represents the Cox proportional hazards model for freedom from cardiac death or MI risk adjusted for age, dyspnea, and coronary risk factors. Patients with early myocardial revascularization were censored from the analysis. No significant statistical differences were observed. (Adapted with permission from J Am Coll Cardiol [3])

of ischemia and with aggressive medical therapy, the adverse event rate in patients with coronary atherosclerosis is low.

10.3 Imaging for Diagnosis

In symptomatic patients with an intermediate likelihood of CAD, imaging is used for diagnosis. Very recently, coronary CT angiography (CTA) has emerged as the most accurate noninvasive method for detecting CAD. Furthermore, an advantage of coronary CTA over stress SPECT or PET methods is that it is highly unlikely to miss very high-risk CAD (**Fig. 10.3**). In patients with left main CAD, while nuclear studies show some abnormality in nearly all of them, the extent of abnormality is generally underestimated [4]. In this patient group, coronary CTA is likely to supersede previously performed nuclear cardiology procedures—as the initial test in symptomatic patients with an intermediate likelihood of CAD. Drawbacks of coronary CTA include inability to judge stenosis in densely calcified plaque,

(a)

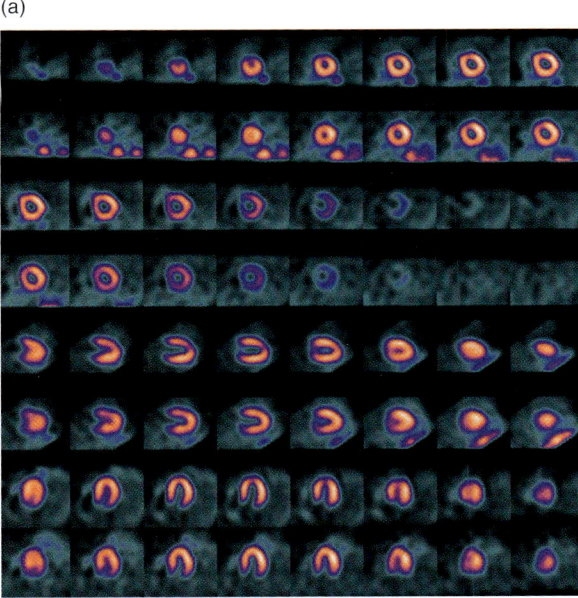

Fig. 10.3 (a) Stress sestamibi (odd-number rows) and rest Tl-201 (even-number rows) SPECT MPI images from a 53-year-old female with recent-onset dyspnea and atypical chest pain showing an equivocal apical anterior stress perfusion defect. The patient also had 1 mm horizontal ST depression early in recovery after treadmill exercise; (b) CCTA obtained with a dual-source 64-slice CT scanner (Siemens, definition) of the patient illustrated in **Fig. 10.8a** showing a >70% narrowing at ostial left main coronary artery stenosis, which subsequently revealed a 90% stenosis by conventional coronary angiography. Coronary calcium score was 0. The patient underwent successful left main coronary artery stenting. CSMC = Cedars-Sinai Medical Center

(b)

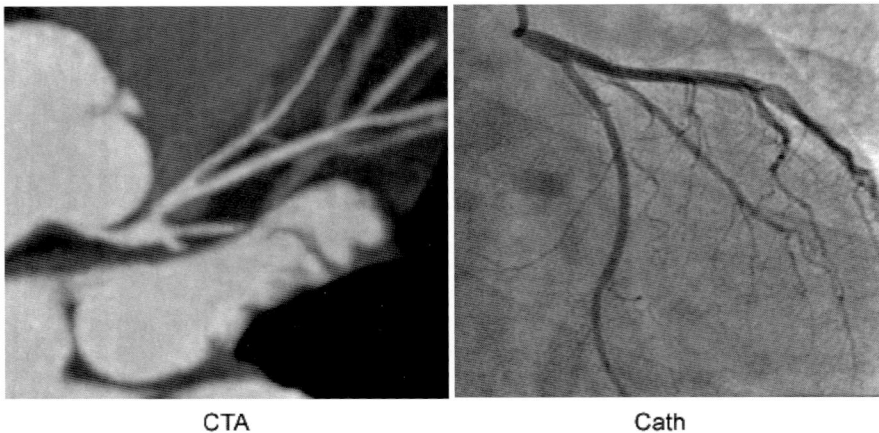

CTA   Cath

Fig. 10.3 (Continued)

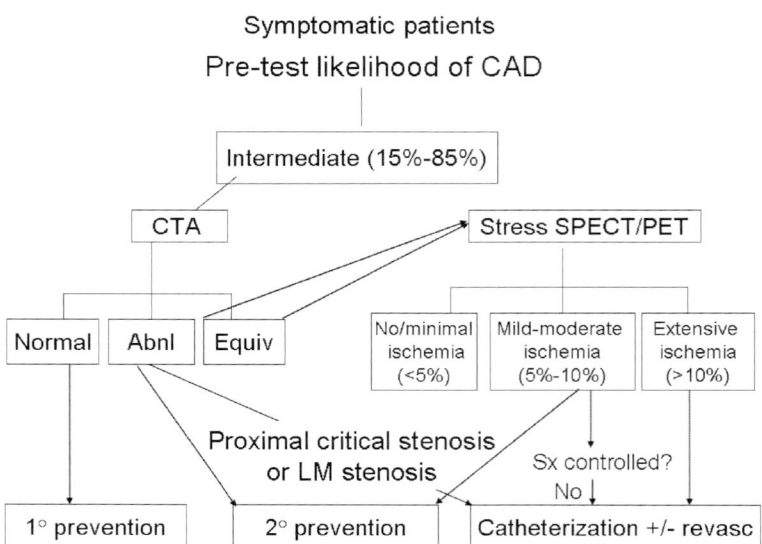

Fig. 10.4 Approach to diagnosis and management of coronary artery disease in *symptomatic* patients with an intermediate pre-test likelihood of CAD. Abnl = abnormal; Equiv = equivocal; LM = left main; CTA = coronary CT angiography; revasc = revascularization. (Adapted with permission from J Nucl Cardiol [5])

dependence on a regular rhythm, limited information regarding coronary plaque activity, and the paucity of outcome data at the present time. There is also no data available as yet that identifies which subgroup of patients will benefit from revascularization identified by coronary CTA alone.

Coronary CTA study is most useful in ruling out CAD in symptomatic patients with an intermediate pre-test CAD likelihood (**Fig. 10.4**) [5]. Patients with normal coronary CTA have an obvious "watchful waiting" treatment plan. When the CTA results are abnormal, the clinical decision making becomes more complex. If there is compelling anatomy by CTA—such as a left main coronary stenosis— catheterization becomes the clear next step, as it is in patients with limiting chest pain or unstable syndromes. However, in those with abnormal CTA, the question often arises regarding the size of the jeopardized myocardial zone, thus providing a role for the complementary information provided by nuclear cardiology methods. We estimate that in approximately 20% of patients with an intermediate pre-test likelihood of CAD who undergo coronary CTA, nuclear testing after CTA will be used to provide functional information to guide management.

10.4 Imaging for Intervention

This application in guiding management becomes the primary concern in patients with known CAD, particularly when they are elderly or otherwise likely to have extensive calcification. In general, the purpose for imaging in these patients more commonly is to determine the need for intervention, rather than to establish a diagnosis. In these groups, patients with limiting symptoms will proceed directly to invasive coronary angiography. In patients for whom the need for revascularization is not clear, nuclear testing is likely to grow as the initial test of choice (**Fig. 10.5**). The COURAGE trial has shown that even invasive coronary angiographic information is limited in its ability to define a subset of patients in whom revascularization provides a benefit with respect to reducing hard cardiac events. In contrast, there is a large and growing body of literature showing that the amount of ischemia plays a pivotal role in guiding management decisions by providing information regarding the likelihood of survival benefit with revascularization (Figs. 10.6 [6] and 10.7 [7]). Thus, in these groups, imaging for ischemia is commonly employed to determine whether invasive intervention is indicated (**Fig. 10.5**). The strength of nuclear cardiology procedures in this regard is both the extensive literature supporting the use of measures of ischemia in guiding management and the fact that automatic quantitative software tools are available to objectively quantify ischemia [8].

Another way of considering the limitations of coronary CTA in patients with known CAD or a high likelihood of CAD is to recognize that the CTA result is highly unlikely to be normal in this setting—and there is little data regarding the appropriate management of patients with coronary CTA findings that are not "compelling" regarding the need for revascularization. Thus, it becomes relatively unlikely in these patients that coronary CTA alone will obviate the need for further testing. In contrast, regarding the effectiveness of nuclear testing in these patients,

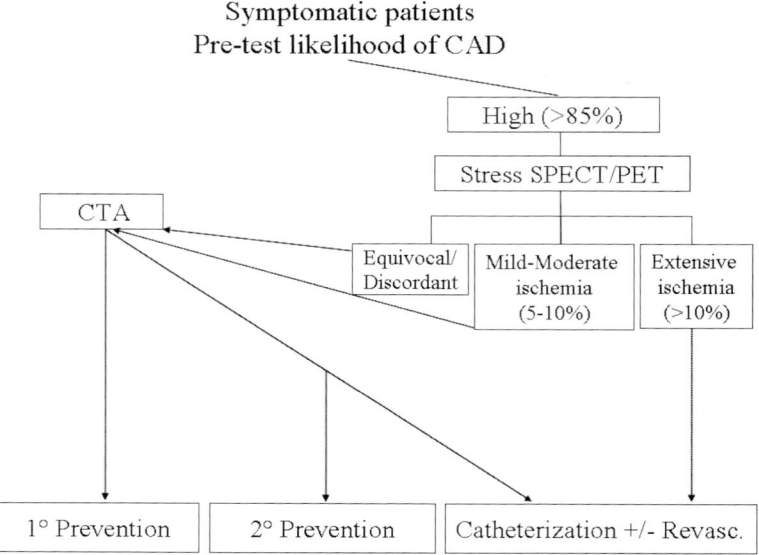

Fig. 10.5 Approach to diagnosis and management of coronary artery disease (CAD) in symptomatic patients with a high pre-test likelihood of CAD, illustrating the complementary role of CTA for management when stress SPECT or PET is equivocal or shows discordant test results with clinical stress testing

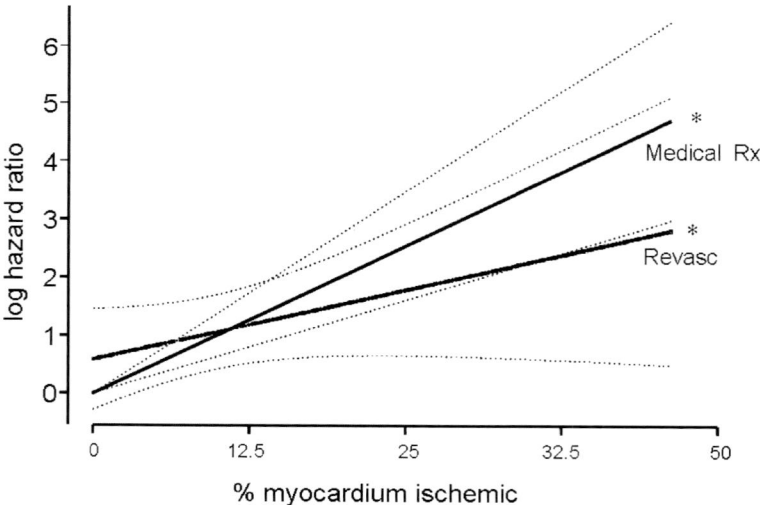

Fig. 10.6 Log hazard ratio for cardiac death with revascularization (revasc) versus medical therapy (Rx) as a function of % myocardium ischemic, after adjustment for predictors of revascularization as well as clinical, historical, and stress SPECT data. Model $p < 0.0001$, interaction $p = 0.0305$. (Adapted with permission from Circulation [6])

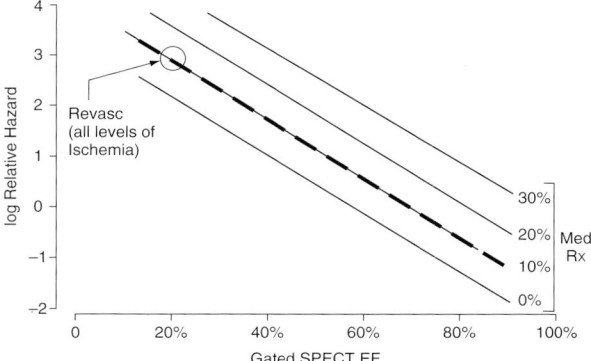

Fig. 10.7 Log hazard ratio for cardiac death in patients treated with medical therapy as a function of gated SPECT EF based on Cox proportional hazards model. Solid lines represent predicted survival for 0%, 10%, 20%, and 30% myocardium ischemic in patients treated medically. Dashed lines represent predicted survival for patients treated with revascularization for all values of % myocardium ischemic. Revasc = revascularization. Model $p < 0.0001$. (Adapted with permission from J Nucl Cardiol [7])

there is data showing that low-risk nuclear studies are found in the majority of patients with a high pre-test likelihood of CAD (**Fig. 10.8**) [9].

Given the speed of technological development, it is a virtual certainty that CT will evolve further and will have expanded capabilities in the future. At the same time, in nuclear cardiology, new developments are occurring that promise to also expand applications for nuclear methods. For example, when patients undergo both

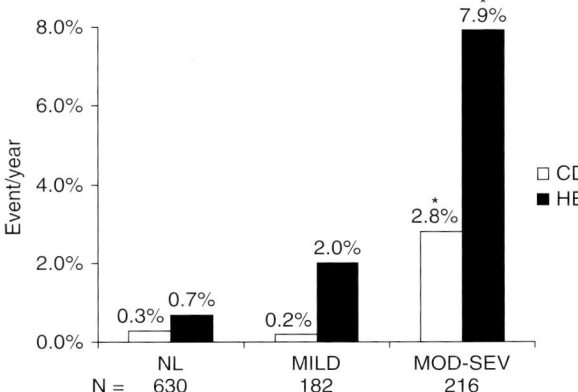

Fig. 10.8 Frequencies of cardiac death (*dark bars*) and hard events (*clear bars*) patients without known CAD but having a high pre-test likelihood of CAD as a function of SPECT scan result—normal (NL), mildly abnormal (MILD), and moderate-to-severely abnormal (MOD-SEV). *$p < 0.05$ for each outcome across scan categories. (Adapted with permission from J Am Coll Cardiol [9])

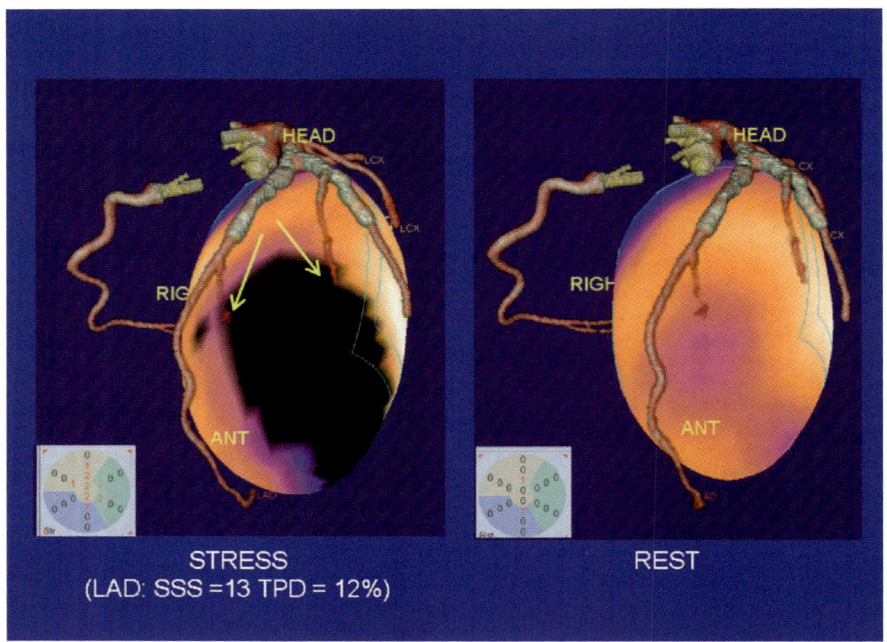

Fig. 10.9 Case example of SPECT/CTA fusion: Volume-rendered 64-slice CTA fused with myocardial perfusion SPECT obtained on a different scanner at a different time. SPECT images show ischemia (3-D blackout region on the *left*). Stress total perfusion (TPD) was 12% in the territory supplied by the diagonal branches of LAD (as anatomically determined by CTA). (Adapted with permission from J Am Coll Cardiol [10])

coronary CTA and nuclear tests, fusion displays of the test results may provide increased information than can be gleaned from separate consideration of test reports (**Fig. 10.9**). Additionally, new SPECT cameras have been introduced that cut short imaging time dramatically, or if desired, markedly reduce the dose of radioactivity employed with cardiac imaging procedures (**Fig. 10.10**) [8]. The possibility of simultaneous dual isotope (or multiple isotope) imaging with these cameras is being explored. Due to their ability to image minute tracer concentrations, both SPECT and PET have great potential in molecular imaging. In this regard for SPECT, tracers that have been used for years in Japan are finally being testing in the United States, potentially allowing the nuclear cardiology field to grow beyond assessment of myocardial perfusion. Advances in cardiac PET suggest great growth potential given the advantages of improved spatial resolution of over conventional SPECT and the inherent use of attenuation correction with PET. Additionally, promising new PET perfusion tracers are under development that may significantly improve the accuracy of CAD detection in nuclear cardiology. Clearly, the use of PET and SPECT methods to assess myocardial viability will continue to provide clinically valuable information in patients with advanced heart disease (**Fig. 10.11**). Finally, the possibility of using PET with CT or SPECT with CT to image vulnerable, rupture-prone plaques offers promise for improving the ability to define which patients with CAD

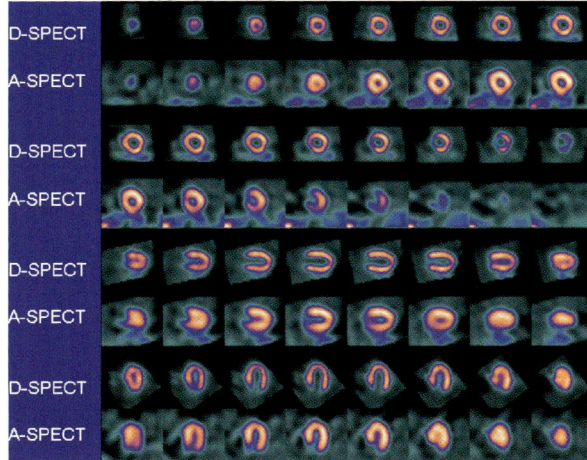

Fig. 10.10 Case example of normal exercise myocardial perfusion scan by D-SPECT (Spectrum-Dynamics) (1st, 3rd, 5th, 7th rows) compared with A-SPECT (E-Cam, Siemens) (alternate rows). D-SPECT images were acquired for 2 min and A-SPECT images were acquired for 16 min. (Adapted with permission from J Nucl Cardiol [8])

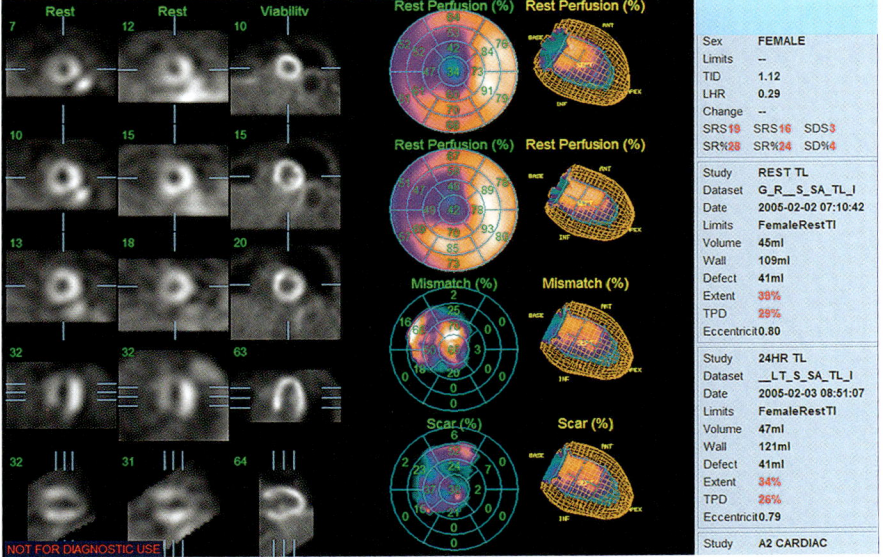

Fig. 10.11 Case example illustrating extensive mismatch by PET in a patient with non-reversible rest/redistribution defect by Tl-201 SPECT. *Left* figures: rest Tl-201 SPECT. *Middle* figures: 24-h redistribution Tl-201 SPECT; *Right* figures: FDG PET; Polar maps (*Top* to *bottom*): Rest Tl-201, redistribution Tl-201, Mismatch (PET viable), Match (PET non-viable). *Right*: surface maps

are at highest risk and in need of invasive management. Quite likely, nuclear and CT methods will be commonly applied over the next decade, with patients often having both procedures. However, what is still not clear at present is whether these procedures will be performed at the same time with hybrid imaging devices, or whether they will be performed separately, with the complementary tests being performed only in selected patient groups.

10.5 Imaging Pearls

10.5.1 Imaging for Prevention

In asymptomatic patients, atherosclerosis imaging is more effective than imaging for ischemia, since it is better suited to defining subclinical disease in need of preventive treatment.

- Approximately 10% of asymptomatic patients undergoing atherosclerosis imaging will be defined as having sufficient subclinical disease that ischemia testing is indicated.
- Patients with extensive atherosclerosis and no ischemia are identified as being at low risk for short- to intermediate-term cardiac events.

10.5.2 Imaging for Diagnosis

- According to Bayes' theorem, coronary CTA is likely to emerge as the test of choice for patients with an intermediate pre-test probability of CAD, due to its highest accuracy for detection of CAD.
- A normal coronary CTA rules out the presence of CAD as a cause of the patient's symptoms.
- In a minority of patients, ischemia testing will be indicated after coronary CTA to determine appropriate management.

10.5.3 Imaging for Intervention

- In symptomatic patients with known CAD, coronary CTA is not the initial test of choice, based on current data, since it may be unable to eliminate the need for further testing with coronary angiography or ischemia testing.
- Testing for ischemia has been shown to be effective in identifying a majority of patients who are not in need of consideration of revascularization, avoiding unnecessary catheterization.

- In selected patients in whom ischemia testing is inconclusive, coronary CTA can be helpful in avoiding unnecessary invasive coronary angiography.
- Viability testing with imaging methods can be effective in patients with ventricular dysfunction for purposes of guiding management decisions.

References

1. Naghavi M, Falk E, Hecht HS, Jamieson MJ, Kaul S, Berman D, et al. From vulnerable plaque to vulnerable patient-part III: executive summary of the screening for heart attack prevention and education (SHAPE) task force report. *Am J Cardiol.* 2006, 98: 2–15.
2. Berman DS, Hachamovitch R, Shaw LJ, Friedman JD, Hayes SW, Thomson L, et al. Roles of nuclear cardiology, cardiac computed tomography, and cardiac magnetic resonance: noninvasive risk stratification and a conceptual framework for the selection of noninvasive imaging tests in patients with known or suspected coronary artery disease. *J Nucl Med.* 2006, 47: 1107–1118.
3. Rozanski A, Gransar H, Wong ND, Shaw LJ, Miranda-Peats R, Polk D, et al. Clinical outcomes after both coronary calcium scanning and exercise myocardial perfusion scintigraphy. *J Am Coll Cardiol.* Mar 27 2007, 49(12): 1352–1361.
4. Berman DS, Kang X, Slomka PJ, Gerlach J, Yang L, Hayes SW, et al. Underestimation of extent of Ischemia by Gated SPECT myocardial perfusion imaging in patients with left main coronary artery disease. *J Nucl Cardiol.* 2007, 14: 521–528.
5. Berman DS. Fourth annual Mario S. verani, MD Memorial Lecture: noninvasive imaging in coronary artery disease: changing roles, changing Players. *J Nucl Cardiol.* 2006, 13: 457–473.
6. Hachamovitch R, Hayes SW, Friedman JD, Cohen I, Berman DS. Comparison of the short-term survival benefit associated with revascularization compared with medical therapy in patients with no prior coronary artery disease undergoing stress myocardial perfusion single photon emission computed tomography. *Circulation.* 2003, 107(23): 2900–2907.
7. Hachamovitch R, Rozanski A, Hayes SW, Thomson LEJ, Germano G, Friedman JD, et al. Predicting Therapeutic benefit from myocardial revascularization procedures: Are measurements of both resting left ventricular ejection fraction and stress-induced myocardial ischemia necessary? *J Nucl Cardiol.* 2006, 13: 768–778.
8. Patton J, Berman DS, Slomka P. Rcent technological advances in nuclear cardiology *J Nucl Cardiol.* 2007, 14: 501–513.
9. Hachamovitch R, Hayes SW, Friedman JD, Cohen I, Berman DS. Stress myocardial perfusion SPECT is clinically effective and cost-effective in risk-stratification of patients with a high likelihood of CAD but No Known CAD. *J Am Coll Cardiol.* 2004, 43: 200–208.
10. Berman DS, Achenbach S, Taylor A, Weigold G, Poon M. Highlights of the Second Annual Scientific Meeting of the Society of Cardiovascular CT 2007. *J Am Coll Cardiol.* 2007, 50: 2329–2335.

Chapter 11
CCT Imaging: Cardiac Electrophysiology Applications

Jerold S. Shinbane

Cardiovascular computed tomography (CCT) can comprehensively assess cardiovascular structure and function relevant to the assessment, treatment, and follow-up of patients with electrophysiologically related disease processes. CT provides 3-D visualization of cardiac chambers, coronary vessels, and thoracic vasculature including structures particularly important to cardiac electrophysiology including the coronary veins, pulmonary veins, and left atrium. This comprehensive technology is extremely useful in identification and characterization of cardiovascular substrates relevant to cardiac electrophysiology, pre-procedure planning, procedural facilitation, and procedural follow-up.

11.1 Cardiovascular Substrates Associated with Sudden Cardiac Death

Sudden cardiovascular death is associated with a variety of cardiovascular structural or primary electrophysiologic abnormalities, often with the first manifestation of disease being sudden death. Vascular anatomies associated with sudden cardiac death can be identified by CCT and can include anomalous coronary arteries, severe coronary artery disease, critical aortic stenosis, and aortic aneurysms and dissections [1, 2, 3, 4, 5, 6]. CCT can identify and characterize cardiomyopathic processes associated with ventricular arrhythmias and sudden cardiac death, including ischemic and non-ischemic dilated cardiomyopathy, hypertrophic cardiomyopathy, and arrhythmogenic right ventricular cardiomyopathy [7, 8, 9]. CCT cine can characterize cardiomyopathy substrates by providing reproducible volumetric quantitative measurement of biventricular volumes and ejection fraction, wall thickness and regional wall motion, and can directly visualize coronary arteries, which may potentially facilitate differentiation between ischemic and non-ischemic cardiomyopathy [7, 10, 11, 12]. The diagnosis of arrhythmogenic right ventricular cardiomyopathy involves criteria including clinical history, family history, ECG criteria, and electrophysiologic testing results [13]. Although cardiovascular magnetic resonance

J.S. Shinbane
Division of Cardiovascular Medicine, USC Keck School of Medicine, Los Angeles, CA, USA
e-mail: shinbane@usc.edu

M.J. Budoff, J.S. Shinbane (eds.), *Handbook of Cardiovascular CT*,
DOI: 10.1007/978-1-84800-091-9_11, © Springer-Verlag London Limited 2008

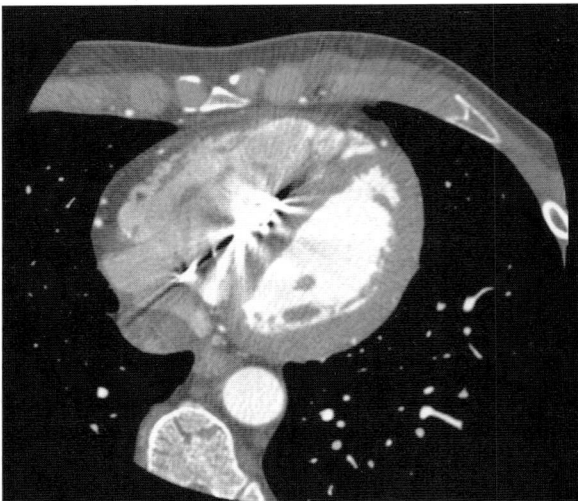

Fig. 11.1 CT angiography axial view demonstrating fibrofatty replacement of right ventricular myocardium, low-attenuation trabeculations, and right ventricular free wall scalloping in arrhythmogenic right ventricular cardiomyopathy. A right ventricular defibrillation lead is present with beam-hardening artifact

imaging has been the diagnostic imaging modality of choice, CT angiography can visualize the anatomic features associated with arrhythmogenic right ventricular cardiomyopathy, such as epicardial and myocardial fat, low-attenuation trabeculations, right ventricular free-wall scalloping, and global and regional right ventricular wall motion abnormalities [9, 14]. This modality is particularly useful in the assessment of patients with preexisting cardiac devices limiting the use of magnetic resonance imaging (**Fig. 11.1**).

11.2 Electrophysiologic Mapping and Radiofrequency Catheter Ablation

11.2.1 Atrial Fibrillation Ablation

Atrial fibrillation ablation requires a detailed understanding of an individual patient's cardiovascular anatomy through 3-D characterization of the relationships between the left atrium, surrounding cardiac structures, and extracardiac thoracic structures. A pre-procedure study serves as a roadmap for procedural planning, a 3-D dataset for intra-procedure electroanatomic mapping and ablation, and a template for the follow-up of atrial remodeling and assessment for complications including pulmonary vein stenosis. There are a variety of approaches to catheter-based ablation for atrial fibrillation. Percutaneous catheter-based approaches access the left atrium via either a single or a double transseptal approach depending on the number of left atrial catheters used. Catheter-based techniques for ablation of atrial fibrillation have focused on segmental ablation or complete circumferential electrical isolation of the pulmonary veins to ablate or isolate ectopic pulmonary vein foci from triggering atrial fibrillation, ablation of other ectopic atrial foci, and long linear lesions providing pathways of preferential conduction [15, 16]. This approach requires that radiofrequency energy applications occur in the left atrium near the pulmonary vein os, while ensuring that they do not enter the os in order to avoid pulmonary vein stenosis.

Characterization of the left atrium and pulmonary veins is achieved through multiple modalities of evaluation including multiplane 2-D views, 3-D volumetric reconstructions, virtual endocardial views, and volumetric quantification of the atria (**Fig. 11.2**). Pulmonary venous anatomy demonstrates great variability regarding vein number, location, size, shape, and os complexity. CT angiography can define the relationship between veins as well as between the left upper pulmonary vein and left atrial appendage [17, 18, 19]. Workstation electrophysiology software can define characteristics of the pulmonary vein os including area, maximum diameter,

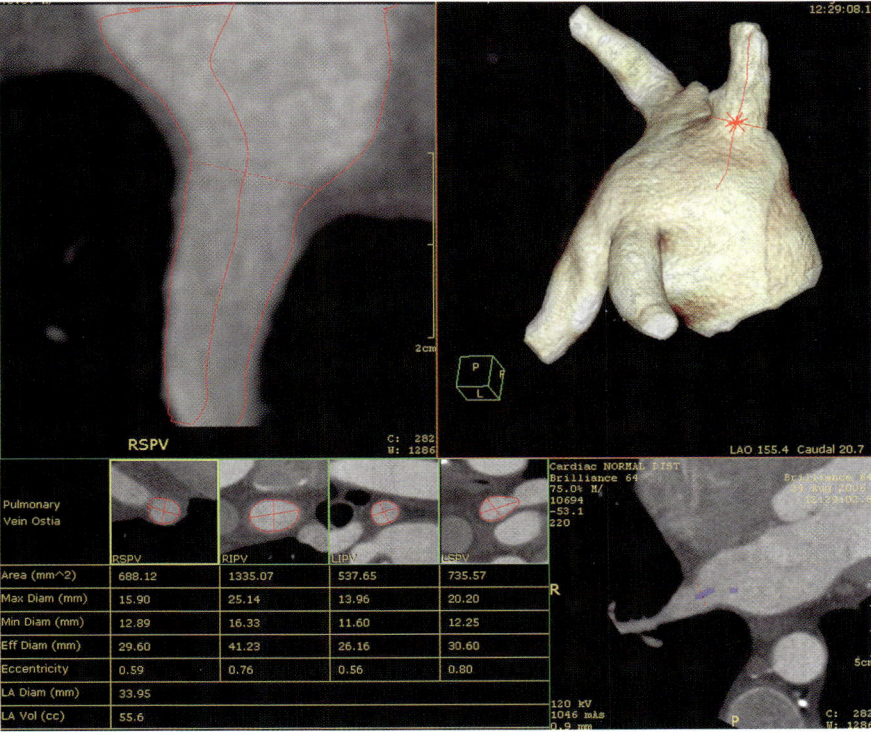

Pulmonary Vein Ostia	RSPV	RIPV	LIPV	LSPV
Area (mm^2)	688.12	1335.07	537.65	735.57
Max Diam (mm)	15.90	25.14	13.96	20.20
Min Diam (mm)	12.89	16.33	11.60	12.25
Eff Diam (mm)	29.60	41.23	26.16	30.60
Eccentricity	0.59	0.76	0.56	0.80
LA Diam (mm)	33.95			
LA Vol (cc)	55.6			

Fig. 11.2 Characterization of the left atrium and pulmonary veins demonstrated through 2-D views (*Panel A*), 3-D volumetric reconstruction (*Panel B*), with definition of characteristics of the pulmonary vein os including area, maximum diameter, minimum diameter, and eccentricity (*Panel C*)

minimum diameter, eccentricity, left atrial diameter, and left atrial volume. Key to these measurements is identification of the left atrial/pulmonary vein interface, determination of the long axis of the vein at the os, and recognition that the vein os is often ovoid in shape rather than circular. Additionally, atrial anatomy can be defined including patent foramen ovale, atrial septal defects, and atrial masses. The recognition of atrial thrombi is extremely important prior to consideration of atrial fibrillation ablation. Trabeculation of the left atrial appendage anatomy makes analysis for left atrial thrombi challenging. Although CCT can visualize the left atrial appendage in detail and has been reported to be able to visualize atrial thrombi, transesophageal echo remains the modality of choice for ruling out left atrial thrombi, as issues of the positive predictive value of identification of CCT remain[20].

Other thoracic anatomy relevant to ablation includes the relationship of the esophagus and aorta to the posterior left atrium and pulmonary veins (**Fig. 11.3**). Left atrial-esophageal fistula has been reported as a fatal complication of atrial fibrillation ablation [21]. There is variability of the course of the esophagus and the degree of contact between the posterior left atrium/pulmonary veins and the esophagus, which can be visualized prior to ablation, and barium swallow has been used during CT to better visualize the esophagus [22, 23]. Esophageal motility, change in position of the esophagus with respiration, patient position, and timing of the CCT in relation to the procedure can cause change in the spatial relationship of the esophagus to the posterior left atrium during procedures. The relationship of the coronary vasculature to the left atrium is also important, especially the relationship between the coronary veins, the circumflex coronary artery, and the posterior

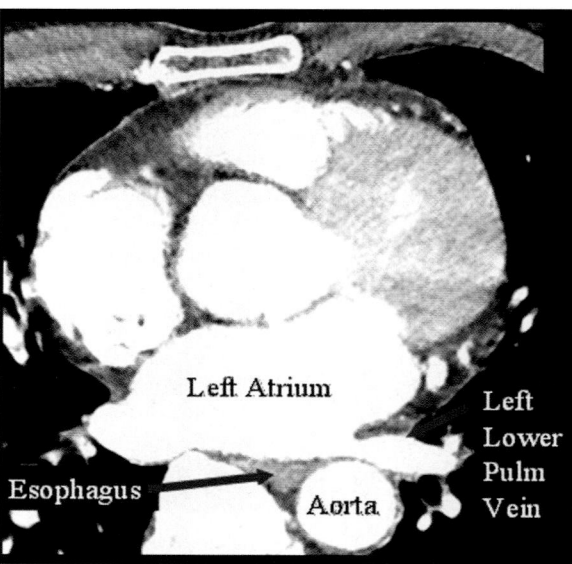

Fig. 11.3 Axial image demonstrating the relationship of the esophagus and aorta to the posterior left atrium and pulmonary veins

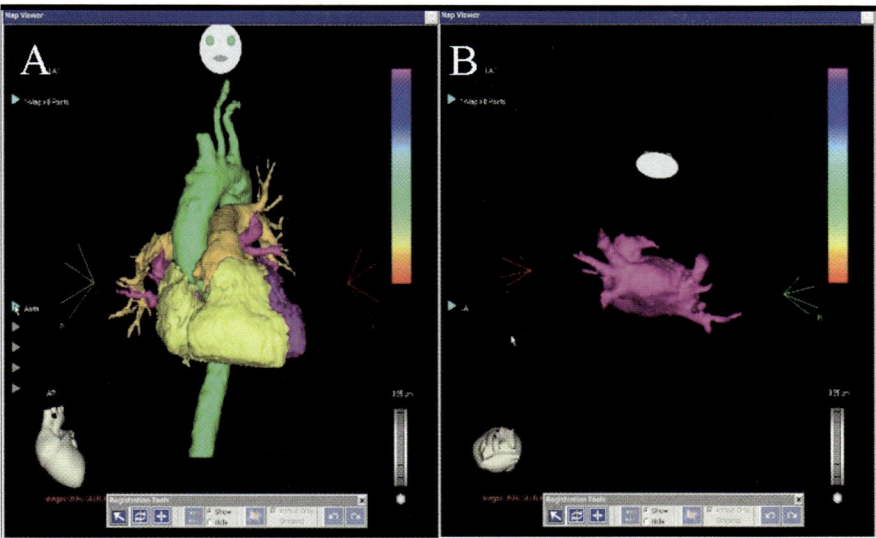

Fig. 11.4 Initial image processing for electroanatomic mapping with CT image integration with segmentation of vascular structures (*Panel A*) and editing of aorta (*green*), pulmonary arteries (*orange*), right atrium and right ventricle (*yellow*), with the left atrium (*purple*) subsequently rotated to demonstrate the posterior left atrium (*purple*) (*Panel B*)

left atrium/AV groove in order to avoid coronary artery complications [24]. Additionally, the relationship of the bronchi and pulmonary veins is important and can be characterized by CCT [25].

Electroanatomic mapping with CCT image integration has revolutionized ablation by allowing for electrical mapping and ablation to occur on a 3-D map of the patient's individual endocardial left atrial anatomy. The process involves import of the unprocessed DICOM images into the mapping system, use of edge detection software to define cardiac vascular structures, and editing of structures relevant to ablation including the left atrium and in some labs the aorta and esophagus (**Fig. 11.4**). Subsequently, a separate catheter-based anatomic map is created using landmark points in the left atrium followed by registration of surface points defining the endocardium of the left atrium. This anatomic catheter-based map is then integrated with the CCT images with assessment of markers of successful integration including definition of an acceptable catheter to endocardium distance and has been demonstrated to be feasible and accurate (**Fig. 11.5**) [26, 27]. If registration is inadequate, catheter-based points are edited and new points registered to ensure that the atrial endocardial surface has been adequately mapped.

Use of electroanatomic mapping with image integration allows catheter position to be tracked on the 3-D cardiac image with mapping of arrhythmias, assessment of electrical activation and propagation, definition of electrically silent areas, assessment of contact with endocardium, and documentation of radiofrequency

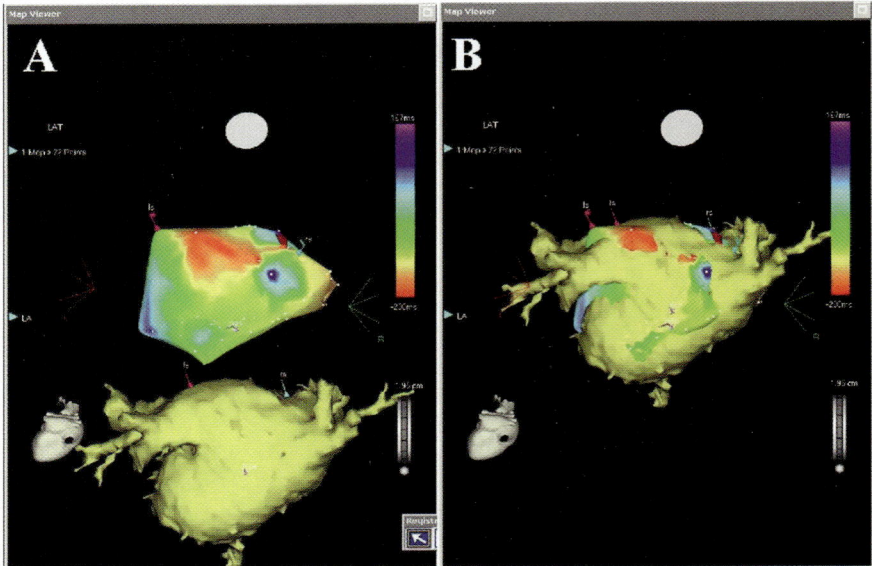

Fig. 11.5 Image processing for electroanatomic mapping with CT image integration with a catheter-based anatomic map of the left atrium (*Panel A, upper image*) and the 3-D volume-rendered CT image of the left atrium (*Panel A, lower image*) with integration of these images (*Panel B*)

applications (**Fig. 11.6**). The localization of the ablation catheter tip on this endocardial left atrial reconstruction helps to ensure that radiofrequency applications are placed in the atrium and not in the actual pulmonary veins or os to avoid pulmonary vein stenosis. Subsequent to ablation, mapping using this system can be performed to ensure electrical isolation of the pulmonary veins. Integration of 3-D images obtained pre-procedure with real-time catheter-based electroanatomic maps has been shown to decrease procedural fluoroscopy time, decrease recurrence of atrial fibrillation, and increase restoration of sinus rhythm compared to electroanatomic mapping alone [28].

Pulmonary vein stenosis is a potential complication of atrial fibrillation ablation (**Fig. 11.7**) [29, 30]. The incidence of stenosis is dependent on technique, definition of significant stenosis, and degree of surveillance [31]. The baseline pre-procedure study can serve as a template for assessment of pulmonary vein stenosis and can identify preexisting pulmonary vein stenoses of other etiologies, preventing misdiagnosis of ablation-related stenosis [32]. Radiation exposure is a major consideration in regard to follow-up considering exposure related to pre-procedure study and fluoroscopy related to the procedure. CCT can also provide comprehensive post-procedure assessment of chest pain or shortness of breath including pulmonary embolus, aortic dissection, pericardial effusion coronary artery complications, and pulmonary vein stenosis.

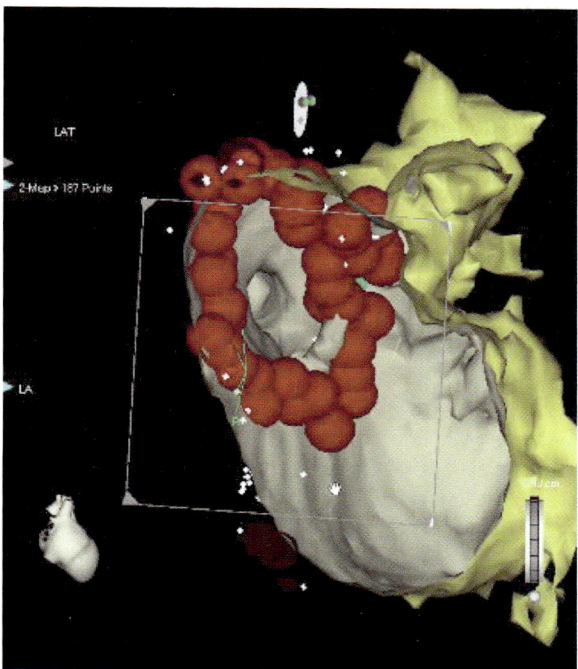

Fig. 11.6 Electroanatomic mapping with image integration demonstrating an endocardial view of the left upper pulmonary vein after radiofrequency catheter isolation of the vein with encircling radiofrequency energy applications (*red spheres*)

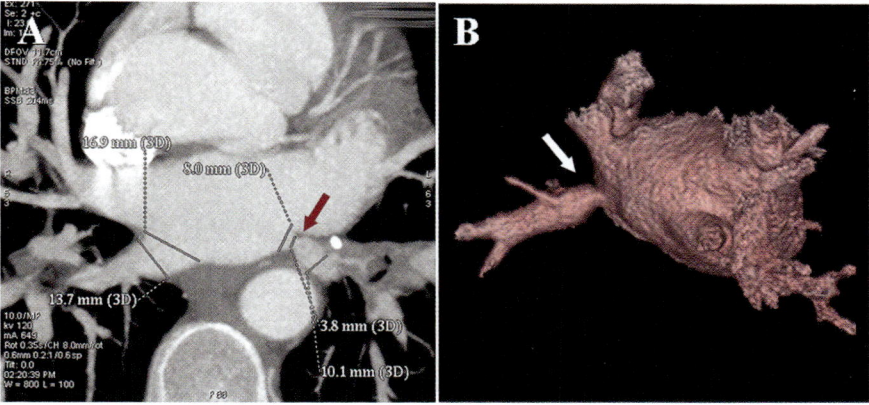

Fig. 11.7 2-D (*Panel A*) and 3-D volume-rendered images demonstrating pulmonary vein stenosis of a left lower pulmonary vein. (Courtesy of Dr. Jeffrey Schussler, Baylor University Medical Center, Dallas, Texas.)

11.3 Cardiac Resynchronization Therapy

CCT can visualize the coronary venous system and may potentially play an important role in the evolution of cardiac resynchronization therapy (**Fig. 11.8**) [33, 34, 35]. CRT is used to optimize cardiac function by resynchronizing ventricular contraction in patients with dilated ischemic and non-ischemic cardiomyopathy, ventricular conduction abnormalities, and moderate-to-severe heart failure [36, 37, 38]. With CRT, a chronic pacing lead is placed in a coronary sinus branch vessel of the coronary venous system to achieve left ventricular pacing. As opposed to the atrial and right ventricular leads that can be actively fixated in many positions in their respective chambers, placement of the coronary venous lead can be challenging, as lead position is limited by the individual location and variation of the existing coronary venous anatomy.

CCT can provide detailed assessment of the coronary venous anatomy, with coronary sinus dimensions, branch vessel locations, branch vessel diameters, and branch vessel angulations off the coronary sinus/great cardiac vein [33]. CCT can also visualize details of coronary veins, which could limit access to the coronary

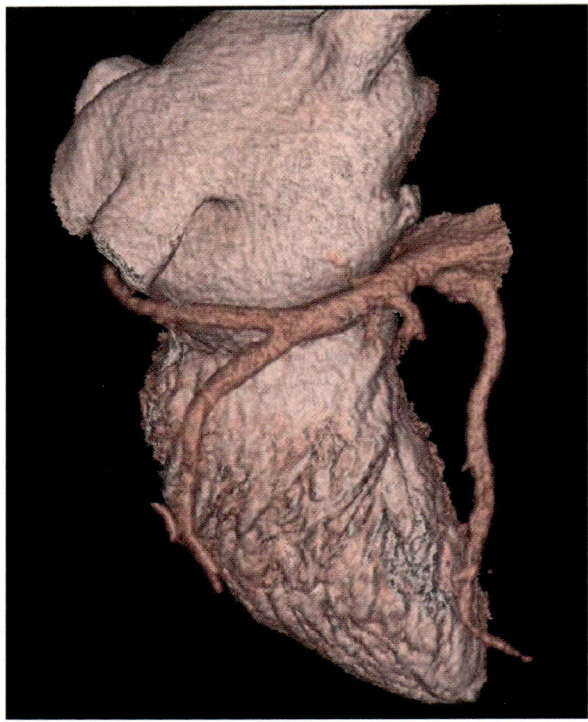

Fig. 11.8 3-D volume-rendered image demonstrating visualization of the coronary venous system and the relationship of the coronary veins to the left atrium, mitral annulus, and left ventricle

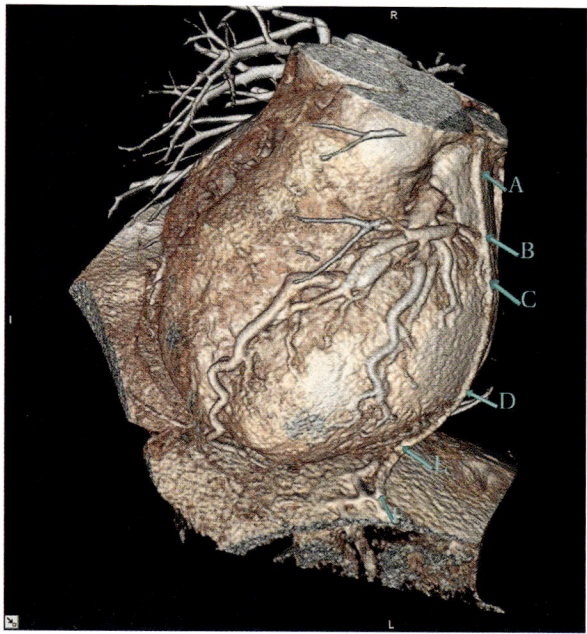

Fig. 11.9 3-D volume-rendered image illustrating visualization of the course (A–E) of the left phrenic nerve. (From Matsumoto Y, Krishnan S, Fowler SJ, et al. (40), by permission of The American Journal of Cardiology)

venous system, such as Thebesian valves (prominent coronary vein os valves) that can obstruct access to the coronary sinus [39]. Other abnormalities such as coronary sinus diverticula and anomalous connections, such as left superior vena cava to coronary sinus, can be visualized. Additionally, visualization of the phrenic nerve and its relation to the coronary venous anatomy may be important for avoidance of diaphragmatic pacing (**Fig. 11.9**) [40]. The advent of systems capable of superimposing CT images with fluoroscopy images may be potentially useful for procedural facilitation and requires further investigation. Additionally, visualization of the relationship between the coronary veins, the coronary arteries, and the mitral annulus may be important for other procedures involving the coronary venous system, such as transvenous mitral annuloplasty.

CCT provides comprehensive assessment important to the diagnosis and treatment of electrophysiologically relevant cardiovascular disease. The ability to rapidly analyze cardiovascular structures relevant to cardiac electrophysiology as well as to use of image sets integrated with real-time mapping systems has revolutionized cardiac electrophysiology procedures and will continue to expand applications of CT imaging in cardiac electrophysiology to mapping and ablation of arrhythmias in the future.

11.4 Imaging Pearls

11.4.1 General

- Many studies are ordered by electrophysiologists and cardiologists managing the patient's arrhythmias issues. Discussion of options for rate and rhythm control prior to the study can help to achieve a more optimal imaging result, including adjustment of pacing parameters to regularize ventricular rates.
- Dose modulation can be problematic with rapid and irregular heart rates, and therefore should be avoided.
- Many patients being studied for electrophysiologic issues have either pacemakers or implantable cardiac defibrillators. Artifacts may be present on study based on type and number of leads, and generator location. Awareness as to the use of appropriate filters during analysis can decrease these artifacts, aiding interpretation of images.

11.4.2 Sudden Death Substrates

- Precise volumetric assessment of ventricular function should be performed as many decisions related to device placement relate to algorithms based on ejection fraction.
- The assessment for left main or three-vessel coronary artery disease is essential prior to consideration of an electrophysiology study with a ventricular stimulation protocol, as these anatomies may contraindicate study.
- Assessment of arrhythmogenic right ventricular cardiomyopathy can be challenging after a device has been placed. CCT can be useful in assessing for depressed global right ventricular ejection fraction, regional wall motion abnormalities, prominent ventricular trabeculation, and low-attenuation signal in ventricular myocardium, and can be helpful in conjunction with the clinical criteria for assessment of this diagnosis.

11.4.3 Atrial Fibrillation Ablation

- The field of view must extend cranially enough to visualize the entirety of the left atrial appendage and left upper pulmonary vein.
- Left atrial analyses should include assessment of atrial volumes, structural abnormalities such as patent foramen ovale, atrial septal defects, and evidence of left atrial thrombus. The assessment of atrial relationships to the esophagus, aorta, bronchi, and coronary arteries is important when ablation of the posterior atrium is being considered.
- Pulmonary venous anatomy is variable, and therefore the baseline study serves as a template for future assessment for pulmonary vein stenoses.

- Perform CCT scanning as soon as possible before electrophysiology study to minimize registration issues when electroanatomic mapping is to be used.
- Barium contrast has been used to better visualize the esophagus for electro-anatomic mapping and ablation procedures for atria fibrillation.
- The actual DICOM files will need to be available to the electrophysiologist for use with electroanatomic imaging systems in the electrophysiology laboratory.

11.4.4 Resynchronization Therapy

- The field of view and scanning timing should encompass thoracic vasculature including venous anatomy to provide assessment of potential catheter routes.
- Attention to circulation time and contrast injection protocol is important for ensuring adequate visualization of the coronary venous and arterial anatomy.
- Assessment of location, size, and angulation of coronary sinus branch veins and of coronary venous anomalies that would affect lead placement should be performed.
- Phrenic nerve location can be visualized with appropriate filtering with information related to location of the nerve in relation to the coronary venous anatomy.

Systems allowing integration of DICOM images with catheterization lab fluoroscopy may provide roadmaps for procedural facilitation.

References

1. Duran C, Kantarci M, Durur Subasi I, et al. Remarkable anatomic anomalies of coronary arteries and their clinical importance: a multidetector computed tomography angiographic study. J Comput Assist Tomogr 2006, 30(6): 939–48.
2. Shabestari AA, Abdi S, Akhlaghpoor S, et al. Diagnostic performance of 64-channel multi-slice computed tomography in assessment of significant coronary artery disease in symptomatic subjects. Am J Cardiol 2007, 99(12): 1656–61.
3. Schuijf JD, Pundziute G, Jukema JW, et al. Diagnostic accuracy of 64-slice multislice computed tomography in the noninvasive evaluation of significant coronary artery disease. Am J Cardiol 2006, 98(2): 145–8.
4. Ropers D, Rixe J, Anders K, et al. Usefulness of multidetector row spiral computed tomography with 64- × 0.6-mm collimation and 330-ms rotation for the noninvasive detection of significant coronary artery stenoses. Am J Cardiol 2006, 97(3): 343–8.
5. Laissy JP, Messika-Zeitoun D, Serfaty JM, et al. Comprehensive Evaluation of Preoperative Patients with Aortic Valve Stenosis. Usefulness of Multi-Detector Cardiac Computed Tomography. Heart 2007.
6. Shiga T, Wajima Z, Apfel CC, Inoue T, Ohe Y. Diagnostic accuracy of transesophageal echocardiography, helical computed tomography, and magnetic resonance imaging for suspected thoracic aortic dissection: systematic review and meta-analysis. Arch Intern Med 2006, 166(13): 1350–6.
7. Cornily JC, Gilard M, Le Gal G, et al. Accuracy of 16-detector multislice spiral computed tomography in the initial evaluation of dilated cardiomyopathy. Eur J Radiol 2007, 61(1): 84–90.

8. Shiozaki AA, Santos TS, Artega E, Rochitte CE. Images in cardiovascular medicine. Myocardial delayed enhancement by computed tomography in hypertrophic cardiomyopathy. Circulation 2007, 115(17): e430–1.

9. Bomma C, Dalal D, Tandri H, et al. Evolving role of multidetector computed tomography in evaluation of arrhythmogenic right ventricular dysplasia/cardiomyopathy. Am J Cardiol 2007, 100(1): 99–105.

10. Kim TH, Ryu YH, Hur J, et al. Evaluation of right ventricular volume and mass using retrospective ECG-gated cardiac multidetector computed tomography: comparison with first-pass radionuclide angiography. Eur Radiol 2005, 15(9): 1987–93.

11. Butler J, Shapiro MD, Jassal DS, et al. Comparison of multidetector computed tomography and two-dimensional transthoracic echocardiography for left ventricular assessment in patients with heart failure. Am J Cardiol 2007, 99(2): 247–9.

12. Andreini D, Pontone G, Pepi M, et al. Diagnostic accuracy of multidetector computed tomography coronary angiography in patients with dilated cardiomyopathy. J Am Coll Cardiol 2007, 49(20): 2044–50.

13. McKenna WJ, Thiene G, Nava A, et al. Diagnosis of arrhythmogenic right ventricular dysplasia/cardiomyopathy. Task Force of the Working Group Myocardial and Pericardial Disease of the European Society of Cardiology and of the Scientific Council on Cardiomyopathies of the International Society and Federation of Cardiology. Br Heart J 1994, 71(3): 215–8.

14. Wu YW, Tadamura E, Kanao S, et al. Structural and functional assessment of arrhythmogenic right ventricular dysplasia/cardiomyopathy by multi-slice computed tomography: comparison with cardiovascular magnetic resonance. Int J Cardiol 2007, 115(3): e118–21.

15. Tamborero D, Mont L, Molina I, et al. Selective segmental ostial ablation and circumferential pulmonary veins ablation. Results of an individualized strategy to cure refractory atrial fibrillation. J Interv Card Electrophysiol 2007, 19(1): 19–27.

16. Oral H, Pappone C, Chugh A, et al. Circumferential pulmonary-vein ablation for chronic atrial fibrillation. N Engl J Med 2006, 354(9): 934–41.

17. Scharf C, Sneider M, Case I, et al. Anatomy of the pulmonary veins in patients with atrial fibrillation and effects of segmental ostial ablation analyzed by computed tomography. J Cardiovasc Electrophysiol 2003, 14(2): 150–5.

18. Wood MA, Wittkamp M, Henry D, et al. A comparison of pulmonary vein ostial anatomy by computerized tomography, echocardiography, and venography in patients with atrial fibrillation having radiofrequency catheter ablation. Am J Cardiol 2004, 93(1): 49–53.

19. Jongbloed MR, Dirksen MS, Bax JJ, et al. Atrial fibrillation: multi-detector row CT of pulmonary vein anatomy prior to radiofrequency catheter ablation–initial experience. Radiology 2005, 234(3): 702–9.

20. Achenbach S, Sacher D, Ropers D, et al. Electron beam computed tomography for the detection of left atrial thrombi in patients with atrial fibrillation. Heart 2004, 90(12): 1477–8.

21. Pappone C, Oral H, Santinelli V, et al. Atrio-esophageal fistula as a complication of percutaneous transcatheter ablation of atrial fibrillation. Circulation 2004, 109(22): 2724–6.

22. Cury RC, Abbara S, Schmidt S, et al. Relationship of the esophagus and aorta to the left atrium and pulmonary veins: implications for catheter ablation of atrial fibrillation. Heart Rhythm 2005, 2(12): 1317–23.

23. Piorkowski C, Hindricks G, Schreiber D, et al. Electroanatomic reconstruction of the left atrium, pulmonary veins, and esophagus compared with the "true anatomy" on multislice computed tomography in patients undergoing catheter ablation of atrial fibrillation. Heart Rhythm 2006, 3(3): 317–27.

24. Lemola K, Mueller G, Desjardins B, et al. Topographic analysis of the coronary sinus and major cardiac veins by computed tomography. Heart Rhythm 2005, 2(7): 694–9.

25. Wu MH, Wongcharoen W, Tsao HM, et al. Close relationship between the bronchi and pulmonary veins: implications for the prevention of atriobronchial fistula after atrial fibrillation ablation. J Cardiovasc Electrophysiol 2007.

26. Kistler PM, Earley MJ, Harris S, et al. Validation of three-dimensional cardiac image integration: use of integrated CT image into electroanatomic mapping system to perform catheter ablation of atrial fibrillation. J Cardiovasc Electrophysiol 2006, 17(4): 341–8.

27. Sra J, Krum D, Hare J, et al. Feasibility and validation of registration of three-dimensional left atrial models derived from computed tomography with a noncontact cardiac mapping system. Heart Rhythm 2005, 2(1): 55–63.

28. Kistler PM, Rajappan K, Jahngir M, et al. The impact of CT image integration into an electroanatomic mapping system on clinical outcomes of catheter ablation of atrial fibrillation. J Cardiovasc Electrophysiol 2006, 17(10): 1093–101.

29. Robbins IM, Colvin EV, Doyle TP, et al. Pulmonary vein stenosis after catheter ablation of atrial fibrillation. Circulation 1998, 98(17): 1769–75.

30. Packer DL, Keelan P, Munger TM, et al. Clinical presentation, investigation, and management of pulmonary vein stenosis complicating ablation for atrial fibrillation. Circulation 2005, 111(5): 546–54.

31. Dong J, Vasamreddy CR, Jayam V, et al. Incidence and predictors of pulmonary vein stenosis following catheter ablation of atrial fibrillation using the anatomic pulmonary vein ablation approach: results from paired magnetic resonance imaging. J Cardiovasc Electrophysiol 2005, 16(8): 845–52.

32. Wongcharoen W, Tsao HM, Wu MH, et al. Preexisting pulmonary vein stenosis in patients undergoing atrial fibrillation ablation: a report of five cases. J Cardiovasc Electrophysiol 2006, 17(4): 423–5.

33. Mao S, Shinbane JS, Girsky MJ, et al. Coronary venous imaging with electron beam computed tomographic angiography: three-dimensional mapping and relationship with coronary arteries. Am Heart J 2005, 150(2): 315–22.

34. Jongbloed MR, Lamb HJ, Bax JJ, et al. Noninvasive visualization of the cardiac venous system using multislice computed tomography. J Am Coll Cardiol 2005, 45(5): 749–53.

35. Van de Veire NR, Schuijf JD, De Sutter J, et al. Non-invasive visualization of the cardiac venous system in coronary artery disease patients using 64-slice computed tomography. J Am Coll Cardiol 2006, 48(9): 1832–8.

36. Saxon LA, De Marco T, Schafer J, Chatterjee K, Kumar UN, Foster E. Effects of long-term biventricular stimulation for resynchronization on echocardiographic measures of remodeling. Circulation 2002, 105(11): 1304–10.

37. Abraham WT, Fisher WG, Smith AL, et al. Cardiac resynchronization in chronic heart failure. N Engl J Med 2002, 346(24): 1845–53.

38. St John Sutton MG, Plappert T, Abraham WT, et al. Effect of cardiac resynchronization therapy on left ventricular size and function in chronic heart failure. Circulation 2003, 107(15): 1985–90.

39. Shinbane JS, Girsky MJ, Mao S, Budoff MJ. Thebesian valve imaging with electron beam CT angiography: implications for resynchronization therapy. Pacing Clin Electrophysiol 2004, 27(11): 1566–7.

40. Matsumoto Y, Krishnan S, Fowler SJ, et al. Detection of phrenic nerves and their relation to cardiac anatomy using 64-slice multidetector computed tomography. Am J Cardiol 2007, 100(1): 133–7.

Chapter 12
Pericardial/Myocardial Disease Processes

Michael D. Shapiro, Ammar Sarwar, and Khurram Nasir

12.1 Introduction

While the current primary clinical use of contrast-enhanced cardiac computed tomography (CCT) remains the exclusion of coronary artery disease in low-to-intermediate risk symptomatic patients, this modality offers a unique opportunity to assess both the pericardium and the myocardium. Given the associated contrast and radiation exposure, CCT presently serves as an adjunct to echocardiography and cardiac MRI for this purpose. However, CCT provides superb delineation of the pericardium and can precisely localize lesions as well as aid in their characterization. Furthermore, CCT can effectively evaluate morphology and function in various myocardial diseases, including the various cardiomyopathies. The volumetric nature of image acquisition with CCT provides an accurate and reproducible method for quantifying ventricular mass, volumes, and function. This chapter will discuss the application of CCT in the assessment of various myocardial and pericardial disease processes.

12.2 CT Imaging of Myocardial Disease

The World Health Organization defines the cardiomyopathies as diseases of myocardial tissue associated with cardiac dysfunction and subdivides them into four categories: dilated, restrictive, hypertrophic, and arrhythmogenic right ventricular cardiomyopathy (ARVC) [1]. Dilated cardiomyopathy is characterized by ventricular enlargement and decreased systolic function. Besides reconstructing the CT data at specific diastolic (and/or systolic) phases of the cardiac cycle for evaluation of the coronary arteries and cardiac morphology, a multiphase dataset, which reconstructs the entire cardiac cycle at 5–10% intervals, allows for viewing images in cine mode. This multiphase reconstruction allows for assessment of left and right

M.D. Shapiro
Cardiac MR PET CT Program, Massachusetts General Hospital and Harvard Medical School, Boston MA, USA
e-mails: mdshapiro@partners.org, shapiromi@gmail.com

M.J. Budoff, J.S. Shinbane (eds.), *Handbook of Cardiovascular CT*,
DOI: 10.1007/978-1-84800-091-9_12, © Springer-Verlag London Limited 2008

ventricular systolic function in any orientation, including all of the standard echocardiographic planes [2]. Thus, CCT can assess myocardial thickness, ventricular shape and volume, and global and regional ventricular function with excellent correlation to echocardiography and cardiac MRI [3, 4]. Additionally, patients with severely reduced left ventricular function are at risk for the development of mural thrombus. Given the inherently high contrast-to-noise ratio and excellent spatial resolution, CCT can readily identify such mural thrombi.

Restrictive cardiomyopathy is characterized by increased ventricular stiffness and associated diastolic dysfunction. Ventricular size and systolic function are usually normal, but the atria and systemic veins (superior and inferior vena cavae, hepatic veins, coronary sinus) are often dilated due to increased filling pressures. These features are easily depicted by CCT but are nonspecific. While CCT is not indicated solely for the evaluation of possible restrictive cardiomyopathy, it is useful in differentiating it from constrictive pericarditis. This distinction leads to important therapeutic consequences.

Hypertrophic cardiomyopathy is a genetic disorder of various sarcomeric proteins resulting in cardiac myocyte disarray and left ventricular hypertrophy with or without obstruction. This most commonly involves asymmetric septal hypertrophy, although other variants exist, including apical and mid-ventricular hypertrophy (**Fig. 12.1**). In patients with dynamic left ventricular outflow obstruction, CCT delineates the systolic anterior motion of the anterior mitral valve leaflet on the multiphase images. While poor acoustic windows may limit echocardiography, CCT can reliably identify all areas of the myocardium and provide accurate measurements of wall thickness.

ARVC is an unusual cardiomyopathy characterized by abnormal right ventricular function, fatty or fibrous deposition of the right ventricular myocardium, and abnormal electrocardiographic changes, which predisposes patients to sudden cardiac death. CCT has an advantage over echocardiography in its ability to visualize the right ventricle and thus to evaluate right ventricular morphology and systolic function, similar to MRI. However, MRI has superior tissue characterization capabilities and remains the modality of choice for evaluating suspected ARVC. When performing CCT in these patients, it is important to ensure adequate opacification of the right ventricle at the time of image acquisition. This can be achieved either by prolonging the contrast administration by several seconds (4–6 s) or by empirically utilizing a shorter delay time. Alternatively, placing a region of interest in the main pulmonary artery and triggering the scan at its peak opacification can consistently achieve preferential right-sided opacification. CCT can reliably characterize right ventricular dimensions as well as focal aneurysms of the myocardium and/or areas of right ventricular dysfunction. More importantly, CCT can also detect fatty infiltration as areas of hypoattenuation, confirmed by CT attenuation measurements. However, the finding of fat is sensitive but not specific for ARVC [5]. Hence, CCT findings must be correlated with clinical and electrocardiographic data to establish the diagnosis of ARVC.

Left ventricular non-compaction is a cardiomyopathy characterized by a two-layered myocardium: a thin compacted layer and a thick non-compacted layer.

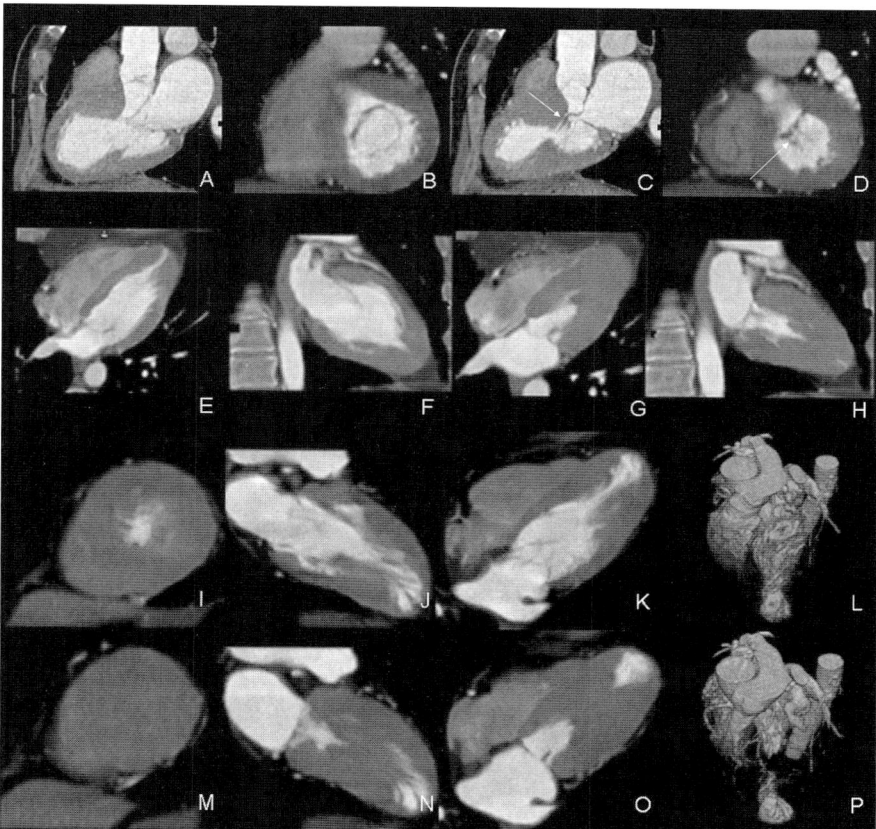

Fig. 12.1 The most common form of hypertrophic cardiomyopathy manifests as asymmetric septal hypertrophy with or without obstruction. This three-chamber view in end-diastole (**A**) demonstrates abnormal thickening of the mid- and basal interventricular septum. The short-axis view in end-diastole (**B**) demonstrates normal mitral valve morphology and opening. In systole, the three-chamber view (**C**) demonstrates systolic anterior motion of the anterior mitral valve leaflet (*arrow*) causing a gradient across the left ventricular outflow tract. This is consistent with hypertrophic obstructive cardiomyopathy. The short-axis view in systole (**D**) also demonstrates systolic anterior motion of the mitral valve as well as incomplete coaptation of the leaflets (*arrow*), causing mitral regurgitation. In the apical form of hypertrophic cardiomyopathy, muscle thickening occurs predominantly at the apex of the left ventricle, as can be seen in end-diastolic images in the four- and two-chamber views (**E, F**). The corresponding end-systolic images demonstrate complete obliteration of the left ventricular apex (**G, H**). When the left ventricular hypertrophy primarily affects the mid-ventricular level, there can be mid-cavitary obliteration with an associated gradient at the level of obstruction. End-diastolic images in the short-axis (**I**), two-chamber (**J**) and four-chamber (**K**) views, and the 3-D volume-rendered image (**L**) demonstrate prominent thickening at the mid-ventricular level. The corresponding end-systolic images (**M–P**) demonstrate complete obliteration of the mid-cavity

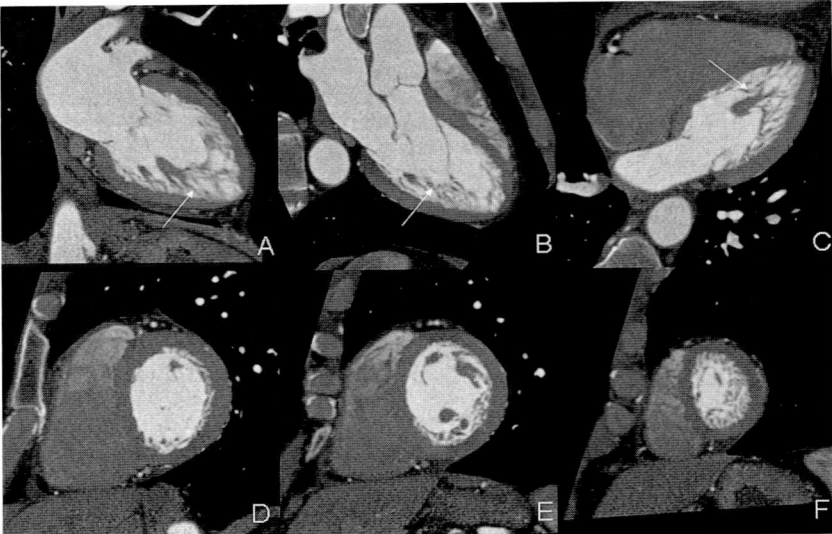

Fig. 12.2 The morphological hallmark of left ventricular non-compaction is the presence of hypertrabeculations. These hypertrabeculations are often most prominent toward the left ventricular apex. End-diastolic images in the two- (**A**), three- (**B**), and four-chamber (**C**) views demonstrate these characteristically prominent trabeculations that form the non-compacted layer (*white arrows*). End-diastolic images in the short-axis view at the base (**D**), mid-ventricular (**E**), and apical levels again demonstrate these hypertrabeculations, most prominently at the apex

The ratio of non-compacted to compacted myocardium has been reported to be 2.3:1 by cardiac MRI [6]. The hypertrabeculations of the non-compacted myocardium, as well as thrombi that may form within the recesses, are easily delineated with CCT due to its favorable contrast-to-noise ratio (**Fig. 12.2**). Left ventricular non-compaction frequently manifests as a dilated cardiomyopathy with reduced left ventricular function, which can also be assessed by CCT.

12.3 CT Imaging of Pericardial Disease

The pericardium is a double-layered membrane measuring <2 mm in thickness, which forms a sac containing 10–50 cc of serous pericardial fluid, surrounding the heart and the origins of the great vessels (**Fig. 12.3**) [7]. While echocardiography is conventionally used for the evaluation of pericardial diseases, CCT offers a number of distinct advantages. CCT provides a larger imaging field allowing assessment of concomitant pathology. In addition, CCT offers superior soft tissue contrast, and thus characterization of specific pericardial processes is sometimes possible. CCT is exquisitely sensitive to the detection of calcium and thus can be useful in identifying pericardial calcification, a finding that can be associated with constrictive pericarditis (**Fig. 12.4**). One of the limitations of CCT in evaluating the pericardium,

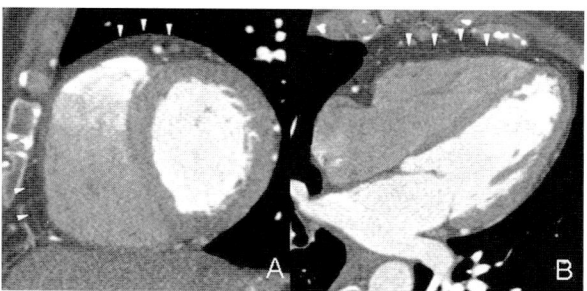

Fig. 12.3 Due to its excellent spatial resolution, cardiac CT can image the pericardium, which is normally <2 mm thick. These short-axis (**A**) and four-chamber (**B**) views demonstrate the normal, thin pericardium (*white arrowheads*). The pericardium is often best visualized over the right side of the heart, as the more abundant epicardial fat located there provides good tissue contrast

however, is its occasional difficulty in differentiating pericardial fluid from a thickened pericardium.

The current reference standard for the non-invasive evaluation of pericardial constriction is cardiac MRI. The characteristic anatomic changes associated with constrictive pericardial disease (elongated and narrow right ventricle, enlargement of the right atrium and inferior cava, and pericardial thickening) are clearly identified with both MRI and CCT. However, since patients with true constrictive pericarditis typically present with orthopnea, it is often difficult for them to lie flat in the MRI scanner for up to 1 h. CCT may offer another option for evaluating constrictive pericarditis, with short examination times representing one of its major advantages. The excellent spatial resolution of CCT allows for accurate measurement of pericardial thickness. Pericardial thickness of >4 mm is considered pathological and in the appropriate clinical context is suggestive of pericardial constriction [8, 9]. However, it is important to note that neither pericardial calcification nor thickening

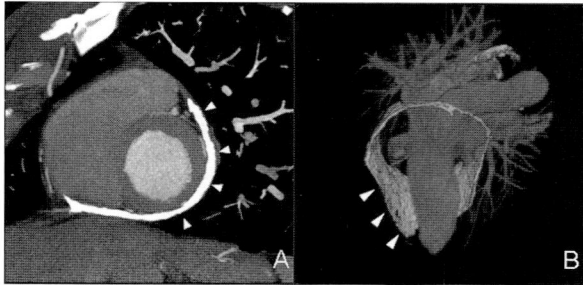

Fig. 12.4 Cardiac CT is exquisitely sensitive for the detection of calcium. In this case of pericardial constriction, the patient was found to have a thickened, heavily calcified pericardium (*white arrowheads*) as noted on the short-axis view (**A**) and 3-D volume-rendered image (**B**). The volume-rendered image demonstrates circumferential pericardial calcification at the base

is diagnostic of constrictive pericarditis. Besides these morphological characteristics, the demonstration of an early diastolic septal bounce on the multiphase cine images is suggestive of pericardial constriction [10].

Pericardial thickening may be found in the absence of constriction (e.g., acute pericarditis, uremia, collagen vascular diseases). Enhancement of the pericardium, indicative of pericardial inflammation, may be found in cases of pericarditis. Pericardial inflammation can be evaluated by performing CCT with and without contrast. The inflamed pericardium will demonstrate a significant increase in CT attenuation after contrast administration.

Rare individuals demonstrate a congenital absence of the pericardium. While this can present as a complete absence of pericardial tissue, most cases demonstrate only partial pericardial defects, typically on the left side (**Fig. 12.5A**). Clues on CCT that suggest this diagnosis are rotation of the heart to the left, interposition of lung tissue in the aorta-pulmonary window, and bulging of the left atrial appendage through the pericardial defect. Infrequently, the left atrial appendage can be incarcerated in the defect, requiring surgical enlargement or closure.

Echocardiography remains the modality of choice for the initial evaluation of pericardial effusion (**Fig. 12.5B**). However, several findings make further evaluation with CCT useful, such as loculated effusion, hemorrhagic effusion, or equivocal findings on echocardiography. Pericardial effusions may be characterized by CCT by measuring their CT attenuation. A CT attenuation close to water (e.g., 0 HU) suggests a simple pericardial effusion. If the CT attenuation is greater than that of water, the effusion may represent hemorrhage, purulence, or a malignant process.

Pericardial masses include cysts and neoplasms. Pericardial cysts are congenital and are usually found at the right costophrenic angle [11]. They tend to be smooth-walled simple cysts that do not enhance after contrast administration (**Fig. 12.5C**). With regard to neoplasms, metastases are far more common than primary pericardial tumors. Neighboring structures, such as lung and breast, are most commonly the source of metastatic disease. Other findings associated with metastatic disease include pericardial effusion and an irregularly thickened pericardium [12]. Primary

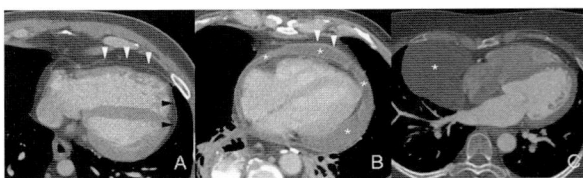

Fig. 12.5 Partial absence of the pericardium (**A**). In this example, normal pericardium is found over the right ventricular free wall (*white arrowheads*), but there is absence of the pericardium over the right ventricular apex and left ventricle (*black arrowheads*). Pericardial effusions (*asterisks*) are often found in the context of pericarditis (**B**). In this case, the pericardium also enhanced after administration of iodinated contrast (*white arrowheads*), suggesting pericardial inflammation. Pericardial cysts (*asterisk*) are benign fluid-filled pericardial masses, typically found at the right cardiophrenic angle (**C**)

neoplasms of the pericardium occur infrequently and may be benign (fibroma, teratoma, lipoma, and hemangioma) or malignant (mesothelioma, lymphoma, sarcoma, and liposarcoma) tumors [13].

This chapter reviewed disease processes of the myocardium and pericardium and their characteristic CCT findings. While echocardiography remains the primary non-invasive imaging modality for evaluation of the myocardium and pericardium, CCT serves as a valuable tool for further evaluation due to its inherently superb spatial resolution and soft tissue contrast. With further improvements in CCT technology, including refinements in temporal resolution and dramatic reductions in radiation exposure, CCT may play a larger role in the evaluation of patients with known or suspected diseases of the myocardium and pericardium.

12.4 Imaging Pearls

- Due to the volumetric nature of image acquisition, cardiac CT provides an accurate and reproducible method for assessing both myocardial and pericardial morphology and function.
- The assessment of right and left ventricular function requires image reconstruction in multiple phases of the cardiac cycle. These multiple datasets can be viewed together in a "cine" mode for assessing both qualitative and quantitative global and regional ventricular function.
- The excellent spatial resolution and contrast-to-noise ratio of CT allows for the detection of mural thrombi in patients with severely reduced left ventricular function.
- While not specific, features such as dilation of the atria and systemic veins, presence of a pericardial effusion, and preservation of systolic ventricular function point toward the diagnosis of restrictive cardiomyopathy.
- Hypertrophic cardiomyopathy is a heterogeneous disorder. The most common form involves asymmetric septal hypertrophy. Systolic anterior motion of the anterior mitral leaflet causing obstruction of the left ventricular outflow tract may be an associated abnormality that can be appreciated on cine images.
- Imaging of the right ventricle, for evaluation of diseases such as ARVC, requires optimal right ventricular opacification. This may be achieved by prolonging the administration of contrast or by reducing the delay time of scan acquisition.
- The normal pericardium is a double-layered membrane that is <2 mm thick. Pericardial thickness >4 mm is considered pathological.
- Pericardial calcification can be easily identified on CT because of its high attenuation. However, neither calcification nor thickening of the pericardium is diagnostic for constrictive pericarditis.
- To evaluate for pericardial inflammation, a non-contrast CT can be performed prior to the contrast-enhanced CT. Enhancement of the pericardium after contrast administration is indicative of pericardial inflammation, and may be seen in cases of pericarditis.

- Findings associated with partial absence of the pericardium include rotation of the heart to the left, interposition of the lung tissue in the aorta-pulmonary window, and bulging of the left atrial appendage through the pericardial defect.
- CT attenuation values may be useful for characterization of pericardial effusions. A value close to water (e.g., 0 HU) suggests a simple effusion, while CT attenuation values greater than water may be indicative of hemorrhage, purulence, or a malignant process.
- Neoplasms affecting the pericardium most commonly represent metastatic lesions, usually originating from the adjacent lung or breast. Findings associated with metastases include pericardial effusions and an irregularly thickened pericardium.

References

1. Richardson P, McKenna W, Bristow M, et al. Report of the 1995 World Health Organization/ International Society and Federation of Cardiology Task Force on the Definition and Classification of cardiomyopathies. Circulation 1996, 93: 841–2.
2. Cerqueira MD, Weissman NJ, Dilsizian V, et al. Standardized myocardial segmentation and nomenclature for tomographic imaging of the heart: a statement for healthcare professionals from the Cardiac Imaging Committee of the Council on Clinical Cardiology of the American Heart Association. Circulation 2002, 105: 539–42.
3. Annuar BR, Liew CK, Chin SP, et al. Assessment of global and regional left ventricular function using 64-slice multislice computed tomography and 2D echocardiography: A comparison with cardiac magnetic resonance. Eur J Radiol 2008, 65: 112–19.
4. Halliburton SS, Petersilka M, Schvartzman PR, Obuchowski N, White RD. Evaluation of left ventricular dysfunction using multiphasic reconstructions of coronary multi-slice computed tomography data in patients with chronic ischemic heart disease: validation against cine magnetic resonance imaging. Int J Cardiovasc Imaging 2003, 19: 73–83.
5. Tandri H, Bomma C, Calkins H, Bluemke DA. Magnetic resonance and computed tomography imaging of arrhythmogenic right ventricular dysplasia. J Magn Reson Imaging 2004, 19: 848–58.
6. Petersen SE, Selvanayagam JB, Wiesmann F, et al. Left ventricular non-compaction: insights from cardiovascular magnetic resonance imaging. J Am Coll Cardiol 2005, 46: 101–5.
7. Roberts WC, Spray TL. Pericardial heart disease: a study of its causes, consequences, and morphologic features. Cardiovasc Clin 1976, 7: 11–65.
8. Soulen RL, Stark DD, Higgins CB. Magnetic resonance imaging of constrictive pericardial disease. Amer J Cardiol 1985, 55: 480–4.
9. Spodick DH. Pericardial disease. JAMA 1997, 278: 704.
10. Himelman RB, Lee E, Schiller NB. Septal bounce, vena cava plethora, and pericardial adhesion: informative two-dimensional echocardiographic signs in the diagnosis of pericardial constriction. J Am Soc Echocardiogr 1998, 1: 333–50.
11. Oyama N, Oyama N, Komuro K, et al. Computed tomography and magnetic resonance imaging of the pericardium: anatomy and pathology. Magn Reson Med Sci 2004, 3: 145–52.
12. Restrepo CS, Largoza A, Lemos DF, et al. CT and MR imaging findings of malignant cardiac tumors. Curr Probl Diagn Radiol 2005, 34: 1–11.
13. Luna A, Ribes R, Caro P, et al. Evaluation of cardiac tumors with magnetic resonance imaging. Eur Radiol 2005, 15: 1446–55.

Chapter 13
Assessment of Cardiac and Thoracic Masses

Patrick M. Colletti, Jabi E. Shriki, and William D. Boswell

13.1 Subject Overview

Excellent spatial and contrast resolution make currently available multislice contrast-enhanced CT an ideal method for the detection and evaluation of cardiac and adjacent masses. CT for cardiac masses is ideally acquired during suspended respiration with cardiac gating. While most cardiac masses are well demonstrated with non-triggered CT, two approaches to cardiac gating may be applied: prospective ECG triggering and retrospective ECG gating [1].

Pre-contrast imaging may help to identify features such as calcium (**Fig. 13.1A**) and hemorrhage. Pre-contrast low attenuation may be helpful for characterizing myxomas (**Fig. 13.1B**). The amount of iodinated contrast agent required for satisfactory CT evaluation of cardiac masses depends on patient mass, with 0.5–1.0 g of iodine per kilogram body mass as the usual dose [2]. Using standard low-osmolality contrast agents with concentrations of 300–400 mg iodine/ml, typically 50–100 ml of contrast agent is administered at 4–5 ml/s via a programmable injector system. This is followed by a bolus flush of 50 ml of normal saline [3].

Timing the CT image acquisition to the contrast agent bolus arrival for left atrial and left ventricular masses is identical to timing used for coronary artery CT examinations [4]. There may be considerable variability in circulation time from patient to patient, particularly in patients with cardiac tumors or thrombi. The time between peripheral contrast injection and appearance of contrast in the aorta can be determined using a small volume test contrast agent bolus of 20 ml and rapid, repeated imaging of a single trans-aortic plane [5]. Alternatively, with bolus tracking, a Hounsfield unit (HU) threshold may be set such that the volume

P.M. Colletti
Professor of Radiology and Medicine, Director Nuclear Medicine Fellowship, USC Keck School of Medicine; Professor of Biokinesiology; Professor of Pharmacology and Pharmaceutical Sciences, Chief of MRI, LAC+USC Imaging Science Center, University of Southern California, CA, USA
e-mail: colletti@usc.edu

M.J. Budoff, J.S. Shinbane (eds.), *Handbook of Cardiovascular CT*,
DOI: 10.1007/978-1-84800-091-9_13, © Springer-Verlag London Limited 2008

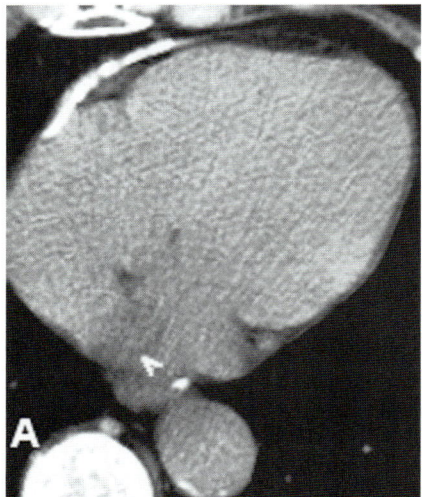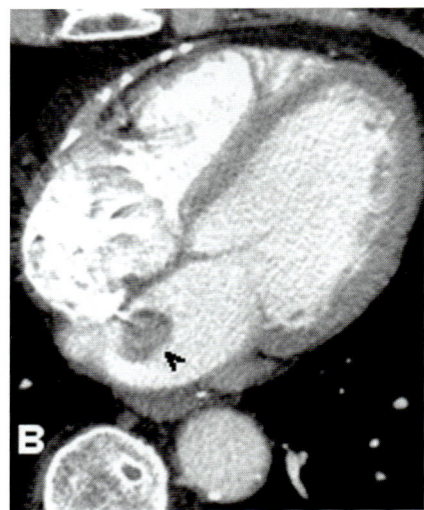

Fig. 13.1 Left atrial myxoma. **A** Pre-contrast CT demonstrates the low-attenuation left atrial mass (*arrowhead*); **B** Post-contrast exam demonstrates the left atrial pedunculated mass (*arrowhead*) attached to the atrial septum. Incidentally noted is anterior pericardial calcification

Table 13.1 Benign cardiac neoplasms

	Location	Features
Myxoma (40% of all benign tumors) (**Figure 13.1**)	LA septum 75%; RA 18%; ventricles 7%; multiple 5%	10% calcified; frequent systemic emboli; may protrude through mitral valve during diastole
Fibroelastoma	Arise from valves; project into aorta or MPA	Derived from endocardium; may be multiple; often an incidental finding at surgery
Lipoma	Varies	Encapsulated adipose tissue (fat attenuation); asymptomatic; negative CT density; 25% are multiple; consider tuberous sclerosis; should not be confused with fat in paracardiac folds
Lipomatous hypertrophy	Atrial septum; protrudes into RA	Fat attenuation
Fibroma	Myocardium	Well delineated, calcified; enhance minimally
Hemangioma	Myocardium	Calcifications; delayed enhancement
Lymphangioma	Myocardium	Diffuse proliferation; minimally enhancing
Paraganglioma, dysembryoma, pheochromocytoma	Paracardiac; AV groove	Sympathetic plexus; hyper-enhancing; correlate with urinary catecholamines; alpha- and beta-blockade for surgery
Teratoma	Pericardial; attach to the aorta or PA roots	Multi-cystic; frequently calcify; moderate enhancement

acquisition is triggered to begin once a certain HU value is detected in the ascending aorta. A uniform programmed injection requires 10–25 s for delivery of intravenous contrast agent and up to 50 additional seconds for the saline flush.

One potential pitfall with automatic bolus detection in cardiac masses is that it is possible to inadvertently locate the bolus detection voxel within a chamber or a vessel with internal thrombus or tumor. Such an error results in failure to detect the bolus as shown in **Fig. 13.1**.

Without appropriate acquisition timing for right heart visualization, there may be insufficient contrast for delineation of right atrial and right ventricular endocardial borders. Optimal timing for right heart examination usually differs from that used for routine coronary CTA. Given the usual relationship of the great vessels and ventricular concordance, right ventricular opacification is optimized by triggering acquisition once the contrast agent reaches the main pulmonary artery. Right ventricular delineation in transposition or other abnormal great vessel–ventricular relationships requires some a priori knowledge of the anatomy and relevant surgical history to select the correct region for timing prescription. As an alternative, prolonged optimal contrast enhancement levels may be achieved with the use of tailored injection protocols with exponentially decelerated profiles [6].

One advantage cardiac magetic resonance imaging (CMR) holdsover cardiac CT for cardiac masses is the ability to obtain excellent contrast for both right ventricle and left ventricle in the same examination due to the ability to image the heart in multiple phases of contrast administration, with no additional radiation dose. This may occasionally occur with CT (usually inadvertently); further investigations are needed to determine how to reliably achieve sufficient contrast in both ventricles.

Clinical [7, 8, 9, 10, 11, 12, 13, 14, 15, 16, 17, 18, 19] and imaging [20, 21, 22, 23, 24, 25, 26, 27, 28] features of cardiac masses are summarized in **Tables 13.1–13.4** and **Figs. 13.1–13.8.**

Table 13.2 Cystic cardiac masses

	Location	Features
Pleuro-pericardial cyst	75% in right paracardiac angle	Asymptomatic (avascular/calcified); unilocular, sharply marginated, 20–40 HU; may communicate with pericardium; change shape with body position
Echinococcal cysts	Myocardial or pericardial	(Avascular/calcific rim); nearly always also in liver, lung, eyes, brain.
Tuberculoma	Myocardial or pericardial	Calcified; constrictive pericarditis
Hematoma	Posterior recesses at the aortic root or left atrium	Acutely hyper-dense; may calcify; traumatic or post-surgical
Thrombosed coronary aneurysm (**Figure 13.2**)	Course of coronary arteries	Calcified rim; thrombus

Table 13.3 Malignant cardiac tumors

	Location	Features
Metastasis (20× as common as primary tumor) (**Figures 13.3, 13.4**)	Pericardial; intravascular; intra-myocardial	Seen in 10% of end-stage cancers; lung (36%), breast (7%), esophagus (6%); lymphoma, melanoma, Kaposi's sarcoma, leukemia (20%); modes of dissemination: direct or lymphatic; hematogenous; direct venous extension (pulmonary veins or inferior vena cava)
Lung, breast, melanoma, sarcoma, leukemia, thyroid, kidney	Pericardial; direct or lymphatic; hematogenous; direct venous extension	Lung cancer may extend to the left atrium along the pulmonary veins
Renal, urothelial, hepatocellular, adrenal, retroperitoneal sarcoma	Extend up the inferior vena cava to the right atrium	Enhancing intravascular mass; primary tumor identified
Lymphoma	Pericardium; myocardium; commonly basal in location	May infiltrate epicardial fat; 50% associated with HIV
Angiosarcoma (**Figure 13.5**)	Pericardium; RV, RA, myocardium	Angiosarcoma of the pericardium or right ventricle is most common; poor prognosis; distribution is similar to lymphoma
Osteosarcoma	RA, RV	Ossification
Rhabdomyosarcoma, fibrosarcoma	Myocardium	Most common primary cardiac malignancy in infants and children. Always involves the myocardium; pericardial involvement is typically in the form of nodular masses rather than sheet-like spread.
Mesothelioma	Pericardium	Intra-pericardial mass; effusions; constrictive physiology

13.2 Interpreting Cardiac Masses

Key descriptors for cardiac masses include the following:

- Location
- Single versus multiple lesions
- Size
- Border description
- Presence of fluid, blood, calcium, or fat
- Contrast enhancement pattern
- Relation to function
- Non-cardiac-related findings

Table 13.4 Other cardiac masses

	Location	Features
Endo-myocardial fibrosis	Pericardium; myocardium	Thickened pericardium; thickened myocardium with patchy enhancement restrictive and constrictive physiology
Erdheim-Chester disease (non-langherans fibrosis)	Pericardium; myocardium	Thickened pericardium; thickened myocardium with patchy enhancement restrictive and constrictive physiology
RA Thrombus (**Figure 13.6**)	Right atrium	Associated with indwelling catheters and devices
RV Thrombus	Right ventricle	Associated with severe coagulopathy; dilated cardiomyopathy
LA Thrombus (**Figure 13.7**)	Left atrium	Seen in atrial fibrillation and mitral stenosis; attached to posterior or superior atrial wall; may be calcified
LV Thrombus (**Figure 13.8**)	Left ventricle	Common complication of myocardial infarction (20–40% of anterior MIs); contiguous to akinetic myocardium; most common at the apex
Vegetations	Valves; catheters	EKG-triggered cine views of valves helpful

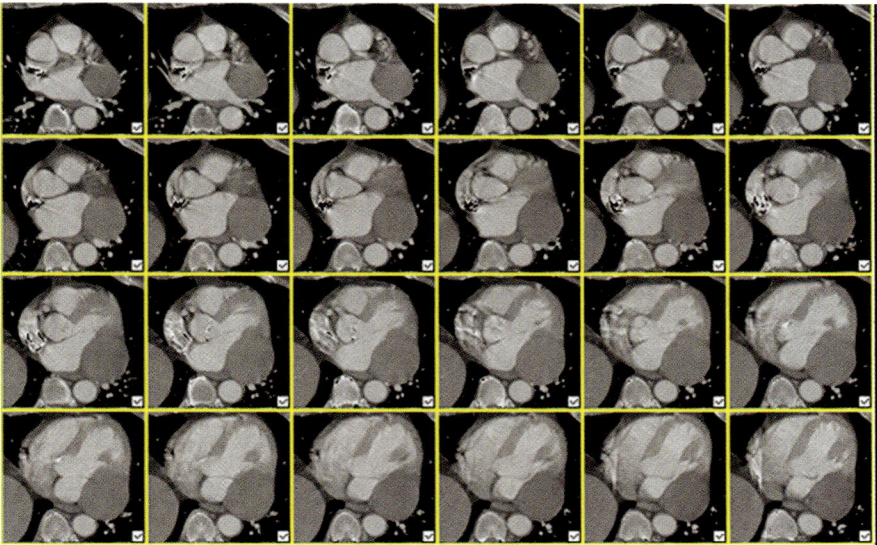

Fig. 13.2 4 × 4 × 8 cm "mass" in the left AV groove. Surgical exploration documented circumflex aneurysm with thrombosis

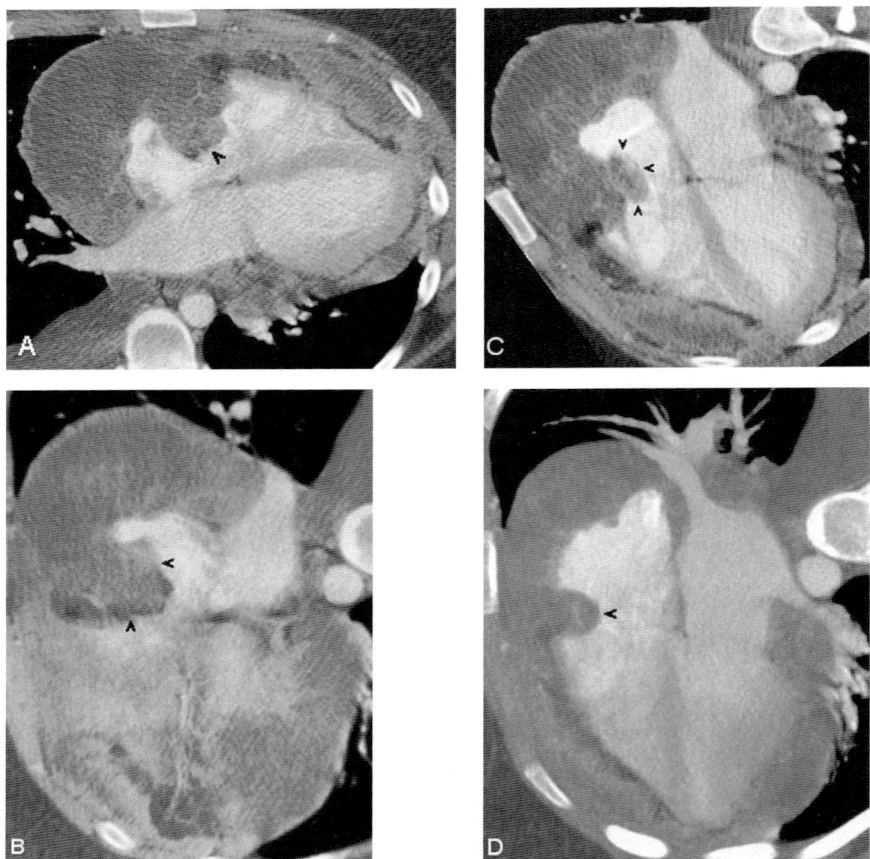

Fig. 13.3A–D This is a 24-year-old woman with increasing dyspnea on exertion. Multiple oblique reformatted enhanced CT views demonstrate a large pericardial mass surrounding her heart. Notice the mass extending into the right atrium (*arrowheads*) Primitive neuro-ectodermal tumor

13.3 Clinical Pearls

- CT is useful to detect and characterize cardiac and paracardiac masses. Key features are location, configuration, attenuation, enhancement, and regional function.
- Location:
  - Paracardiac and Pericardium
    - Direct invasion from lung or esophageal cancer, lymphoma
  - Vena cava
    - SVC: catheter-related thrombus or vegetation
    - IVC: renal, adrenal, hepatic cancer

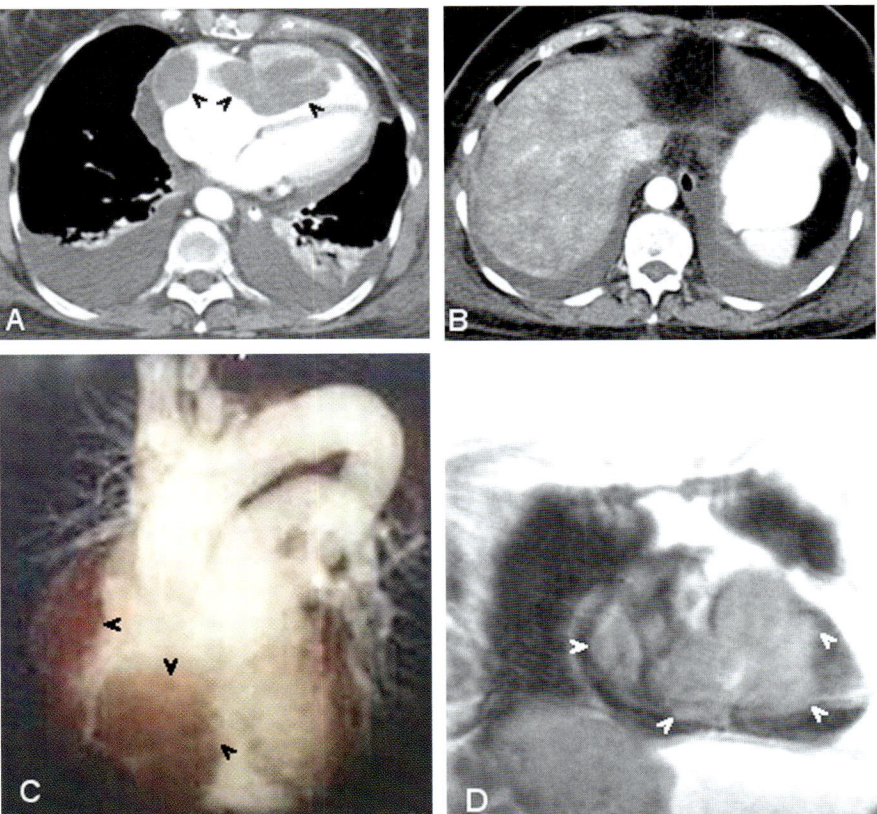

Fig. 13.4 Colon cancer metastasis. **A** Axial contrast-enhanced CT demonstrates a large tumor in the right atrium and the right ventricle (*arrowheads*). A small pericardial effusion is noted; **B** CT in the upper abdomen demonstrates heterogeneity typical for "nutmeg" liver associated with passive venous congestion; **C** A 3-D oblique projection image demonstrates tumor in the right atrium and the right ventricle (*arrowheads*); **D** Coronal MRI confirms the tumor in the right atrium and the right ventricle (*arrowheads*). The small pericardial effusion is again noted

- Right atrium
    - Intraluminal from SVC: catheter-related thrombus or vegetation
    - Intraluminal from IVC: renal, adrenal, hepatic cancer
    - Right atrial myxoma
- Right ventricle
    - Intraluminal: thrombus
    - Mural: angiosarcoma
- Left atrium
    - Left atrial appendage, posterior and superior wall: thrombus
    - Atrial septum: myxoma

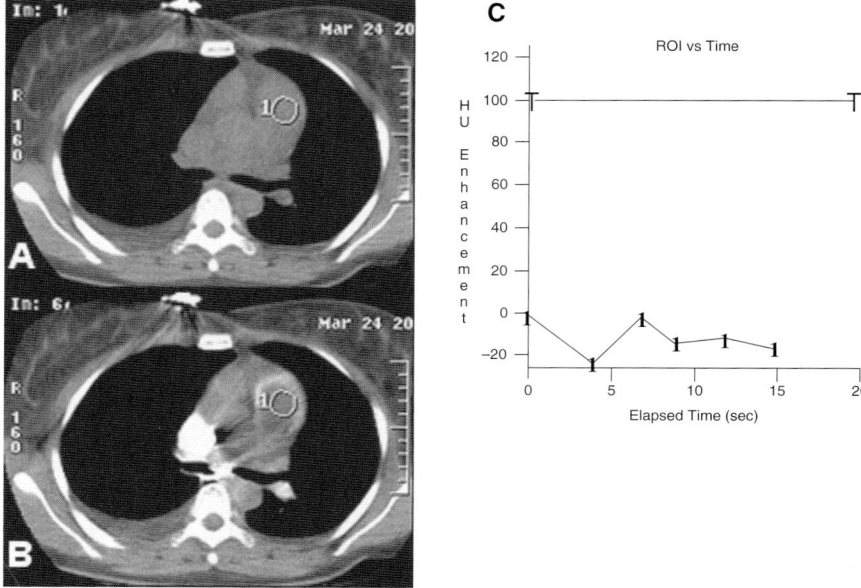

Fig. 13.5A–C Automatic bolus detection fails due to tumor replacing the blood pool in the selected region-of-interest in the main pulmonary artery

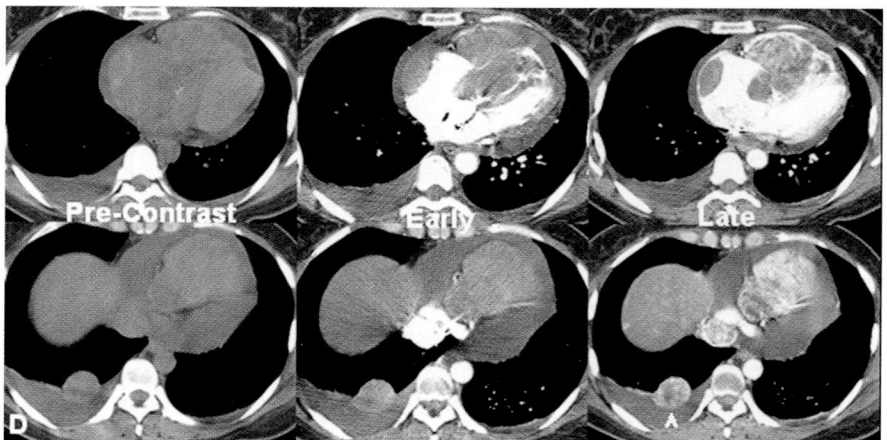

Fig. 13.5D Sequential pre-contrast, early, and late contrasted images demonstrate vascular enhancement within the angiosarcoma. Note the enhancing right lower lobe pulmonary nodule (*arrowhead*)

- Left ventricle

  – Luminal: thrombus (adjacent to aneurysm)
  – Mural: hypertrophic cardiomyopathy

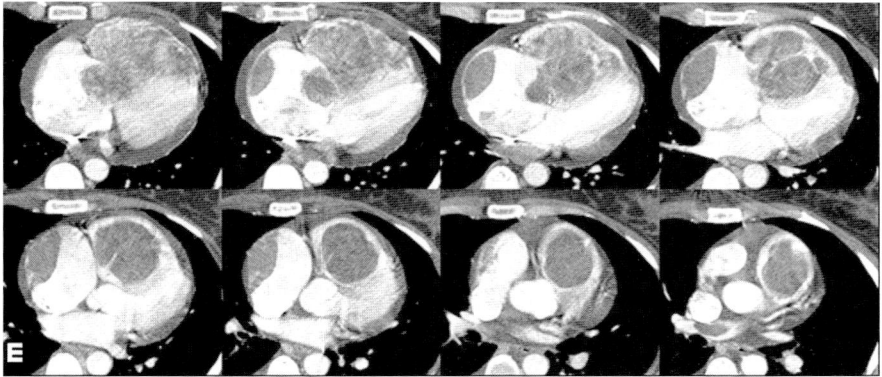

Fig. 13.5E Right atrial and right ventricular angiosarcoma extending into the main pulmonary artery

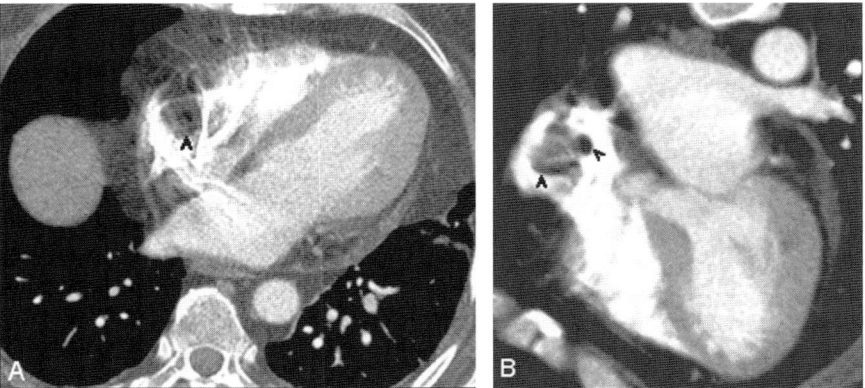

Fig. 13.6 Right atrial thrombus (*arrowheads*) is noted on axial (**A**) and four-chamber (**B**) views

- Configuration
    - Broad based: more suggestive of an aggressive neoplastic process such as a sarcoma or metastasis
    - Pedunculated/narrowly attached: More suggestive of thrombus or a benign mass such as a myxoma
- Attenuation (pre-enhanced)
    - Low attenuation
        - Fat (<−10 HU)
        - Fluid (0–20 HU)
    - Intermediate attenuation: blood (40–70 HU)
    - High attenuation: calcium (>130 HU)

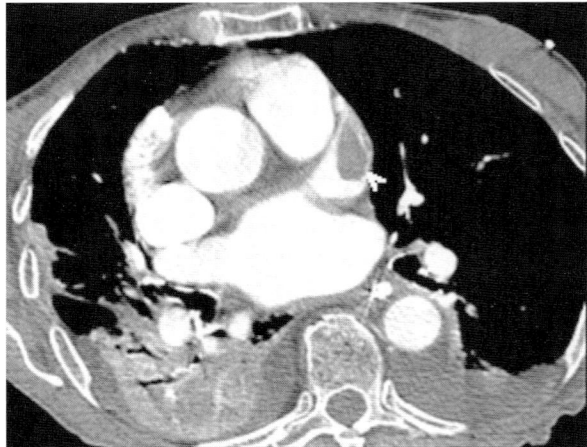

Fig. 13.7 Left atrial appendage thrombus (*arrowheads*)

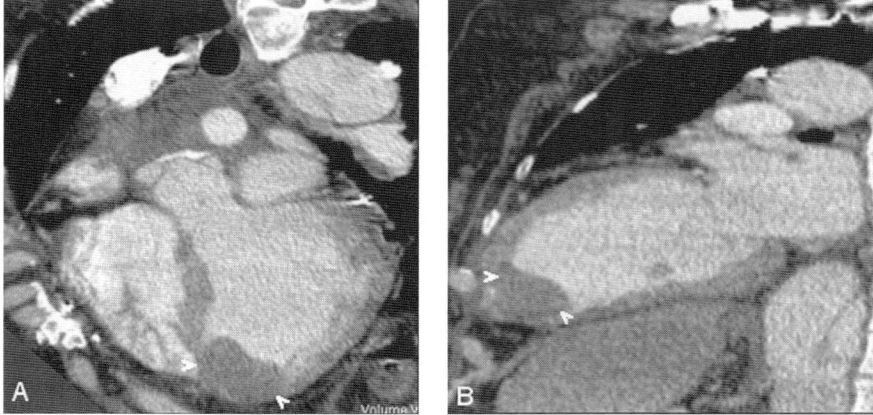

Fig. 13.8 This is a 45-year-old woman with recent surgery for a type-A dissection. She has had a prior apical infarction. Left ventricular apical aneurysm with thrombus (*arrowheads*) is noted on the five-chamber (**A**) and the vertical long-axis (**B**) views

- Enhancement
  - Thrombi generally do not enhance
  - Neoplasms demonstrate variable degrees of enhancement
  - Myxomas enhance mildly
  - Enhancement of metastasis varies with grade and cell type
  - Angiosarcoma enhances strongly, with a prominent vascular prominence
  - Some tumors enhance early; that is, sarcoma, some metastasis
  - Late enhancement is noted with dilated veins, aneurysms, and hemangiomas

- Function

  - Evaluated with cardiac-gated multiphase cardiac CT
  - Usually preserved with small neoplasms
  - Thrombi occur at sites of akinesis and stasis
  - Embolization (30–45% of left atrial myxomas; 50% of left ventricular myxomas)
  - Conduction defects with arrhythmia
  - Diastolic dysfunction

    - Predominates with extensive myocardial or pericardial tumor
    - Ventricular size is often reduced by tumors
    - Dilated atria, vena cava
    - Prominent septal "bounce"

  - Systolic dysfunction

    - Luminal incursion with volume reduction
    - Outlet obstruction
    - Valvular dysfunction
    - Reduced ejection fraction "compressive" heart failure

References

1. Desjardins B, Kazerooni. EA ECG-Gated Cardiac CT. Am. J. Roentgenol. April 2004, 182: 993–1010.
2. Newhouse JH, Murphy RX. Tissue distribution of soluble contrast: effect of dose variation and changes with time. Am J Roentgenol 1981, 136: 463–467[Medline].
3. Cademartiri F, Mollet N, van der Lugt A, et al. Non-invasive 16-row multislice CT coronary angiography: usefulness of saline chaser. Eur Radiol 2004, 14: 178–183
4. Awai K, Hiraishi K, Hori S. Effect of Contrast Material Injection Duration and Rate on Aortic Peak Time and Peak Enhancement at Dynamic CT Involving Injection Protocol with Dose Tailored to Patient Weight. Radiology, January 1, 2004, 230(1): 142–150.
5. Cademartiri F, Nieman K, van der Lugt A, et al. Intravenous contrast material administration at 16-detector row helical CT coronary angiography: test bolus versus bolus-tracking technique. Radiology 2004, 233: 817–823
6. Bae KT, Tran HQ, Heiken JP. Uniform Vascular Contrast Enhancement and Reduced Contrast Medium Volume Achieved by Using Exponentially Decelerated Contrast Material Injection Method. Radiology 2004, 231: 732–736.
7. Boyd DB. Computerized transmission tomography of the heart using scanning electron beams. In: Higgins CH, ed. Computed tomography of the heart and great vessels. Mount Kisco, New York: Futura Publishing Company, 1983, 45–55.
8. Newhouse JH. Fluid compartment distribution of intravenous iothalamate in the dog. Invest Radiol 1977, 12: 364–367[Medline].
9. Prichard RW. Tumors of the heart. Arch Pathol 1951, 51: 98–128
10. Glancy DL, Morales JB, Roberts WC. Angiosarcoma of the heart. Am J Cardiol 1968, 21: 413–419
11. McAllister HA, Fenoglio JJ Jr. Tumors of the cardiovascular system: atlas of tumor pathology, second series. In: Washington, DC: Armed Forces Institute of Pathology. 1978

12. Lund JT, Ehman RL, Julsrud PR, et al. Cardiac masses: assessment by MR imaging. AJR Am J Roentgenol 1989 Mar, 152(3): 469–73

13. Burke AP, Cowan D, Virmani R. Primary sarcomas of the heart. Cancer 1992, 69:387–395

14. Tazelaar HD, Locke TJ, McGregor CG. Pathology of surgically excised primary cardiac tumors. Mayo Clin Proc 1992 Oct, 67(10): 957–65

15. Lam KY, Dickens P, Chan AC. Tumors of the heart. A 20-year experience with a review of 12,485 consecutive autopsies. Arch Pathol Lab Med 1993 Oct, 117(10): 1027–31.

16. Marx GR: Cardiac Tumors. In: Emmanouilides GC, Gutgesell HP, Riemenschneider TA, Allen HD, eds. Moss and Adams Heart Disease in Infants, Children, and Adolescents: Including the Fetus and Young Adult. Vol. 2. 5th ed. Baltimore: Williams & Wilkins, 1995: 1773–1786.

17. Burke A, Virmani R. Tumors of the heart and great vessels: Atlas of tumor pathology. Fasc 16, ser 3. Washington, D.C.: Armed Forces Institute of Pathology, 1996

18. Takach TJ, Reul GJ, Ott DA, Cooley DA. Primary cardiac tumors in infants and children: immediate and long-term operative results. Ann Thorac Surg 1996 Aug, 62(2): 559–64.

19. Ludomirsky A. Cardiac tumors. In: Bricker JT, Fisher DJ, eds. The Science and Practice of Pediatric Cardiology. Vol 2. 9th ed. Williams & Wilkins; 1998: 1885–1893.

20. Araoz PA, Eklund HE, Welch TJ, Breen JF. CT and MR imaging of primary cardiac malignancies. Radiographics 1999 Nov–Dec, 19(6): 1421–34

21. Chiles C, Woodard PK, Gutierrez FR, Link KM. Metastatic involvement of the heart and pericardium: CT and MR imaging. RadioGraphics 2000, 20: 1073–1103

22. Grebenc ML, Rosado de Christenson ML, Burke AP, Green CE, Galvin JR. Primary cardiac and pericardial neoplasms: radiologic–pathologic correlation. RadioGraphics 2000, 20: 1073–1103; quiz 1110–1071, 1112

23. Grebenc ML, Rosado-de-Christenson ML, Green CE, Burke AP, Galvin JR. Cardiac myxoma: imaging features in 83 patients. RadioGraphics. 2002, 2(3): 673–89.

24. Piazza N, Chughtai T, Toledano K, et al. Primary cardiac tumours: eighteen years of surgical experience on 21 patients. Can J Cardiol 2004 Dec, 20(14): 1443–8.

25. Tatli S, Lipton MJ. CT for intracardiac thrombi and tumors. Int J Cardiovasc Imaging 2005 Feb, 21(1): 115–31.

26. Butany J, Nair V, Naseemuddin A, et al. Cardiac tumours: diagnosis and management. Lancet Oncol 2005 Apr, 6(4): 219–28.

27. Leipsic JA, Heyneman LE, Kim RJ. Cardiac masses and myocardial diseases. In: McAdams HP, Reddy GP, eds. Cardiopulmonary imaging syllabus—2005. Leesburg, VA: American Roentgen Ray Society, 2005: 1–13

28. Sparrow PJ, Kurian JB, Jones TR, Sivananthan MU. MR imaging of cardiac tumors. RadioGraphics 2005, 25: 1255–1276

Chapter 14
Computed Tomography Evaluation in Valvular Heart Disease

Javier Sanz, Susanna Prat-González, and Mario J. García

14.1 Introduction

Valvular heart disease (VHD) affects 2.5% of US adults and predominantly involves the left cardiac valves. Regurgitant lesions are more common than stenoses, and mitral regurgitation (MR) is the most prevalent abnormality [1]. Doppler echocardiography is the initial imaging modality of choice, allowing for a complete diagnosis in the majority of patients [2]. In cases of poor acoustic window and/or disparate results regarding disease severity, additional tests may be required. Cardiac catheterization is a time-honored modality, but limited by its invasive nature. Magnetic resonance imaging (MRI) has become an excellent noninvasive alternative for both valvular insufficiency and stenosis. Due to the need for radiation and contrast, computed tomography (CT) has a limited role for the evaluation of VHD as the primary indication. It may occasionally be employed as such when echocardiographic results are incomplete and the patient is not a good candidate for MRI. However, CT is increasingly used for noninvasive coronary angiography, and useful information on valve anatomy and function can simultaneously be obtained from a coronary examination.

14.2 General Considerations

A diagram summarizing the potential applications of CT for the evaluation of patients with VHD is shown in **Fig. 14.1**. Valvular assessment includes the detection of calcification in non-contrast scans and of other aspects of valvular anatomy and cardiac function using contrast enhancement. Quantification of valve calcification follows the same principles as coronary calcium scoring, and the "Agatston" volumetric and mass scores have been proposed. Electron-beam CT (EBCT) has been

M.J. García
The Zena and Michael A. Wiener Cardiovascular Institute and Marie-Josee and Henry R. Kravis Center for Cardiovascular Health, Mount Sinai Hospital, One Gustave Levy Place, Box 1030, New York, NY 10029, USA
e-mail: mario.garcia@mountsinai.org

M.J. Budoff, J.S. Shinbane (eds.), *Handbook of Cardiovascular CT*,
DOI: 10.1007/978-1-84800-091-9_14, © Springer-Verlag London Limited 2008

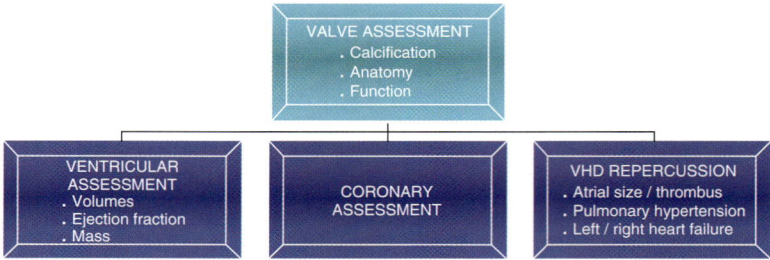

Fig. 14.1 Comprehensive evaluation of valvular heart disease (VHD) with CT

traditionally the reference standard for coronary calcium quantification, although multi-detector CT (MDCT), particularly using scanners with more than 16 slices, has proven comparable in terms of accuracy and reproducibility. Regarding contrast-enhanced CT, detailed evaluation of valvular function and anatomy is possible for both regurgitant and, particularly, stenotic lesions (planimetry of the valve area). Visualization is usually better with MDCT due to its superior spatial resolution and the ability to image all phases of the cardiac cycle with the use of retrospective gating.

CT allows for accurate quantification of ventricular volumes, ejection fraction, and mass [3], all of which carry important prognostic and therapeutic implications in patients with VHD [2]. In isolated regurgitant lesions, the regurgitant volume (and fraction) can be derived from the difference between the left and right stroke volumes [4]. Stenosis or regurgitation of the atrioventricular valves usually results in atrial enlargement. Significant regurgitation of any valve eventually causes ipsilateral ventricular dilatation, often accompanied by eccentric hypertrophy. Stenotic lesions of the semilunar (aortic and pulmonary) valves lead to concentric hypertrophy and, in rare instances, may also lead to ventricular dilatation. Post-stenotic dilatation of the pulmonary trunk or the ascending aorta may be present as well.

CT can provide important information regarding hemodynamic repercussions of valvular lesions. Enlargement of the right-heart chambers can be caused by tricuspid/pulmonary abnormalities or secondary pulmonary hypertension, and it typically leads to posterior rotation of the cardiac axis. Pulmonary vein dilatation and interstitial and alveolar lung edema are all signs of increased left atrial pressures and left-sided heart failure. Similarly, dilatation of the pulmonary arteries, right-heart chambers, superior and inferior vena cava, and pleuro-pericardial effusions and ascitis are suggestive of pulmonary hypertension and/or right ventricular heart failure [5].

As mentioned before, the most common primary indication for CT is the assessment of the coronary tree. The accuracy of CT coronary angiography has been reported in recent studies, with slightly lower diagnostic yield in cases of aortic stenosis (AS) due to the frequent co-existence of both aortic and coronary calcification [6, 7]. These studies have demonstrated high negative predictive value, although lower positive predictive value for the detection of significant coronary stenosis. Thus, patients who are referred for surgical repair of valvular lesions and demonstrate absence of significant coronary stenosis by CT may safely avoid the need for invasive coronary angiography. On the other hand, patients who appear to have greater than mild degree of luminal stenosis or extensive calcifications need to have a confirmatory catheterization. For this reason, it is prudent to consider CT for this application only in selected patients with low or intermediate pre-test probability.

A typical imaging protocol is summarized in **Table 14.1**. Contrast infusion is routinely followed by saline, resulting in a more compact bolus and easier evaluation of the right coronary artery; however, it may also impair the visualization of right chambers and valves. This can be overcome by employing a dual-phase contrast infusion protocol. In addition, tube current modulation with maximal output in diastole may lead to suboptimal image quality during systole. This could limit the assessment of both ventricles and valves, particularly in obese patients. If such evaluation is intended, it may be necessary to avoid the use of tube current modulation.

Table 14.1 Imaging protocol

Scanning protocol (for a 32-detector scanner)	
Tube voltage (kV)	120
Tube output (eff mAs)	700–800
Detector number	32
Detector collimation (mm)	0.6
Helical pitch	0.2
Rotation time (ms)	330
Tube current modulation	
(HR $\leq$ 65)	On
(HR > 65	Off
Contrast protocol (370 mmgI/cc)	
Contrast amount (cc)	80–100
Contrast infusion rate (cc/s)	4–5
Saline amount (cc)	50
Saline infusion rate (cc/s)	4–5
Image reconstruction	
Kernel	Intermediate (B35f)
Reconstruction algorithm (HR $\leq$ 65)	Single-segment
Reconstruction algorithm (HR > 65)	Dual-segment
Slice width (mm)	0.75
Increment (mm)	0.4 mm
Matrix	512 × 512
Reconstruction interval	Every 10%
Image analysis: Axial images, MPR, MIP (cine loops and still frames)	

Typical scanning protocol for MDCT coronary angiography employed in our institution (*Sensation 64*®, Siemens). HR: heart rate; MPR: multiplanar reformation; MIP: maximum intensity projection.

14.3 Specific Valvular Abnormalities

14.3.1 Aortic Stenosis

AS is often accompanied by cusp calcification and tends to occur in patients above 65 years with tri-leaflet valves or in younger patients with congenital leaflet abnormalities. Severe calcification is associated with faster rates of stenosis progression and increased cardiac event rates. Aortic valve calcification can be accurately quantified using CT (**Fig. 14.2**), and interscan reproducibility is >90% [8, 9, 10]. The amount of calcification is directly correlated with the severity of AS [11], although the relationship is curvilinear (the increment in stenosis degree with increasing scores is more rapid at lower calcium loads than at higher ones). The incremental value of the information derived from the aortic valve calcium score may be particularly useful to evaluate stenosis severity in patients with low cardiac output and reduced transvalvular gradients.

Contrast-enhanced CT can precisely evaluate valve morphology, accurately differentiating tri-leaflet from bicuspid valves (**Fig. 14.3A,B**). Planimetric determinations of the aortic valve area (**Fig. 14.3C**) have shown excellent correlation with echocardiographic measurements [12, 13].

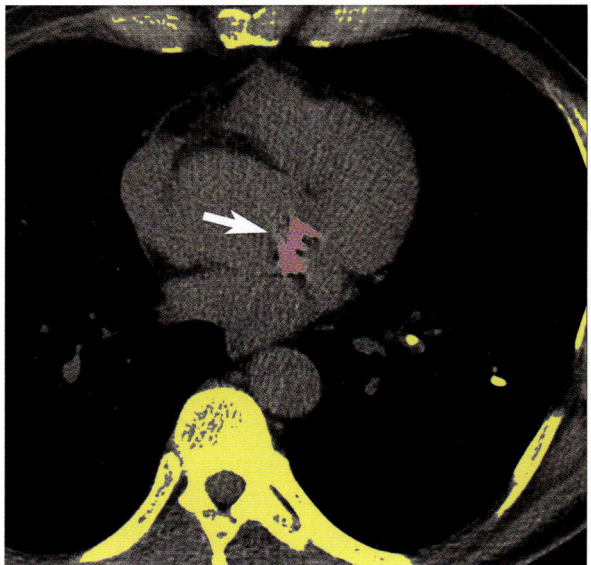

Fig. 14.2 Axial, non-contrast CT image in a patient with moderate aortic stenosis, demonstrating the quantification of aortic valve calcium (*arrow*) using the same approach as for coronary calcium scoring. The valvular calcium score ("Agatston") was 2227

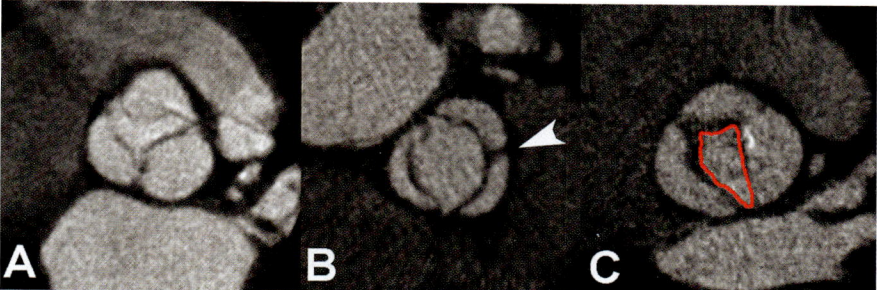

Fig. 14.3 Double oblique systolic reconstructions of contrast-enhanced CT scans showing a tri-leaflet (*Panel A*) and a bicuspid aortic valve (the *arrowhead* indicates the fusion of the right and left coronary sinuses; *Panel B*). Planimetry of the valve can be performed subsequently (*red contour*, *Panel C*): the figure shows a bicuspid aortic valve with moderate stenosis (valve area = 1.2 cm^2)

14.3.2 Aortic Regurgitation

CT may be useful in evaluating the mechanism leading to aortic regurgitation (AR). Aortic regurgitation caused by degenerative valve disease is characterized by increased leaflet thickness and calcification, and the area of lack of coaptation may be visualized in diastolic-phase reconstructions centrally or at the commissures. In cases of AR secondary to enlargement of the aortic root, the regurgitant orifice is typically located centrally (**Fig. 14.4**). Other etiologies that can be depicted include interposition of an intimal flap in cases of dissection, valve distortion or perforation in cases of endocarditis, or leaflet prolapse (observed in dissection and in Marfan syndrome). The severity of AR cannot be accurately established by CT, since this modality cannot visualize flow. However, in cases of severe regurgitation, CT may demonstrate left ventricular dilatation and/or a significant difference between the left and right ventricular stroke volumes.

14.3.3 Mitral Stenosis

As in the case of aortic valve calcification, the presence of calcium in the mitral annulus is associated with systemic atherosclerosis and carries negative prognostic implications. The amount of mitral annular calcium can also be quantified with CT, although reproducibility appears to be somewhat lower [10]. In rheumatic mitral stenosis (MS), calcification can extend to the leaflets, commissures, subvalvular apparatus, or even the left atrial wall. MS is often accompanied by marked atrial enlargement involving the appendage. The presence or absence of thrombus can be determined after contrast administration with very high sensitivity although lower specificity, since slow flow may often impair contrast opacification in the left atrial appendage. Planimetry of mitral opening by CT provides accurate assessment of MS severity [14].

Fig. 14.4 Contrast-enhanced
MDCT in a patient with an
aneurysmal aorta and aortic
insufficiency. The valvular
plane (*yellow line*; *left lower
panel*) is oriented
perpendicular to two
orthogonal planes aligned
with the ascending aorta (*red
and green lines*). A large,
central area of insufficient
leaflet coaptation during
diastole (*right lower panel*;
arrowhead) can be visualized

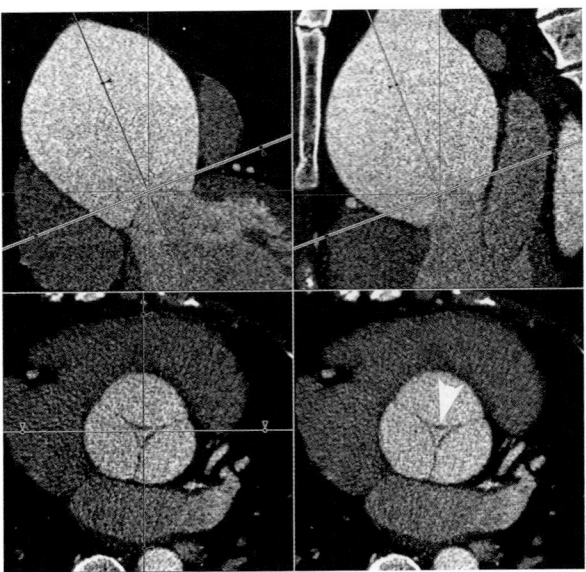

14.3.4 Mitral Regurgitation

In patients with mitral valve prolapse, CT can demonstrate the presence of leaflet thickening or the degree and location of prolapse. In cases of MR secondary to annular enlargement (often accompanying dilated cardiomyopathy), dimensions of the annulus can be accurately quantified, and a central area of insufficient leaflet coaptation may be observed. Although quantifying MR severity may be difficult, a recent study suggested that planimetry of the regurgitant orifice by CT correlates well with echocardiographic grading of MR severity [15]. An alternative approach validated for EBCT includes quantification of cardiac output with the flow mode by the indicator dilution method, and volumetric left ventricular calculations in the cine mode. The regurgitant fraction is obtained from the difference between these two measurements [16].

14.3.5 Infective Endocarditis

The diagnosis of infective endocarditis usually relies on the visualization of vegetations, and transthoracic and transesophageal echocardiography are usually superior to CT due to higher temporal resolution. Vegetations are often mobile and tend to be on the atrial aspect of the atrioventricular valves, and the ventricular aspect in semilunar valves (**Fig. 14.5**). However, CT can be particularly useful in the demonstration of perivalvular abscesses as fluid-filled collections (**Fig. 14.5**) [17].

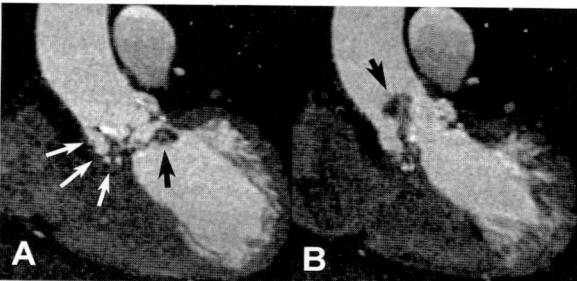

Fig. 14.5 Diastolic (*Panel A*) and systolic (*Panel B*) reconstructions of a contrast-enhanced MDCT study in a patient with a bioprosthesis in the aortic position. A large, mobile vegetation that prolapses into the ascending aorta in systole can be noted (*black arrows*). In addition, perivalvular thickening and fluid-filled collections can be noted (*white arrows*), indicating the presence of a perivalvular abscess

In patients with aortic valve endocarditis with highly mobile vegetations, CT offers an alternative to invasive coronary angiography for evaluation of the coronary arteries.

14.3.6 Prosthetic Valves

Many of the aforementioned features of native VHD apply also to the evaluation of cardiac bioprostheses. CT is particularly useful for the evaluation of some types of mechanical valves. In prosthesis with two discs, these should open symmetrically (**Fig. 14.6**). In those with a single disc, the angle of opening can also be measured. Finally, heterografts and homografts can be evaluated completely, including the distal anastomosis and the patency of the coronary arteries if these were reimplanted.

14.3.7 Imaging Pearls

Plan ahead; this will allow for imaging protocol optimization if valvular evaluation will be attempted.

- If assessment of the right-heart structures is intended, an initial contrast bolus of 80–100 cc followed by a mixture of contrast and saline (1:1) at 4–5 cc/s will result in adequate coronary evaluation and sufficient right-heart opacification without excessive enhancement. Alternatively, a biphasic infusion may be used with the second infusion of contrast administered at a slower rate (2–3 cc/s).
- Quantification of ventricular end-systolic volumes and the degree of MR and AS requires adequate image quality during systole. It may be necessary to avoid tube current modulation in these cases. Alternatively, the maximal tube output can be timed to end-systole, which will provide adequate depiction of mitral closure and

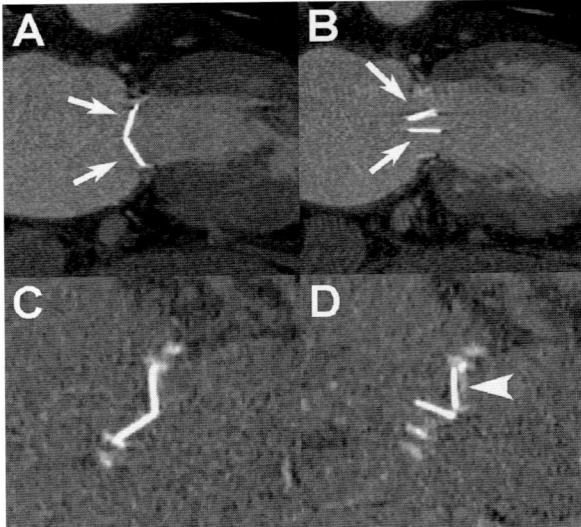

Fig. 14.6 Evaluation of mechanical prostheses by CT. The top row shows contrast-enhanced images (systole, *Panel A*; diastole, *Panel B*) of a normal-functioning mechanical prosthesis in the mitral position. The two discs close and open completely and symmetrically (*white arrows*) during the cardiac cycle. Comparable systolic (*Panel C*) and diastolic (*Panel D*) reconstructions of a non-contrast CT evaluation of a dysfunctional mitral prosthesis. One of the discs does not open in diastole (*white arrowhead*). Subsequent surgical intervention demonstrated prosthetic thrombosis

aortic opening, as well as potentially motionless coronary images (particularly at higher heart rates).

- If the whole thoracic aorta needs to be imaged (i.e., in cases of aneurysm with associated AR) and the coronary evaluation is not required, using thicker detector collimation will enable reductions in radiation dose and breath-hold duration.
- Most patients with VHD can tolerate beta blockers for optimal coronary evaluation. However, caution and smaller doses are recommended in cases with severe degrees of left ventricular dysfunction/dilatation, AS, AR, or pulmonary hypertension.
- Atrial fibrillation is common in patients with VHD. It may lead to decrease in image quality and accuracy of valvular and ventricular assessment, although this is typically more significant for evaluation of the coronary arteries.
- For the evaluation of ventricular or valvular function with MDCT, reconstructions at every 10% of the RR interval are usually sufficient. In specific cases, a more detailed evaluation of the valve can be obtained by reconstructing images at smaller intervals (i.e., every 5%) in the cardiac phase of interest (e.g., during systole for AS).
- The combination of cine loops and still frames facilitates the detection of valvular abnormalities.
- Variability of the quantification of aortic valve calcium is lowest in mid-diastole.

- A valvular "Agatston" score ≥ 1100 results in respective sensitivity and specificity of 93% and 82% for the diagnosis of severe AS [9]. A score >3700 has a positive predictive value of near 100% [18].
- The optimal plane to perform planimetry of the valvular area is parallel to the annulus as determined from two orthogonal double-oblique views perpendicular to the valve plane. The optimal level of that plane is the one showing the smallest area during the phase of maximum valve opening (**Fig. 14.4**).
- Quantification of the regurgitant volume/fraction from the difference in right and left stroke volumes is only accurate for isolated regurgitant lesions.
- A score evaluating leaflet mobility and thickening, subvalvular thickening and calcification, as well as the presence of left atrial thrombus may determine whether MS can be treated percutaneously or surgically. CT can provide useful information of all of these features.
- The mitral valve is divided into the anterolateral commissure, posteromedial commissure, anterior leaflet, and posterior leaflet. The leaflets are subdivided into three segments each (A1, A2, and A3; and P1, P2, and P3; from lateral to medial). Determination of which segments are affected and to what degree determines the likelihood of successful surgical repair in mitral valve prolapse.
- Sharper reconstruction filters and increasing window level of the image display facilitate evaluation of mechanical prosthetic valves (**Fig. 14.6**).

References

1. Nkomo VT, Gardin JM, Skelton TN, Gottdiener JS, Scott CG, Enriquez-Sarano M. Burden of valvular heart diseases: a population-based study. The Lancet 2006, 368: 1005–1011.
2. Bonow RO, Carabello BA, Kanu C, et al. ACC/AHA 2006 guidelines for the management of patients with valvular heart disease: a report of the American College of Cardiology/American Heart Association Task Force on Practice Guidelines (writing committee to revise the 1998 Guidelines for the Management of Patients With Valvular Heart Disease): developed in collaboration with the Society of Cardiovascular Anesthesiologists: endorsed by the Society for Cardiovascular Angiography and Interventions and the Society of Thoracic Surgeons. Circulation 2006, 114: e84–231.
3. Orakzai SH, Orakzai RH, Nasir K, Budoff MJ. Assessment of cardiac function using multidetector row computed tomography. J Comput Assist Tomogr 2006, 30: 555–63.
4. Reiter SJ, Rumberger JA, Stanford W, Marcus ML. Quantitative determination of aortic regurgitant volumes in dogs by ultrafast computed tomography. Circulation 1987, 76: 728–35.
5. Boxt LM. CT of valvular heart disease. The International Journal of Cardiovascular Imaging (formerly Cardiac Imaging) 2005, 21: 105–113.
6. Meijboom WB, Mollet NR, Van Mieghem CA, et al. Pre-operative computed tomography coronary angiography to detect significant coronary artery disease in patients referred for cardiac valve surgery. J Am Coll Cardiol 2006, 48: 1658–65.
7. Gilard M, Cornily J-C, Pennec P-Y, et al. Accuracy of Multislice Computed Tomography in the Preoperative Assessment of Coronary Disease in Patients With Aortic Valve Stenosis. J Am Coll Cardiol 2006, 47: 2020–2024.
8. Koos R, Mahnken AH, Kuhl HP, et al. Quantification of aortic valve calcification using multislice spiral computed tomography: comparison with atomic absorption spectroscopy. Invest Radiol 2006, 41: 485–9.

9. Messika-Zeitoun D, Aubry M-C, Detaint D, et al. Evaluation and Clinical Implications of Aortic Valve Calcification Measured by Electron-Beam Computed Tomography. Circulation 2004, 110: 356–362.
10. Budoff MJ, Takasu J, Katz R, et al. Reproducibility of CT measurements of aortic valve calcification, mitral annulus calcification, and aortic wall calcification in the multi-ethnic study of atherosclerosis. Acad Radiol 2006, 13: 166–72.
11. Koos R, Kuhl HP, Muhlenbruch G, Wildberger JE, Gunther RW, Mahnken AH. Prevalence and Clinical Importance of Aortic Valve Calcification Detected Incidentally on CT Scans: Comparison with Echocardiography. Radiology 2006, 241: 76–82.
12. Alkadhi H, Wildermuth S, Plass A, et al. Aortic Stenosis: Comparative Evaluation of 16-Detector Row CT and Echocardiography. Radiology 2006, 240: 47–55.
13. Feuchtner GM, Dichtl W, Friedrich GJ, et al. Multislice computed tomography for detection of patients with aortic valve stenosis and quantification of severity. J Am Coll Cardiol 2006, 47: 1410–7.
14. Messika-Zeitoun D, Serfaty JM, Laissy JP, et al. Assessment of the mitral valve area in patients with mitral stenosis by multislice computed tomography. J Am Coll Cardiol 2006, 48: 411–3.
15. Alkadhi H, Wildermuth S, Bettex DA, et al. Mitral Regurgitation: Quantification with 16-Detector Row CT–Initial Experience. Radiology 2005, 238: 454–463.
16. Lembcke A, Borges AC, Dushe S, et al. Assessment of Mitral Valve Regurgitation at Electron-Beam CT: Comparison with Doppler Echocardiography. Radiology 2005, 236: 47–55.
17. Gilkeson RC, Markowitz AH, Balgude A, Sachs PB. MDCT evaluation of aortic valvular disease. AJR Am J Roentgenol 2006, 186: 350–60.
18. Cowell SJ, Newby DE, Burton J, et al. Aortic Valve Calcification on Computed Tomography Predicts the Severity of Aortic Stenosis. Clin Radiol 2003, 58: 712–716.

Chapter 15
The Aorta and Great Vessels

David M. Shavelle

15.1 Introduction

Technological improvements with 64-multislice CT have greatly advanced its role for diagnostic imaging in patients with vascular disease. CT angiography has thus become a useful tool in evaluating patients with various diseases of the aorta and the great vessels, such as aortic dissection, aortic aneurysm, and carotid artery disease.

15.2 Normal Anatomy

The thoracic aortic is commonly divided into three anatomic segments: (1) the ascending aorta, (2) the aortic arch, and (3) the descending aorta. The aortic arch gives rise to three branches: (1) the brachiocephalic, (2) the left common carotid, and (3) the left subclavian artery. Approximately 35% of patients will have a variation in this normal branching pattern, such as the "bovine arch" where the origin of the left common carotid artery arises from the brachiocephalic trunk as opposed to the aortic arch (**Fig. 15.1A**). In patients being evaluated for carotid artery stenting, it is also useful to classify the overall shape of the aortic arch as level I, II, or III. A horizontal line is drawn across the top of the aortic arch and a second horizontal line is drawn two times the diameter of the common carotid artery inferior to this (**Fig. 15.1B**). A level I arch describes each of the great vessels originating along this horizontal line. A level II arch has the great vessels originating below this line, and a level III arch has the origin of the great vessels arising more than two times the diameter of the common carotid artery below this line. The normal size of the aorta varies at different anatomic locations and decreases in size with distance from the aortic valve (**Table 15.1**).

D.M. Shavelle
David Geffen School of Medicine at UCLA, Division of Cardiology, Harbor-UCLA Medical Center, Torrance, CA 90509, USA
e-mail: dshavelle@hotmail.com

M.J. Budoff, J.S. Shinbane (eds.), *Handbook of Cardiovascular CT*,
DOI: 10.1007/978-1-84800-091-9_15, © Springer-Verlag London Limited 2008

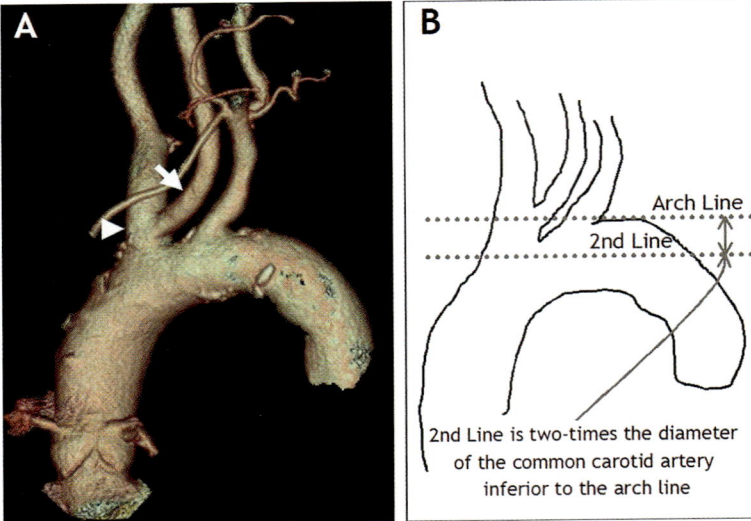

Fig. 15.1 A. Bovine aortic arch with left common carotid artery (*white arrow*) originating from the right brachiocephalic artery (*white arrowhead*). Volume rendering. **B**. To classify the shape of the aortic arch, a horizontal line is drawn along the top of the arch (*arch line*). A second line is drawn two times the diameter of the common carotid artery, inferior to the arch line. This is an example of a level II arch

Table 15.1 Normal diameters referenced to body surface area (m^2) of the ascending, descending, and abdominal aorta

Location	Normal size	Comments
Ascending aorta	<2.1 cm/m^2	Surgery recommended for aneurysms >5.5 cm in those with Marfan's syndrome and >6.0 cm in those without connective tissue disease
Descending aorta	<1.6 cm/m^2	
Abdominal aorta	<3.0 cm	

15.3 Diseases of the Aorta

Common diseases that involve the aorta include aneurysm, dissection, and athero-sclerosis.

15.3.1 Aortic Aneurysm

Aneurysms commonly involve the abdominal and thoracic aorta. Aortic endovas-cular stenting is gaining acceptance as an alternative to traditional open surgical

Table 15.2 Essential CT measurements in the evaluation of an abdominal aortic aneurysm for possible aortic stent graft placement; see **Fig. 15.1**

Measurement	Description of measurement
D1	Aortic diameter at lowest renal artery
D2	Maximal aortic diameter
D3	Diameter at right iliac artery landing zone
D4	Diameter at left iliac artery landing zone
L1	Length of aortic neck below renal arteries
L2	Length of aorta from beginning of aneurysm to bifurcation
L3	Length of aneurysmal right iliac artery
L4	Length of nonaneurysmal right iliac artery
L5	Length of aneurysmal left iliac artery
L6	Length of nonaneurysmal left iliac artery

repair for abdominal aortic aneurysms. CT imaging is the predominant method used for preoperative planning to assess the feasibility of endovascular aortic stenting. In addition, following endovascular aortic stenting placement, CT is commonly used to assess for device complications that include endoleaks, aneurysm expansion, rupture, and graft migration that may occur in up to 10% of cases [1].

CT imaging of abdominal and thoracic aneurysms should assess the proximal and distal extent of the aneurysm, size of the aneurysm, and involvement of adjacent vessels. Axial CT images (raw data) should be the primary source to accurately size the aneurysm and obtain preoperative measurements for selecting the appropriate aortic stent graft (**Table 15.2**, **Fig. 15.2**). The most accurate measurement

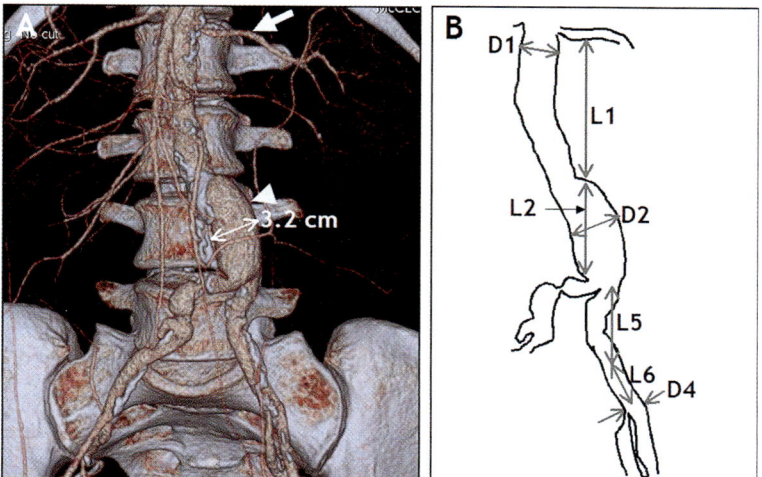

Fig. 15.2 A. Infra-renal abdominal aortic aneurysm (*white arrowhead*) measuring approximately 3.2 cm at the largest diameter. *White arrow* shows left renal artery. Volume rendering. **B**. Essential measurements used in the evaluation of an abdominal aortic aneurysm for possible aortic stent graft placement. See **Table 15.2**

of aneurysm size should be obtained in a plane perpendicular to the center line of the vessel. Maximum intensity projection (MIP) provides images similar to those obtained with conventional angiography and is useful to visualize calcification and the relationship of the aneurysm to adjacent vessels. Volume rendering (VR) provides an accurate anatomic representation of the aneurysm to adjacent vessels and helps to define vessel tortuosity.

15.3.2 Aortic Dissection

The main CT feature of an aortic dissection is the presence of an intimal flap that separates the true and false lumen (**Figs. 15.3** and **15.4**). The ability to establish this diagnosis relies heavily upon a good-quality CT scan with optimal vascular enhancement. The extent of the dissection (proximal entry and distal re-entry sites), involvement of adjacent branch vessels, and potential comprise of the true lumen should be evaluated. Potential imaging artifacts include insufficient contrast enhancement of the lumen (improper timing of contrast), streak artifacts (adjacent surgical staples, vascular calcification), periaortic structures (soft tissue masses, residual thymus), and congenital aortic diverticulum (residual ductus tissue) [2]. Two disease processes that can be confused with an aortic dissection include intramural hematoma (focal dissection of blood within the aortic wall) and penetrating aortic ulcer.

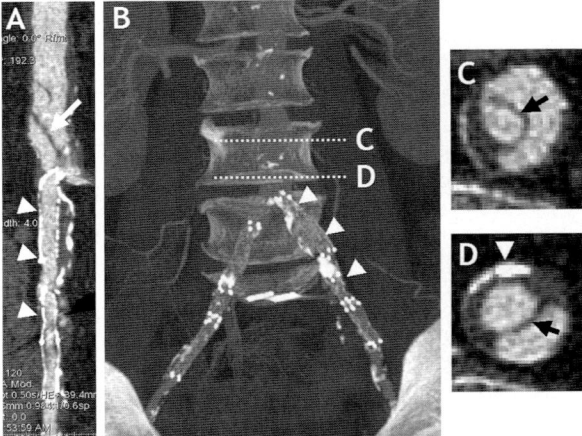

Fig. 15.3 Dissection of the distal abdominal aorta. **A**. A clear dissection flap is present (*white arrow*). Three stents are seen in the right and left iliac (*white arrowheads*) arteries. **B**. Frontal image showing the location of the left iliac stents (*white arrowheads*) and location of the cross sections (*axial cuts*) shown in *Panels C* and *D*. **C**. Cross-sectional image showing dissection (*black arrow*). **D**. Cross-sectional image showing dissection (*black arrow*) with calcification within aortic wall (*white arrowhead*)

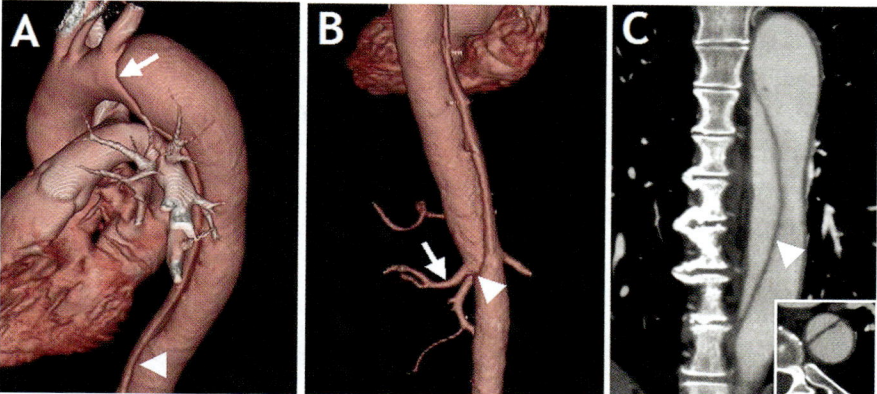

Fig. 15.4 Type B aortic dissection. **A.** Dissection begins just distal to the origin of the left subclavian artery (*white arrow*) and extends into the abdominal aorta (*white arrowhead*). Volume rendering. **B.** Dissection ends (*white arrowhead*) just inferior to the left renal artery (*white arrow*). Note that this is a posterior projection, so the left renal artery is on the left side of the image. Volume rendering. **C.** MIP in a sagittal section through the dissection (*white arrowhead*) in the thoracic and abdominal aorta. The true and false lumens are clearly seen. Inset shows MIP cross section of dissection within the abdominal aorta

15.3.3 Atherosclerosis

CT findings of aortic atherosclerosis include thickening or raised lesions of the aortic wall and the presence of calcification (**Fig. 15.5**). The presence of thoracic aortic calcification by CT is associated with coronary calcification and both the severity and the extent of angiographic coronary artery disease [3–4].

15.4 Disease of the Great Vessels

The most common disease process that involves the great vessels is atherosclerosis. Atherosclerosis typically affects the carotid artery system at the bifurcation of the common carotid into the internal carotid artery (ICA) and the external carotid artery (ECA).

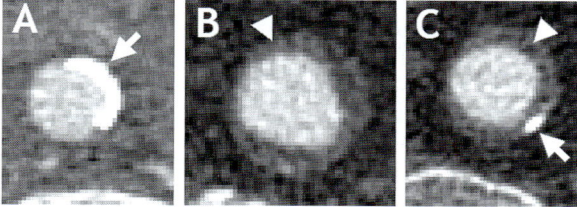

Fig. 15.5 Aortic atherosclerosis. **A.** Raw axial image showing calcification of the aortic wall (*white arrow*). **B.** Raw axial image showing thickening of the aortic wall (*white arrowhead*). **C.** Raw axial image showing both calcification of the aortic wall (*white arrow*) and thickening of the aortic wall (*white arrowhead*)

The common carotid artery should be followed from its aortic origin, through the carotid bifurcation, and into the skull base using the raw data in axial imaging cuts. The ECA can usually be easily differentiated from the ICA because of multiple side branches arising from the ECA within the neck region (the ICA lacks branches within the neck, **Fig. 15.6**). In the setting of complete occlusion of the ICA, the ECA may occasionally be mistaken for the ICA. The presence of near-occlusion of the ICA (so-called angiographic 'string sign') may result in a reduction in the caliber of the distal ICA relative to its expected size, and an increase in size of

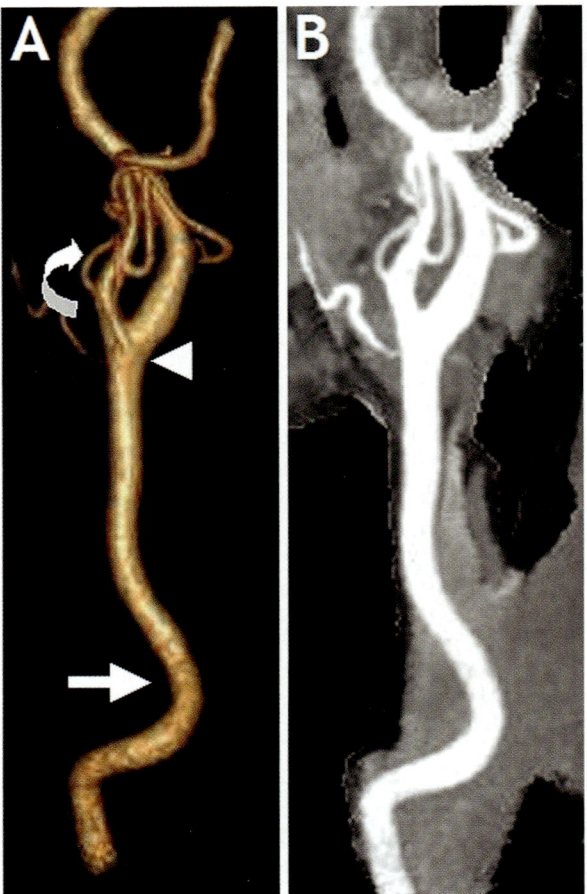

Fig. 15.6 Normal left carotid artery. **A**. Volume-rendering projection showing normal left carotid artery. The proximal common carotid artery is tortuous (*white arrow*), and there is no disease at the carotid bifurcation (*arrowhead*). The external carotid artery can be differentiated from the internal carotid artery because of its multiple branches (*curved arrow*). **B**. Maximum intensity projection (MIP) with a slice thickness of 7 mm in the same projection as shown in *Panel A*

both the contra-lateral ICA and the ipsilateral ECA. The right ICA can be separated from the right ECA using a right anterior oblique or lateral projection. Similarly, the left ICA can be separated from the left ECA using a left anterior oblique or lateral projection.

In order to accurately evaluate the carotid arteries, a spatial position perpendicular to the carotid axis should be chosen. VR is useful as the initial post-processing option to assess the general course of the carotid arteries and the shape and configuration of the aortic arch. Sagittal MIP with a slab thickness of 7–10 mm and multiplanar reconstruction (MPR) with a slice thickness of 1 mm should be applied to completely evaluate disease severity. Cross-sectional images should be used to assess lumen diameters and stenosis severity [5] MIP appears to be the most accurate reformatting technique to assess stenosis severity (**Fig. 15.7**) [6]. A steep left anterior oblique or left lateral, as opposed to an anterior, projection is useful to show the origins of the common carotid arteries (**Fig. 15.8**). Although various window/level settings can be used based on operator preference, a setting of 700/200 HU will suffice in majority of the cases, and 1100/200 HU can be used in the setting of significant calcification. Significant calcification often precludes the use of MIP formatting and in this setting, VR and axial raw data should be used.

Given that a large proportion of patients with carotid artery disease will be evaluated for potential carotid artery stenting, CT imaging should focus on the assessment of the following: (1) stenosis severity, (2) disease within the aortic arch and at the origin of the common carotid arteries, (3) size of the common carotid artery at lesion

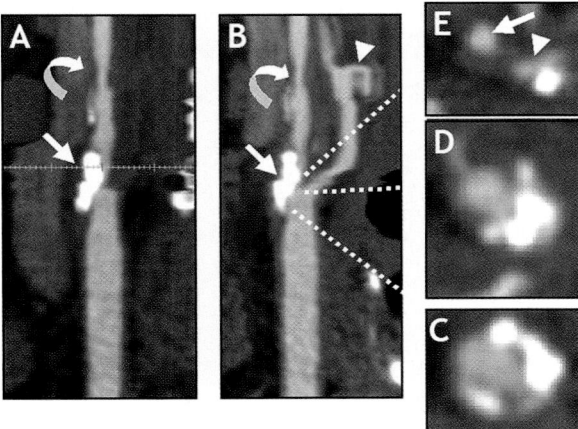

Fig. 15.7 Severe left carotid artery disease. **A.** Maximum intensity projection showing severe calcification (*white arrow*) at the carotid bifurcation and moderate disease of the internal carotid artery, distal to the bifurcation (*curved arrow*). **B.** A slightly different section as in *Panel A* that includes the origin of the external carotid artery (*white arrowhead*) and shows locations of the cross-sectional images shown in *Panels C, D*, and *E*. **C.** Severe calcification with mild adjacent stenosis. **D.** Severe calcification at the carotid bifurcation with moderate adjacent stenosis. **E.** Location of this section is immediately distal to the carotid bifurcation with calcification and severe adjacent stenosis of the internal carotid artery (*arrowhead*). External carotid artery (*white arrow*)

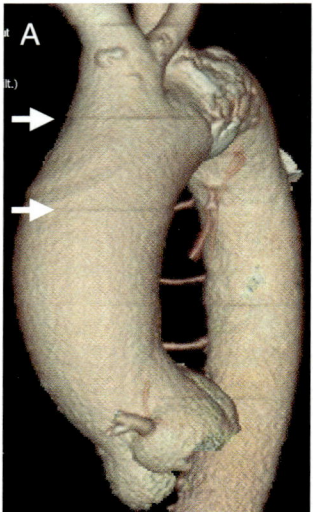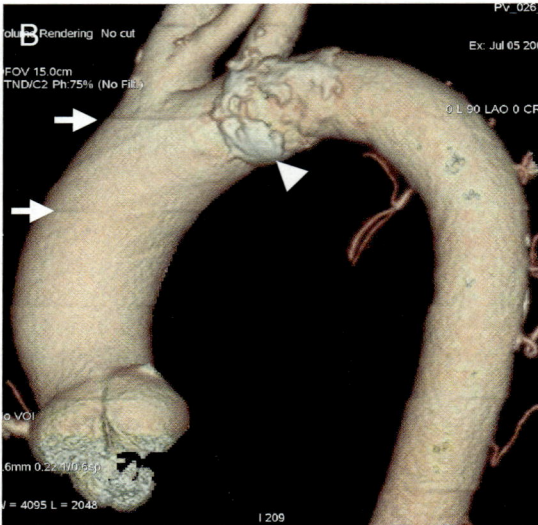

Fig. 15.8 **A.** Anterior projection (AP) of the ascending aorta, aortic arch, and descending aorta. Calcification within the aortic arch (*white arrowhead*). Note that in the AP, the origins of the great vessels are not well visualized. White arrows show misalignment artifact. Volume rendering. **B.** Lateral projection clearly showing the origin of the great vessels. Calcification within the aortic arch (*white arrowhead*), adjacent to the origin of the left subclavian artery. White arrows show misalignment artifact. Volume rendering

location, (4) size of the distal ICA, and (5) the presence of contra-lateral disease (**Table 15.3**). A recent meta-analysis found the sensitivity and specificity for CT angiography to detect severe carotid artery stenosis (>70%) to be 85% and 93%, respectively [7]. CT angiography is also highly accurate in assessing carotid plaque morphology, particularly ulcerated plaques [8–9].

Table 15.3 Essential information to be obtained during CT imaging of carotid artery disease

	Comments
Stenosis severity	NASCET classification using the distal internal carotid artery as the reference segment to assess disease severity [10]
Disease within the aortic arch and origins of common carotid arteries	Placement of catheters and sheaths in diseased segments could result in embolic events to the central nervous system
Size of common carotid artery at lesion location	Useful for choosing correct size of endovascular stent
Size of distal internal carotid artery	Useful for choosing correct size of distal protection device

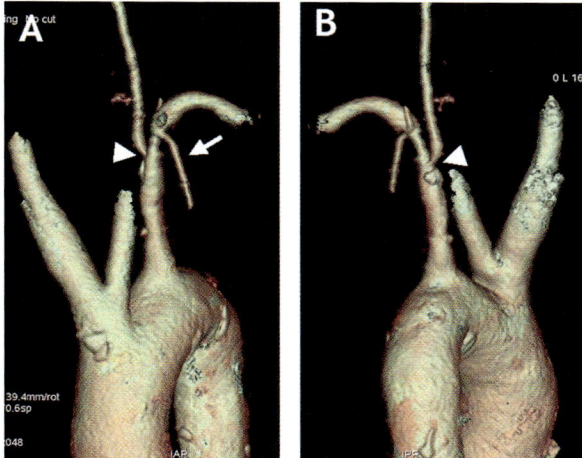

Fig. 15.9 Subclavian artery stenosis. **A**. Stenosis is located in the proximal subclavian artery, adjacent to the origin of the left vertebral artery (*white arrowhead*). The left internal thoracic artery originates distal to the stenosis (*white arrow*). Volume rendering. **B**. Different orientation to *Panel A* showing moderate stenosis of the proximal left subclavian artery and severe stenosis at the origin of the left vertebral artery (*white arrowhead*). Volume rendering

Atherosclerosis can also involve the subclavian artery, commonly at its origin and therefore proximal to the origin of the internal thoracic arteries. CT imaging of the subclavian artery follows the same principles as outlined above for the carotid arteries. In patients being considered for endovascular treatment for subclavian artery stenosis, CT imaging can be useful to evaluate the reference vessel diameter and length of disease so that the appropriately-sized stent can be chosen. For subclavian artery lesions that extend into the origin of the vertebral artery, endovascular treatment may pose significant risk (compromise of the vertebral artery during stent placement), and alternative forms of therapy (conservative versus surgical) should be considered (**Fig. 15.9**).

15.5 Imaging Pearls

15.5.1 Carotid Artery Disease

- To evaluate patients for possible carotid stenting, CT imaging should focus on assessment of the following: [8, 9, 10]
  - ○ Stenosis severity (NASCET criteria is widely used)
  - ○ Disease within the aortic arch and at the origin of the common carotid arteries
  - ○ Size of common carotid artery at lesion location

    ○ Size of the distal ICA
    ○ The presence of contra-lateral disease

- A window/level setting of 700/200 HU will suffice in majority of the cases, and 1100/200 HU can be used in the setting of significant calcification
- VR and axial raw data can be useful in the setting of significant calcification

15.5.2 Aortic Atherosclerosis

- CT findings include thickening or raised lesions of the aortic wall and the presence of calcification

15.5.3 Aortic Dissection

- The main CT finding is an intimal flap that separates the true and false lumen
- CT imaging should assess the following:
  - ○ Extent of the dissection (proximal entry and distal re-entry sites)
  - ○ Involvement of adjacent branch vessels
  - ○ Potential comprise of the true lumen
- Imaging artifacts include insufficient contrast enhancement of the lumen, streak artifacts, periaortic structures, and congenital aortic diverticulum

15.5.4 Aortic Aneurysm

- CT imaging should focus on assessment of the following:
  - Proximal and distal extent of the aneurysm
  - Size of the aneurysm
    - ○ Axial CT images (raw data) should be the primary source to accurately size the aneurysm and obtain preoperative measurements for selecting the appropriate aortic stent graft
  - Involvement of adjacent vessels
  - MIP provides images similar to those obtained with conventional angiography and is useful to visualize calcification and the relationship of the aneurysm to adjacent vessels
  - VR provides an accurate anatomic representation of the aneurysm to adjacent vessels and helps to define vessel tortuosity

References

1. Hobo R, Buth J. Secondary interventions following endovascular abdominal aortic aneurysm repair using current endografts. A EUROSTAR report. *J Vasc Surg* 2006 May, 43(5): 896–902.
2. Batra P, Bigoni B, Manning J, Aberle DR, Brown K, Hart E, Goldin J. Pitfalls in the diagnosis of thoracic aortic dissection at CT angiography. *Radiographics* 2000 March, 20(2): 309–320.
3. Yamamoto H, Shavelle D, Takasu J, Lu B, Mao SS, Fischer H, Budoff MJ. Valvular and thoracic aortic calcium as a marker of the extent and severity of angiographic coronary artery disease. *Am Heart J* 2003 July, 146(1): 153–159.
4. Wu MH, Chern MS, Chen LC, Lin YP, Sheu MH, Liu JC, Chang CY. Electron beam computed tomography evidence of aortic calcification as an independent determinant of coronary artery calcification. *J Chin Med Assoc* 2006 September, 69(9): 409–414.
5. Lell M, Fellner C, Baum U, Hothorn T, Steiner R, Lang W, Bautz W, Fellner FA. Evaluation of carotid artery stenosis with multisection CT and MR imaging: influence of imaging modality and postprocessing. *AJNR Am J Neuroradiol* 2007 January, 28(1): 104–110.
6. Sparacia G, Bencivinni F, Banco A, Sarno C, Bartolotta TV, Lagalla R. Imaging processing for CT angiography of the cervicocranial arteries: evaluation of reformatting technique. *Radiol Med (Torino)* 2007 March, 112(2): 224–238.
7. Koelemay MJ, Nederkoorn PJ, Reitsma JB, Majoie CB. Systematic review of computed tomographic angiography for assessment of carotid artery disease. *Stroke* 2004 October, 35(10): 2306–2312.
8. Saba L, Sanfilippo R, Pirisi R, Pascalis L, Montisci R, Mallarini G. Multidetector-row CT angiography in the study of atherosclerotic carotid arteries. *Neuroradiology* 2007 July 3.
9. Saba L, Caddeo G, Sanfilippo R, Montisci R, Mallarini G. CT and Ultrasound in the Study of Ulcerated Carotid Plaque Compared with Surgical Results: Potentialities and Advantages of Multidetector Row CT Angiography. *AJNR Am J Neuroradiol* 2007 June, 28(6): 1061–1066.
10. Beneficial effect of carotid endarterectomy in symptomatic patients with high-grade carotid stenosis. North American Symptomatic Carotid Endarterectomy Trial Collaborators. *N Engl J Med* 1991 August 15, 325(7): 445–453.

Chapter 16
Adult Congenital Heart Disease

Louise E.J. Thomson, Ronald P. Karlsberg, John D. Friedman,
Sean W. Hayes, Rola Saouaf, and Daniel S. Berman

Heart defects are the most common birthdefects, with 1/120 babies born with some kind of heart defect and an estimated 1 million adults in the USA suffering from heart defects. Adults with complex congenital heart disease (CHD) are increasing in number with the improved longer term survival of modern correction techniques, so that today, there are more adults than children living with heart defects. With modern surgical approaches, 90% of children born with heart defects are now expected to live up to adulthood, and thus the number of adults with CHD is likely to continue to increase as a function of this improved childhood care [1, 2] (**Table 16.1**).

Echocardiography is the established noninvasive test of choice for evaluation of CHD, and cardiac magnetic resonance imaging (CMR) is favored as a validated second-line test, particularly for imaging of chest vascular anomalies and right ventricular function, and for the noninvasive quantitation of shunts. CMR cannot usually be performed in patients with pacemakers and remains contraindicated in patients with defibrillators.

The evolution of MDCT systems leads invariably to increased application of this technology for assessment of cardiovascular structure and function in adult patients with CHD. CTA has an advantage over both CMR and catheter cardio-angiography in being a gated 3-D volumetric acquisition providing data that can be reformatted to view the beating heart in any image plane. CTA is an excellent noninvasive test for defining the presence and nature of coronary anomalies (**Fig. 16.1**) and is a second-line noninvasive test of choice for adult and pediatric patients with other forms of CHD, who cannot have CMR due to the above-mentioned contraindications.

The speed of data acquisition and recent improvements in spatial and temporal resolution of modern MDCT systems are also advantages of CTA. Radiation dose considerations and exposure to iodinated contrast media are the frequently cited disadvantages of CTA compared to CMR. It should also be noted that if physiologic data, such as flow velocity measurements, are required, this information should be obtained by CMR or echo.

L.E.J. Thomson
Department of Imaging, Cedars Sinai Medical Centre, Los Angeles, CA, USA
e-mail: Louise.Thomson@cshs.org

M.J. Budoff, J.S. Shinbane (eds.), *Handbook of Cardiovascular CT*, 153
DOI: 10.1007/978-1-84800-091-9_16, © Springer-Verlag London Limited 2008

Table 16.1 Classification of congenital cardiac and chest vascular anomalies

Congenital cardiac anomalies

Simple
Atrial septal defects
    Secundum (70%)
    Venosus
    Patent foramen ovale
    (Primum—AVCD)
Ventricular septal defects
    Perimembranous (80%)
    Supracristal (outlet)
    Muscular (trabecular)
    Posterior (inlet)
Patent ductus arteriosus
Bicuspid aortic valve
Pulmonary valvular stenosis

Complex
Transposition of the great arteries (TGA)
Tetralogy of Fallot
Tricuspid atresia
Pulmonary atresia
Ebstein's anomaly
"Univentricular" heart
Atrioventricular canal defect
    (aka endocardial cushion defect)
Truncus arteriosus

Coronary anomalies
Anomalies of origin and course
    Absent left main
    High, low or commissural ostial position
    Ostium outside sinus
    Coronary origin from facing sinus
    Single coronary artery
Anomalies of intrinsic coronary arterial anatomy
    Congenital ostial stenosis
    Intramural coronary artery course
    Absent PDA (split RCA)
    Absent LAD (split LAD)
Anomalies of coronary termination
    Fistulous connections
Anomalous collateral vessels

Chest vascular anomalies
Aortic arch anomalies
    Right arch with mirror branching
    Right arch with aberrant origin left subclavian
    Double arch
    Left arch with Aberrant origin right subclavian
Anomalies of the great veins
    Persistent left SVC- coronary sinus
    Interrupted IVC
Pulmonary venous anomalies and abnormal connections
    Middle veins
    Common trunk – right or left
    Anomalous pulmonary venous connections
Pulmonary arterial anomalies
    Pulmonary artery stenosis

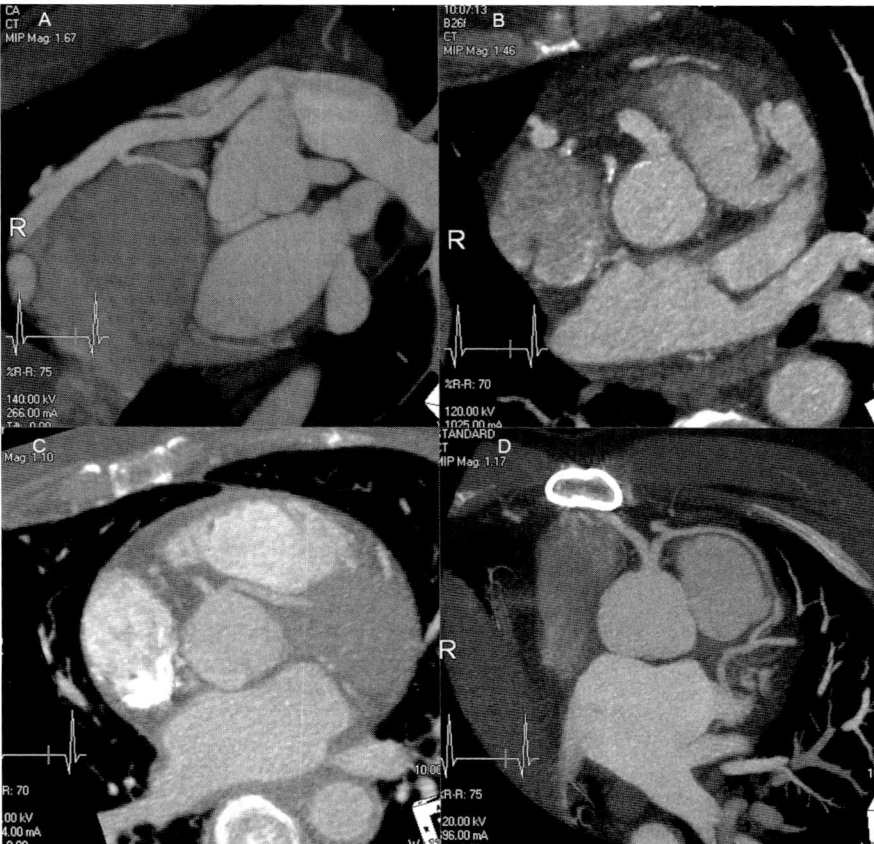

Fig. 16.1 Panel images: coronary artery anomalies (**A**) Origin of the right coronary artery from the pulmonary artery. Note the large size of the coronary, (**B**) Origin of the right coronary artery from the left coronary sinus, (**C**) Origin of the left coronary artery from the pulmonary artery, (**D**) Origin of the left coronary artery from the right coronary sinus, with course of the left coronary anterior to the main pulmonary artery

In adult patients with known CHD, CTA is most likely to be requested for evaluation of long-term sequelae of disease or prior surgical correction. Guidelines for care of adult CHD recommend that patients with complex CHD should be cared for in specialist centers because of the complicated nature of the anatomy, and the corrections (**Table 16.2**) and complications that ensue [3,4]. However, these patients may present for care and require imaging at non-specialist centers—when it becomes important that a systematic approach to scan performance and interpretation be used.

Successful performance of CTA in adult patients with complex CHD is dependent on clearly defining the pre-test clinical question in order to adequately plan the CT acquisition protocol. For example, in a patient with a Fontan procedure and a univentricular heart, whether the CTA being performed for detection of pulmonary

Table 16.2 Palliative and corrective surgical procedures in congenital heart disease

- **Bentall procedure**
  Replacement of the ascending aorta and aortic valve with a composite valve-graft device and re-implantation of the coronary artery ostia into the conduit.

- **Damus–Kaye: Stansel operation**
  The MPA is transected and surgically connected to the proximal ascending aorta to provide the systemic ventricle–aortic connection. A conduit from the right ventricle to the distal pulmonary artery delivers venous blood to the lungs. The aortic orifice and any VSD are closed, and coronary arteries are left in place and perfused retrogradely. (Procedure for patients with abnormal ventriculo-arterial connection who are not suitable for a switch, e.g., TGA with non-suitable coronary anatomy).

- **Fontan operation**
  The systemic venous return is directly and passively to the pulmonary arteries. This is performed in the setting of univentricular circulation, with the single ventricle functioning as the systemic pump.

- **Glenn shunt**
  SVC-PA anastamosis to increase pulmonary blood flow, usually as a step before a Fontan operation.

- **Jatene–Arterial switch**
  The arterial switch operation for TGA. Coronary arteries are re-implanted after reattachment of the transposed great arteries to the contralateral ventricles.

- **Mustard or Senning procedure**
  Atrial-level correction for TGA with a conduit (Mustard) or baffle (Senning) to redirect systemic venous return to the left ("new right") atrium and pulmonary venous return to the right ("new left") atrium.

- **Rastelli procedure**
  Operative repair in TGA with pulmonary stenosis and a large VSD. The LV is connected to the aorta via a baffle through the VSD. The RV is connected to the PA by a valved conduit. The native LV-PA connection is closed.

- **Ross procedure**
  This procedure for aortic valve replacement places the native pulmonary valve, annulus, and root in the aortic position and reconstructs the right ventricular outflow with a valved homograft conduit. The coronary arteries are re-implanted into the neo-aorta.

thromboemboli is for assessment of systemic ventricular outflow and function or for detection of pulmonary arterial or venous collateral formation?

Contrast timing, duration, and even the chosen site of contrast administration may all be influenced by the clinical question and pre-scan knowledge of the nature of the CHD. Interpretation of data requires knowledge of the congenital pathology, the type of surgical corrections that are usually performed and the spectrum of complications that are known occur with various types of CHD and subsequent to procedures/repair performed.

This extends to familiarity with the "normal" imaging characteristics of implanted defect closure devices, prosthetic cardiac valves, shunts and the surgical corrections performed (**Fig. 16.2 and Fig. 16.3** provide example images from two patients with palliated or repaired complex CHD).

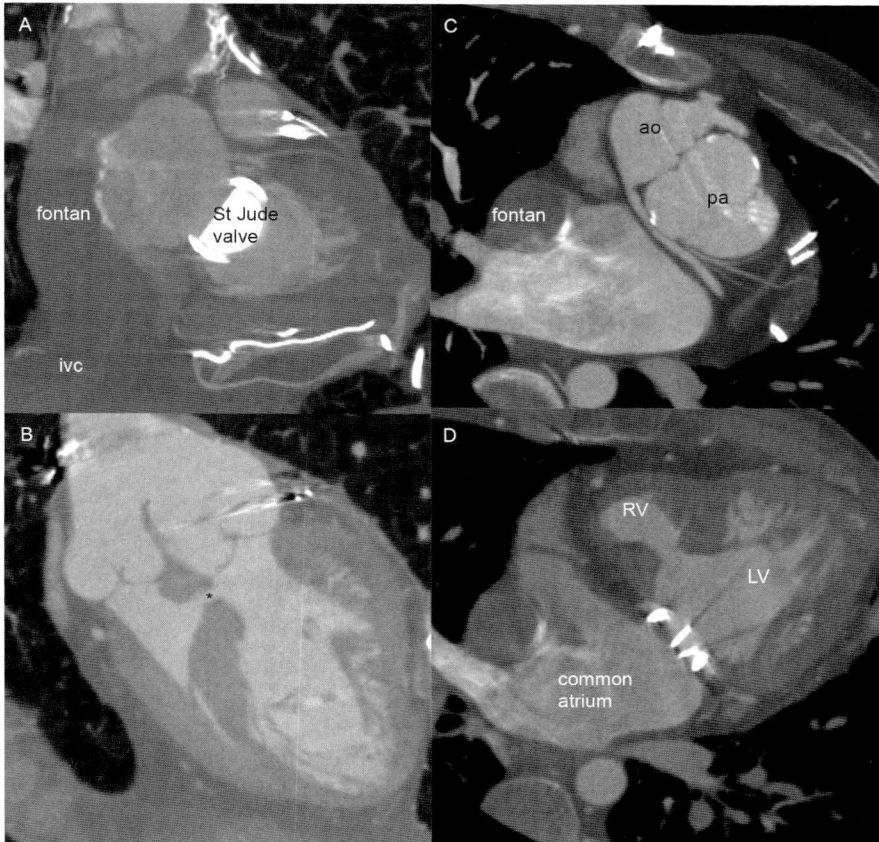

Fig. 16.2 Panel images: 26-year-old man with transposition of the great arteries, tricuspid atresia, VSD, and a hypoplastic right ventricle, who had prior PA band followed by Glen shunt followed by completion of Fontan with Damus procedure and mitral valve replacement. He also has an extra-cardiac pacemaker/defibrillator. (**A**) The IVC connection to the Fontan channel is seen with connection to the pulmonary arteries. The St Jude mitral valve and an inferiorly positioned extrac-ardiac defibrillator pad can be seen, (**B**) There is a small right ventricle VSD, and the pulmonary trunk is anastomosed to the proximal ascending aorta, (**C**) The aortic valve with coronary origins is anterior to the larger pulmonary valve. The circumflex coronary courses posterior to the pulmonary valve, (**D**) The ventricular septal defect and hypoplastic right ventricle are seen in this "four chamber view" of the heart. It can also be appreciated that there is no tricuspid valve and a prosthetic valve (St Jude) is seen in the mitral position. The Fontan channel lies to the right of the contrast-opacified atrium

Some patients present in adult life with more simple forms of CHD—such as coronary anomalies, atrial and ventricular septal defects, congenital bicuspid aortic valve, thoracic aortic anomalies, and chest venous anomalies. It is estimated that 10% of all cases seen at an adult CHD clinic (particularly with ASD, Ebstein's anomaly, and corrected transposition) are not diagnosed until adulthood [2].

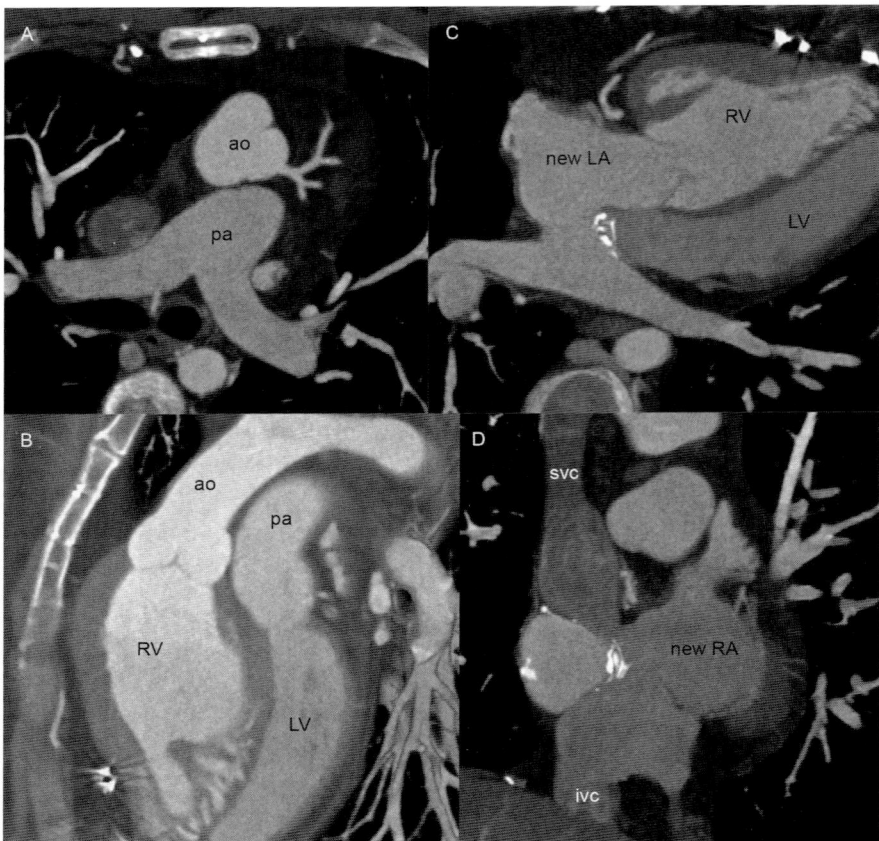

Fig. 16.3 Panel images: 27-year-old man with D-transposition of the great arteries, who had an atrial switch at 18 months of age and presence of fatigue and shortness of breath with exertion. (**A**) The aortic valve with left coronary artery origin lies anteriorly to the pulmonary trunk, with the pulmonary bifurcation seen. The sagittal oblique view demonstrates the aorta arising from the trabeculated right ventricle and the pulmonary artery arising from the smooth-walled left ventricle, (**B**) The pulmonary venous return is to the morphologic right atrium (the "new left atrium") with the broad-based appendage demonstrated. Calcification is seen at the surgical site in the mid-atrium, (**C**) The SVC and IVC are directed into the morphologic left atrium (the "new right atrium") with the narrow-based and trabeculated appendage demonstrated

Congenital anomalies may present "late" as a consequence of late development of symptoms (e.g., small atrial septal defects causing symptoms as a patient ages), because of complications related to the presence of a small defect (e.g., paradoxical embolism), or may be detected incidentally in asymptomatic individuals having CTA for another reason (**Fig. 16.4**).

Anomalies should always be reported, regardless of symptoms or the incidental nature of the discovery. Small defects may be managed conservatively or considered for elective percutaneous approaches to closure (in the case of secundum ASD,

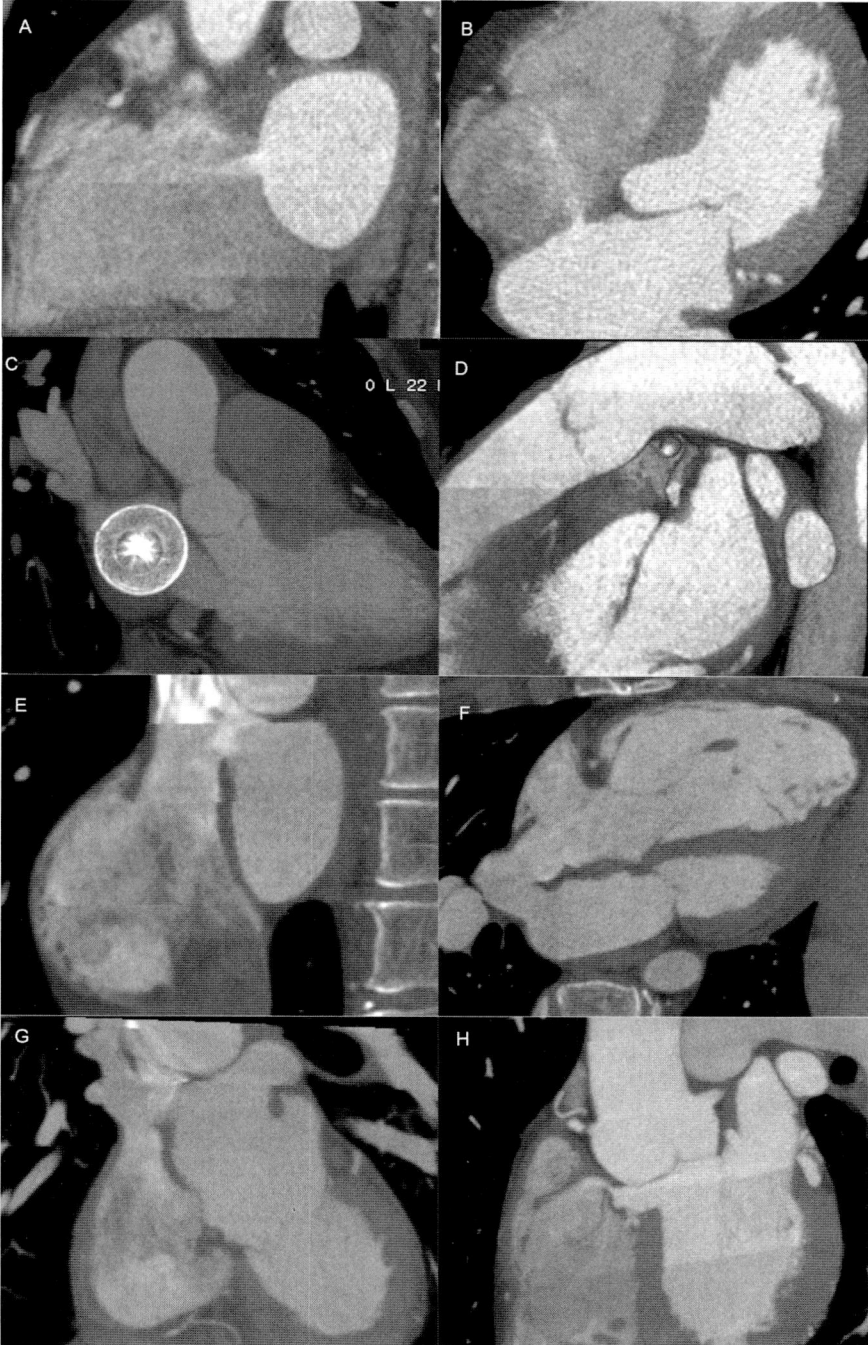

Fig. 16.4 (Continued)

muscular VSD, or PDA), with management often influenced by the presence of complications such as paradoxical embolism (**Fig. 16.5**).

As the utilization of CTA for coronary artery disease indications increases, it is probable that there will be increased recognition of "incidental" mild CHD. Although there is diversity in approaches to interpretation and reporting of CT coronary angiography, most will agree that a reader has a responsibility to detect the presence of incidental cardiac pathology. It is recommended that, in all studies, a systematic approach to CT data be used and that readers should avoid assuming that any heart is anatomically "normal" until this has been proved by inspection of the data (**Table 16.3**).

One such systematic approach is to consider the heart in segments and to routinely inspect each segment in turn, to define that the heart is normal (and to systematically define abnormalities) [5]. Familiarity with cardiac anatomy in the axial plane may be sufficient for a reader to identify all anatomic features that define the "normal heart," but routine reformatting of data is recommended to demonstrate normal cardiac chamber relationships and normal inflow and outflow from each cardiac chamber and to adequately inspect the relative size of chambers. This approach of visualizing multiple standard cardiac imaging planes has been defined by echo and mimicked by CMR. This approach permits ready comparison between modalities in terms of the features being described and the location and size of abnormal structures. Viewing the heart in this manner requires familiarity with double oblique reformation of 3-D data and can be performed on all commercially available workstations (**Table 16.4**).

Demand for CTA in adult CHD is likely to increase as a consequence of increased availability and awareness of this technology and as a consequence of the increasing numbers of children with complex disease surviving to adult age. Cardiac CTA has an important role to play in these patients, and the challenge for the reader is to approach these studies in a systematic manner in order to maximize the quality of the information obtained from the test.

Fig. 16.4 Panel images: atrial and ventricular septal defects and PDA. (**A**) Incidental discovery in a 46-year-old man with atypical chest pains referred for detection of coronary artery disease. Small atrial septal defect with left-to-right contrast flow—oblique sagittal view, (**B**) Small atrial septal defect with left-to-right contrast flow—four-chamber view, (**C**) Double oblique reformation of data to demonstrate the enface view of an Amplatzer Septal Occluder (AGA medical corporation) in a 70-year-old woman with atypical chest pain following percutaneous closure of a 17 mm ASD detected by echo in adulthood, (**D**) Small patent ductus arteriosus with calcification of the ductus diverticulum found incidentally in a 50-year-old man having coronary artery CTA for evaluation of chest pain, (**E**) Large superior venosus atrial septal defect—oblique sagittal view—in a 48-year-old woman with a known heart murmur since age 13. Recent increasing tiredness and subtle exertional dyspnea led to echocardiography, which demonstrated significant cardiac enlargement, (**F**) Large superior venosus atrial septal defect—four-chamber view, (**G**) Anomalous pulmonary venous connections to the SVC associated with the superior venosus ASD seen in E, F, (**H**) Small perimembranous ventricular septal defect, immediately inferior to the right coronary cusp in a 45-year-old man with chest pain and risk factors for coronary artery disease, who had CTA

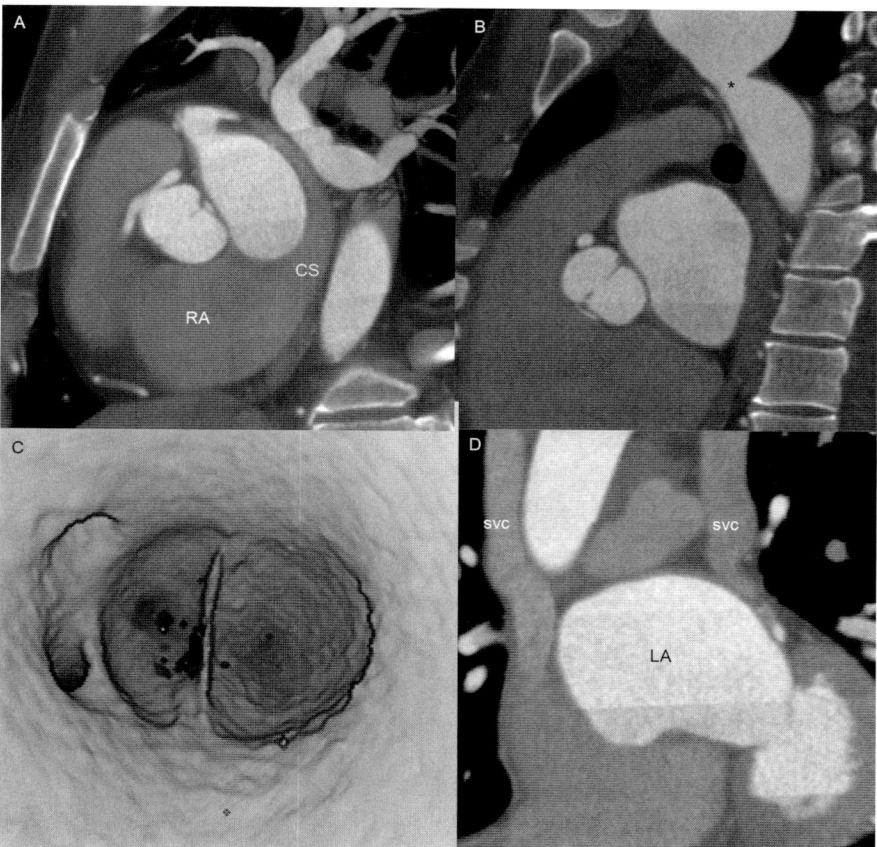

Fig. 16.5 Panel images: aortic coarctation with bicuspid aortic valve, anomalous coronary origin, and persistent left SVC in a 43-year-old woman. (**A**) Right and left coronary arteries arise from the anterior sinus of Valsalva, and the dilated coronary sinus is visualized entering the right atrium, (**B**) Aortic coarctation is present in addition to a left-sided SVC, visualized coursing posterior to the left atrium, (**C**) Navigator view of the aortic sinuses confirming the presence of a bicuspid aortic valve and origin of the coronary arteries from the anterior sinus, (**D**) Coronal view demonstrating right- and left-sided SVC

16.1 Clinical Pearls

1. The value of *pre-scan planning* in adults with CHD should not be underestimated. Pre-scan knowledge of the cardiac anatomy, prior surgical procedures, the presence of ventricular dysfunction, and the primary clinical question to be answered by imaging should guide decisions regarding scan protocol and assist in interpretation of data.
2. What about *contrast delivery timing*? Hounsfield unit–triggered acquisitions reduce the need for unnecessary contrast and radiation exposure. In patients

Table 16.3 Segmental approach to inspection of cardiac anatomy in congenital heart disease

1. Define the atrial segment:

RA   Wide neck triangular appendage

LA   Narrow neck and shaped appendage

Coronary sinus location and connection to RA

2. Define the ventricular segment:

Each ventricle has inlet, outlet and trabecular portions.

RV: Trabecular wall, with infundibular region separating inlet and outlet valves.

LV: Smooth walled, with a fibrous continuity between the inlet and outlet valves.

Inspect the atrio-ventricular junction. The atrio-ventricular valves follow their associated ventricles

Inspect the ventriculo-arterial connection.

3. Define the arterial segment:

Coronary arteries arise from the aortic sinus and the aortic arch branches to supply the head, neck and arms.

Pulmonary artery bifurcates

with complex disease for whom pre-scan anatomic information is not available, non-contrast chest CT will aid the identification of cardiac chambers and chest vascular structures. Bolus tracking may also be of value in planning acquisitions when contrast opacification of systemic arterial but not venous structures is desired, but the overall cardiovascular circulation is either prolonged (ventricular failure) or abnormal (shunt).

3. What about the use of a *saline chase bolus*? The use of a saline chasing bolus in coronary CTA is primarily to minimize contrast opacification of the right heart and systemic venous return structures and to maximize contrast opacification of the left-sided structures. In the clinical settings when visualization of right-sided structures is desired, an imaging and contrast delivery protocol should be chosen to produce either steady-state contrast imaging or differential contrast in right and left sides of the heart. Contrast-related artifacts can be reduced by minimizing the total contrast amount or by use of a diluted contrast second-phase infusion [6].

Table 16.4 Imaging protocols and post-processing

Adult cardiac-gated CCT

Pre-scan beta-blocker for HR < 65 if possible.

120 kVp, 350 mA/rotation.

Collimation 0.6–0.75 mm for coronary imaging.

  1—2 mm for larger cardiovascular structures.

Pitch for gated CT—determined by heart rate: 0.28–0.44.

Dose modulation on for regular HR (50–80% of the RR).

Scan time: 10–15 s.

Contrast—left opacification greater than right opacification.

  90 ml at the rate of 5 ml/s, then 30:70 mix, 40 ml at the rate of 5 ml/s

  saline 40 ml at the rate of 5 ml/s.

For greater right ventricular opacification, consider decreasing rate of delivery of the second-phase contrast mix or omission of the saline chase.

Delivery: via dual-chamber power injector, antecubital 18 g IV.

Region of interest: determined by anatomy.

Pediatric

Weight-based protocol (ALARA).

80—120 kVp, 30—80 mA/rotation.

Cardiac gated with dose modulation for coronary and function evaluations.

Contrast 2 ml/kg, triggered with aortic region.

1.5—2 ml/s for 22 g, 3 ml/s for 20 g.

Manual injection for supervised sedated patient.

Image post-processing

A. 2-D Standard cardiac anatomic views

Ventricular short- and long-axis images.

RVOT, RV inflow, LVOT, perpendicular to LVOT.

Aortic valve, aortic arch sagittal view.

Proximal pulmonary artery views.

SVC and IVC.

B. 2-D Non-standard anatomic imaging

Double oblique images of shunts, surgical connections.

For example, ASD, VSD, baffle, Fontan channel etc.

C. 2-D Gated imaging

Ventricular short axis.

RV views for dysplasia detection.

Aortic valvular thin slice for valve area measurement.

Prosthetic valve short-axis systolic and diastolic imaging.

D. 3-D Volume rendering

Overview of vascular connections.

Visualize anatomic relationship for shunts.

Overview of endovascular stent location.

4. Which *osmolality* of contrast is appropriate? Relatively high osmolality nonionic contrast agents are routinely utilized for CT angiography. For adults with CHD, who have cardiac dysfunction, lower-osmolality contrast or isosmolar contrast agents may provide sufficient image quality for visualization of cardiac structure and function, with reduced likelihood of adverse chemotoxic reactions [7].

5. Is contrast CT safe in the setting of *Eisenmenger* syndrome? Special consideration should be given to safety of CTA in CHD when there may be a risk of paradoxical air embolism, and patients with right-to-left shunt are at increased risk. Use of an air-filtered intravenous line will protect against paradoxical air bubble embolism. Patients with pulmonary hypertension and Eisenmenger syndrome have a very high rate of pulmonary arterial thrombus formation, and this is particularly seen in women and in the setting of low oxygen saturation [8].

6. *Radiation exposure* should be the minimum required for diagnostic images (ALARA). Radiation dose varies with the square of the kilovoltage. A small reduction in kVp in addition to the use of ECG-dependent dose modulation can reduce the magnitude of estimated exposure by 50–65% in gated contrast CT. Image noise increases as tube energy decreases, but this may be offset by use of increased tube current, when possible, depending on the CT manufacturer. ECG-dependent dose modulation may not be appropriate in arrhythmic patients, in whom image quality needs to be optimized throughout the cardiac cycle [9].

7. *Double oblique reformation of image planes* is crucial for demonstration of normal and abnormal relationships between structures and for determination of the true short axis of any structure. This technique should be applied for accurate measurement of any structural narrowing in a "true" short axis, for example, subaortic narrowing, shunt or conduit narrowing, aortic coarctation, in recognition that long-axis views may be misleading. On gated CT data, the presence of dynamic narrowing of pulsatile and contractile tissue should be considered (e.g., systolic outflow tract obstruction).

8. *Coronary anomalies* are defined by considering the origin, course, and termination of the coronary artery. Presence of high flow (e.g., due to fistulous connection to the RV or origin of a coronary from the pulmonary artery) leads to marked dilation of the entire coronary arterial tree. If the LCA arises from the right coronary sinus (anterior sinus of Valsalva), the anomalous passage of this artery between the MPA and aorta is associated with risk of sudden cardiac death [10].

9. *Prosthetic valves*, implanted metal devices, metal stents, and surgical clips are all associated with beam-hardening artifacts that may distort surrounding structures. Inspection of the device itself may be achieved through windowing and leveling images in order to obtain clear visualization of device components and possibly function (e.g., prosthetic valve leaflet motion). In gated CT, systolic and diastolic positions of prosthetic leaflets may be clearly demonstrated.

10. *Atrial septal defects*. Occluder device closure suitability is defined by the size and location of the ASD. Defects associated with anomalous venous connections or defects without a surrounding rim of atrial septal tissue are not suitable for closure by device. Complications of device placement include erosion of neighboring structures (aortic root), obstruction of venous return and embolization due to malpositioning or inadequate rim tissue.

11. *Late complications after the Fontan* operation can be considered in terms of the Fontan circuit itself, the systemic arterial system, and the non-cardiovascular

complications. CT data should be inspected to exclude the presence of narrowing of the Fontan pathway, pathway leak, presence of thromboembolism, or evidence of marked dilation of a residual systemic venous atrium (and associated hepatic congestion). The systemic ventricular size, overall function, and both pulmonary venous return and ventriculo-aortic outflow should be evaluated, noting that a morphologic right ventricle is prone to failure when it functions for long term at systemic arterial pressure. Systemic venous collateralization (systemic or hepatic veins connecting to pulmonary veins or left atrium) and pulmonary arteriovenous malformations are potential causes of progressive hypoxia and may be amenable to transcatheter closure, and should be reported if seen by CT [11].

12. *Late complications of repaired TGA* are dependent on the type of repair procedure performed and the presence or absence of an associated VSD. With an atrial switch repair (Mustard and Senning), check the systemic right ventricular function and look for baffle obstruction or leak. With a Rastelli repair, there is long-term risk of biventricular dysfunction and attention should be given to possible (relatively common) RV-PA conduit stenosis. With a Jatene arterial switch, the more common long-term problems are with supravalvular or peripheral pulmonary arterial stenosis and stenosis or occlusion of re-implanted coronary arteries [12].

13. *Late complications after correction of Tetralogy of Fallot* include right ventricular dilation and dysfunction (often a consequence of severe chronic pulmonary regurgitation), and right ventricular outflow tract obstruction either at the infundibular level or potentially at any level of the pulmonary arterial tree. Aortic root dilation with aortic valvular regurgitation and left ventricular dysfunction may also occur [13].

14. What are *rings and slings*? In the setting of abnormal thoracic aortic anatomy, the arch-branching pattern and the relationship of pulmonary arterial, systemic arterial, esophageal, and tracheal structures should be carefully inspected. Aberrant origin of the left subclavian artery in a right-sided aortic arch is associated with aneurysmal dilation of the diverticulum of Kommerel and may present with a mediastinal mass or chest pain. Vascular rings may require surgical intervention due to the presence of tracheal and esophageal constriction from aberrant vessels and the fibrous remnant of ductus arteriosus.

References

1. Marelli AJ, Mackie AS, Ionescu-Ittu R, Rahme E, Pilote L. Congenital heart disease in the general population: changing prevalence and age distribution. Circulation. 2007 Jan 16, 115(2): 163–72. Epub 2007 Jan 8.
2. Warnes CA, Liberthson R, Danielson GK, Dore A, Harris L, Hoffman JI, Somerville J, Williams RG, Webb GD. Task force 1: the changing profile of congenital heart disease in adult life. J Am Coll Cardiol. 2001 Apr, 37(5): 1170–5.
3. Webb GD, Williams RG. Summary of recommendations- Care of the adult with congenital heart disease 32nd Bethesda conference, J Am Coll Cardiol 2001, 37(5): 1161–98

4. Therrien J, Dore A, Gersony W, Iserin L, Liberthson R, Meijboom F, Colman JM, Oechslin E, Taylor D, Perloff J, Somerville J, Webb GD. CCS Consensus conference 2001 update: recommendations for the management of adults with congenital heart disease Part 1. Can J Cardiol 2001, 17(9): 944–959

5. Tynan MJ, Becker AE, Macartney FJ, Jimenez MQ, Shinebourne EA, Anderson RH. Nomenclature and classification of congenital heart disease, Br Heart J 1979, 41(5): 544–53

6. Leschka S, Oechslin E, Husmann L, Desbiolles L, Marincek B, Genoni M, Pretre R, Jenni R, Wildermuth S, Alkadhi H. Pre- and postoperative evaluation of congenital heart disease in children and adults with 64-section CT. Radiographics. 2007 May–Jun, 27(3): 829–46.

7. Bush WH, Swanson DP. Acute reactions to intravenous contrast media: types, risk factors, recognition and specific treatment. AJR 1991 157: 1153–1161

8. Silversides CK, Granton JT, Konen E, Hart MA, Webb GD, Therrien J. Pulmonary thrombosis in adults with Eisenmenger syndrome. J Am Coll Cardiol. 2003 Dec 3, 42(11): 1982–7.

9. Hausleiter J, Meyer T, Hadamitzky M, Huber E, Zankl M, Martinoff S, Kastrati A, Schomig A. Radiation dose estimates from cardiac multislice computed tomography in daily practice. Impact of different scanning protocols on effective dose estimates. Circulation 2006, 113: 1305–1310

10. Dodd JD, Ferencik M, Liberthson RR, Cury RC, Hoffmann U, Brady TJ, Abbara S. Congenital anomalies of coronary artery origin in adults: 64-MDCT appearance. AJR Am J Roentgenol. 2007 Feb, 188(2): W138–46.

11. Varma C, Warr MR, Hendler AL, Paul NS, Webb GD, Therrien J. Prevalence of "silent" pulmonary emboli in adults after the Fontan operation. J Am Coll Cardiol. 2003 Jun 18, 41(12): 2252–8.

12. Cook SC, McCarthy M, Daniels CJ, Cheatham JP, Raman SV. Usefulness of multislice computed tomography angiography to evaluate intravascular stents and transcatheter occlusion devices in patients with d-transposition of the great arteries after mustard repair. Am J Cardiol. 2004 Oct 1, 94(7): 967–9.

13. Raman SV, Cook SC, McCarthy B, Ferketich AK. Usefulness of multidetector row computed tomography to quantify right ventricular size and function in adults with either tetralogy of Fallot or transposition of the great arteries. Am J Cardiol. 2005 Mar 1, 95(5): 683–6.

Chapter 17
Cardiovascular CT: Assessment of the Lower Extremity Vasculature

John R. Lesser, Bjorn P. Flygenring, Alan T. Hirsch, Thomas Knickelbine, Terrance F. Longe, and Robert S. Schwartz

Reliable non-invasive CT imaging of the peripheral arterial vasculature has been possible since the advent of four-row multidetector CT angiography (MDCTA) [1, 2, 3, 4, 5]. MDCTA evaluation of the peripheral arteries provides specific anatomic diagnoses and allows better targeted interventional therapeutic procedures. Four-row studies using a 2.5 mm collimator with 3 mm reconstructed slices [1, 3] compared diagnostic accuracy against digital subtraction angiography (DSA). The sensitivity, specificity, and accuracy for stenosis detection using four-row MDCTA was greater than 90% at the aortoiliac and femoropopliteal levels but was significantly worse in the infrapopliteal vessels [5]. Four-row MDCTA may thus falsely indicate a total occlusion (false positive), or miss an occlusion because of well-developed collaterals (false negative). Problems with the four- and eight-slice CT include a longitudinal (z-axis) spatial resolution of 1 mm, which is inadequate for the small size of the infrapopliteal vessels. Moreover, it does not match the in-plane (x and y axes) resolution of 0.5–0.7 mm [6]. As a result, reconstructed images off the axial dimension degrade image quality because the voxel is non-isotropic, or unequal in all three spatial dimensions, which yields image distortion [6].

By increasing the detector rows from 4 to 16 and by using smaller detector elements combined with smaller collimation, the spatial resolution improved to ~ 0.6 mm along the longitudinal (z) axis with isotropic voxels. The 16- and higher row MDCT scanners permit image reconstruction in any orientation with large-volume coverage from the diaphragm to the feet along with a short breath-hold time. Compared to DSA, a 16-MDCT scanner had a sensitivity of 96 % and a specificity of 85% using a 2 mm slice width for detection of significant stenosis. By decreasing the slice thickness to 0.75 mm, the sensitivity and the specificity improved to 98% and 95%, respectively. The advantage was seen most in the infrapopliteal vessels [7]. Another study using 2–3 mm slice widths showed that additional non-CT imaging was more often required in those whose arteries were more calcified [8] because of non-diagnostic arterial segments. Thinner slices such as those present in 64-row MDCT scanners result in smaller voxels (z-axis spatial resolution <0.4 mm), which

J.R. Lesser
Minneapolis Heart Institute Foundation and the University of Minnesota, Minneapolis, MN, USA
e-mail: john.lesser@allina.com

M.J. Budoff, J.S. Shinbane (eds.), *Handbook of Cardiovascular CT*,
DOI: 10.1007/978-1-84800-091-9_17, © Springer-Verlag London Limited 2008

lessen the partial volume effects from calcium and improve luminal visualization. No trials have measured the impact of 64-row MDCTA imaging in patients with heavy calcification. Overall, MDCTA provides very high diagnostic accuracy for the assessment of vascular stenoses [5, 20].

17.1 Alternative Anatomic Test: MRA

Peripheral vascular MRA and MDCTA have an equivalent ability relative to the DSA gold standard for evaluating aortoiliac and renal artery stenoses when using scans with similar voxel dimensions and slice width (2–3 mm) [9, 10]. Current 64-row MDCT scans have better z-axis spatial resolution (<0.4 mm) than the best 3D MRA exams (∼1 mm), but time-resolved images of often calcified infrapopliteal vessels offer an advantage with MRA. A head-to-head comparison is not yet available. The ability of either test to identify and quantify aneurysmal disease is equivalent. These tests are also similarly valuable in visualizing vascular bypass grafts. MRA is preferred in patients with heavy vascular calcification [8], and MDCTA is preferable in patients with prior metallic device implants (e.g., stents, stent grafts) [11, 12]. In younger patients, MRA may be the preferred technique because of the lack of ionizing radiation. An MDCTA scan involves much less time in the scanner than MRA, allowing adequate scans in patients who have difficulty lying still. Patients with renal insufficiency represent a problem for either scan type because of CTA-related iodinated contrast or MR gadolinium–related nephrogenic systemic fibrosis [13]. The decision to use one test or the other is often dependent on the degree of local expertise or the presence of a relative or absolute contraindication for a specific test.

17.2 Alternative Anatomic Test: DSA

Lower extremity MDCTA is nearly equivalent to DSA in accurately measuring stenosis severity (see above) and may be better at visualizing collateralized distal infrapopliteal vessels in patients with multiple proximal vessel occlusions. MDCTA is clearly superior to DSA in determining the presence and size of aneurysmal disease. As a cross-sectional imaging technique, MDCTA shows both the vascular lumen and the wall, allowing an accurate assessment including intramural thrombus, hematoma, and/or a false lumen. Its greatest advantage is avoiding invasive complications of DSA, including groin site bleeding, femoral pseudoaneurysm, AV fistulae, and catheter-related cholesterol embolization [5]. Using automatic radiation dose reduction techniques, the MDCTA radiation dose is slightly lower than DSA [14]. The iodinated contrast dose is comparable but is dependent on the vascular beds examined. MDCTA can only assess anatomy. However, during DSA, an interventionalist can measure a translesional pressure with and without papaverine or nitroglycerine provocation in order to assess the physiologic significance of a stenosis.

DSA also has better spatial resolution (~0.2 mm) but only provides limited 2D views relative to the 3D capability of MDCT scanners with isotropic voxels.

17.3 Indications (Lower extremity MDCTA) [15]

- Assess peripheral arterial anatomy for location and severity of stenoses. (This most often follows a lower extremity Doppler and/or pressure-pulse volume recording.)

  ○ Thigh and/or calf claudication in the setting of an abnormal Doppler or abnormal (or pseudonormalized) ABI rest/rest–exercise test
  ○ Buttock claudication (assess internal iliac arteries)
  ○ Critical limb ischemia (non-healing ulcers, gangrene)

- Evaluate possible acute or chronic mesenteric ischemia [12]

  ○ Assess mesenteric arterial stenoses (**Fig. 17.1**) and the bowel wall for ischemic changes
  ○ Assess mesenteric venous occlusion

- Assess renal arteries (mostly searching for a correctable secondary cause of hypertension)

  ○ Evaluate fibromuscular dysplasia (**Fig. 17.2**)
  ○ Atherosclerotic vascular stenosis
  ○ Renal artery and venous anatomy for renal donor evaluation

- Provide associated soft tissue diagnostic information connected with peripheral arterial disease (e.g., location of the medial head of the gastrocnemius with popliteal entrapment, cystic advential disease) [15, 16]
- Assess precise aneurysm size and location (particularly useful in identifying the frequent presence of multiple aneurysms otherwise unrecognized from a screening ultrasound) [15, 16] (**Figs. 17.3–17.5**)

  ○ Use for surveillance of aneurysm size in those with unreliable ultrasound information or as an alternative to ultrasound
  ○ Pre-op stent graft or surgical planning
  ○ Post-stent graft surveillance for aneurysm size and presence of stent graft endoleaks [11, 17] (**Fig. 17.11**)
  ○ Surveillance of prior aortic dissection to assess total aortic size and status of vascular branch perfusion to end-organs

- Evaluate vascular stent stenosis in those with suspected restenosis based on ultrasound and/or symptoms (**Figs. 17.7, 17.8**)
- Assess surgical bypass graft stenosis or patency in those with abnormal surveillance ultrasound or symptoms (**Figs. 17.5, 17.9**)

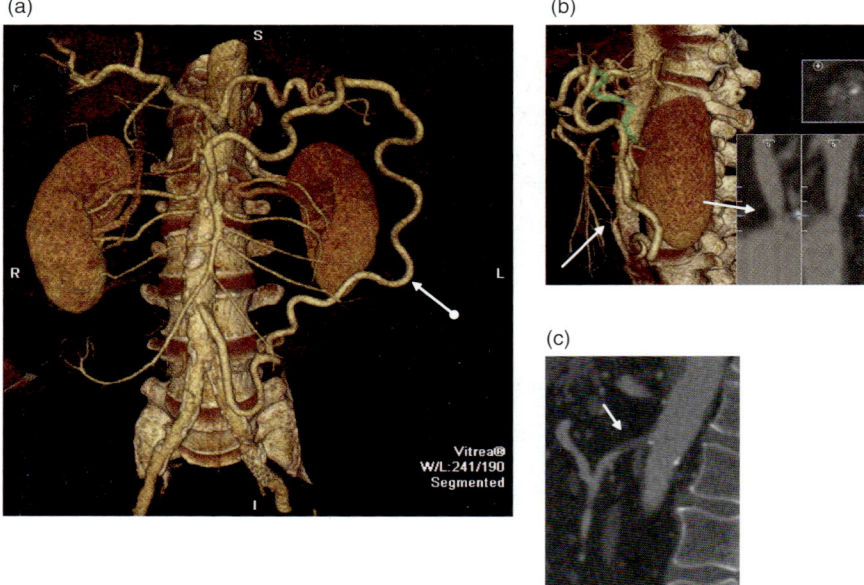

Fig. 17.1 In a patient with abdominal angina, the coronal VR image (**a**) demonstrates a large IMA to SMA (L colic a.) collateral called the "arc of Riolan" (*arrow*). A centerline image (**b**) of the celiac a. and the VR image of the IMA ostia show significant lesions (*white arrows*). A sagittal MPR (**c**) image documents a well-collateralized SMA occluded at its ostium (*arrow*)

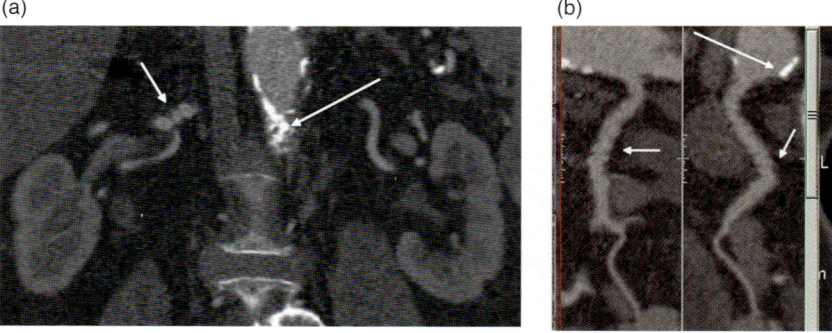

Fig. 17.2 Fibromuscular dysplasia of the mid-R renal artery is seen in an MPR coronal image (**a**), (*short arrow*) using the minimum 0.6 mm slice width. The same R renal artery is seen using a centerline technique (**b**) in orthogonal views (*short arrows*). Note the characteristic beaded appearance. The patient has concomitant aortic atherosclerosis (*long arrows*)

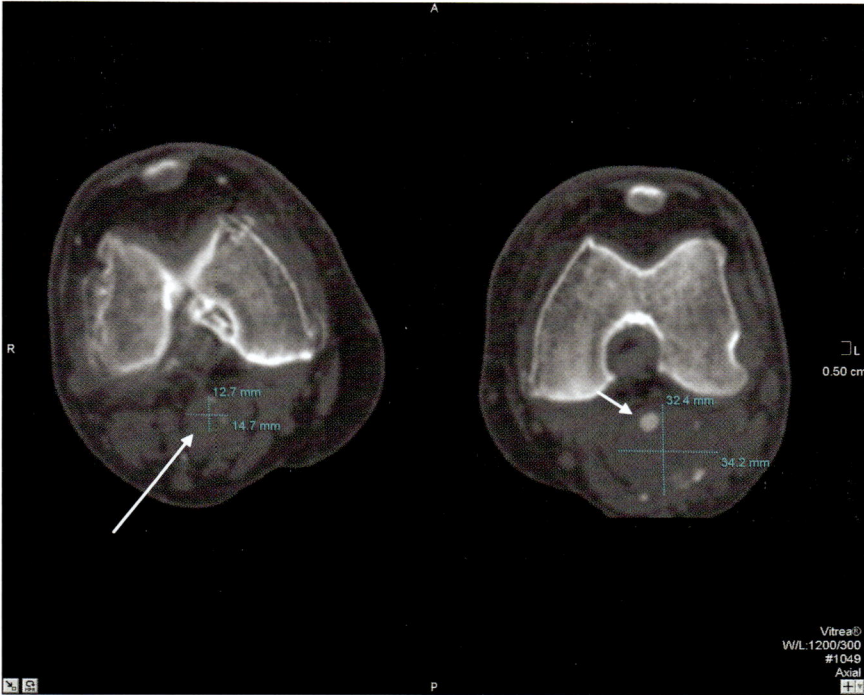

Fig. 17.3   An axial multiplanar reconstruction view shows bilateral popliteal aneurysms. (>0.7 cm). The smaller R-sided aneurysm is occluded (*long arrow*). The left is large with an eccentric lumen (*arrow*). Elective surgery is indicated for a popliteal aneurysm >2 cm [15] to prevent future thrombosis or embolization

(a)   (b)   (c)

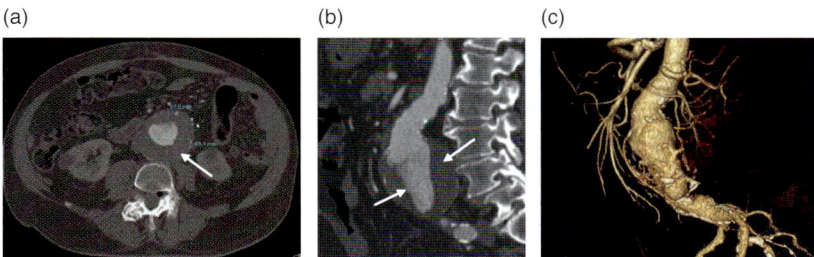

Fig. 17.4 Asymptomatic AAA. The axial (**a**) and sagittal (**b**) measurements show the aneurysm to be much larger than seen on the sagittal VR image (**c**). The large amount of intramural thrombus within the aneurysm sac (**a**), (*arrows*) has low HU and is not seen in the VR reconstruction (**c**). Detailed diagnoses and measurements should not be taken from the VR images alone

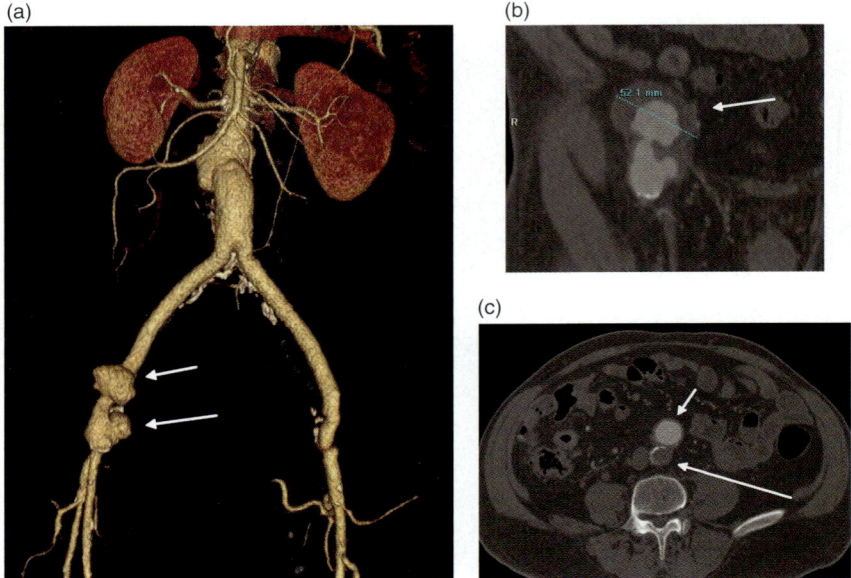

Fig. 17.5 The patient presented with a pulsatile R groin mass. Pseudoaneurysms are noted in a VR (**a**) and MRP (**b**) view at the R femoral distal anastamosis of an aortobifemoral bypass graft (*arrows*, **a** and **b**). An axial slice (**c**) shows the typical appearance of an occluded and calcified native aorta posteriorly (*long arrow*) with a patent aortic component of the graft (*short arrow*). Surgical revision was required

17.4 Contraindications

- Significant renal insufficiency—assess risk versus benefit of contrast load

  - Minimize contrast volume
  - Pre-treat with saline, bicarbonate, and N-acetylcysteine

- Contrast allergy

  - Pre-treat with prednisone, and H1 and H2 antihistamines

- Relatively radiation sensitive—assess risk versus benefit of exposure

  - Woman of child-bearing age

    - Check pregnancy test, if sexually active

  - Young woman
  - Child

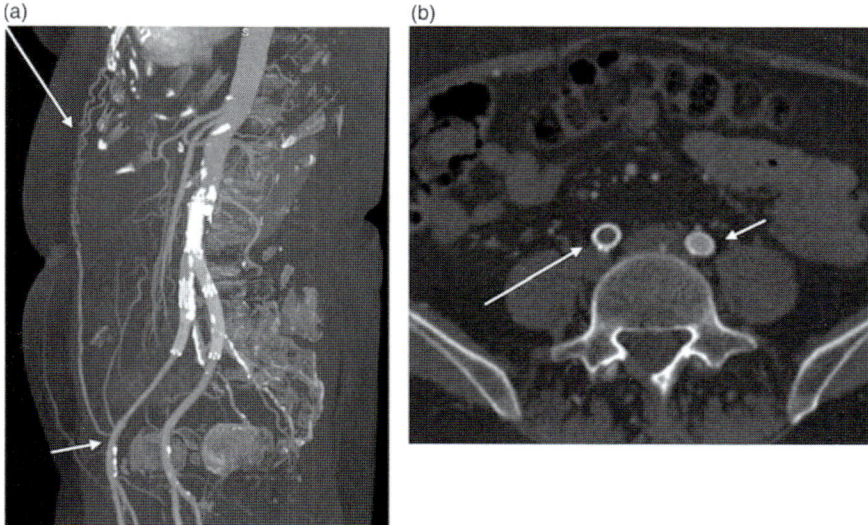

Fig. 17.6 Well-developed abdominal wall collaterals (**a**), (*long arrow*) communicate with the R common femoral a. (**a**), (*short arrow*). The thick MIP (**a**) obscures a totally occluded R common iliac stent. The axial MPR view (**b**) demonstrates an occluded R (*long arrow*) and patent L common iliac a. stent (*short arrow*)

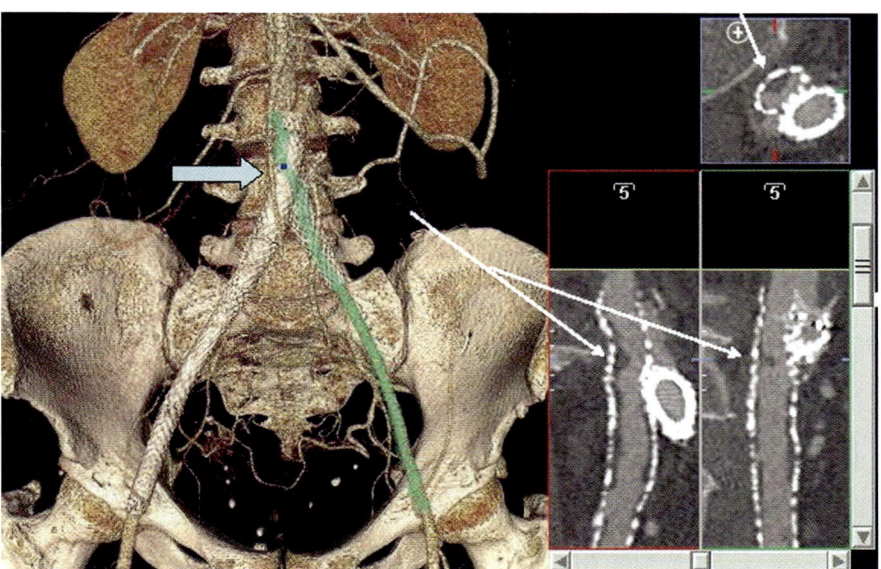

Fig. 17.7 L LE claudication 8 months after bi-iliac stents. The thinnest slice of 0.6 mm, window widened from 1200 to 1800 and the level increased from 300 to 400. A discreet L common iliac stent stenosis was seen above using a centerline technique with orthogonal long axis view (*long white arrows*) and a short-axis view (*short white arrow*). The blue dot (*blue thick arrow*) on the VR corresponds to the short-axis view. A 40 mmHg translesional gradient was present prior to intervention

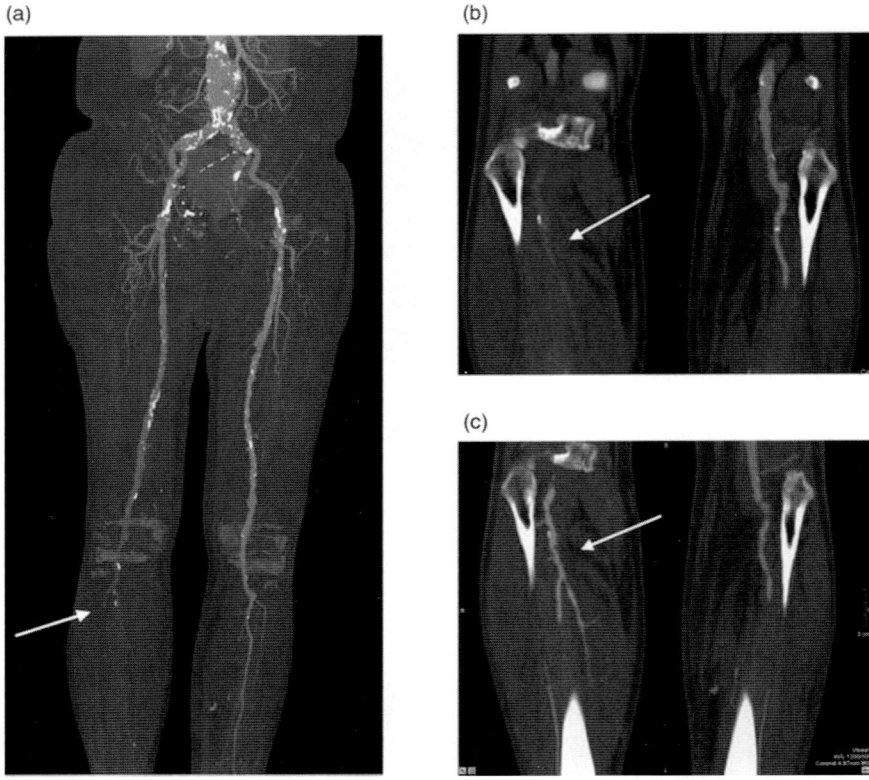

Fig. 17.8 A patient with abdominal aortic and iliac a. aneurysms had his scan "outrun the contrast" on the R leg (*arrow* **a**, **b**), despite using a slow scan. A second scan automatically followed from the suprapopliteal region to the feet and allowed an assessment of the R infrapopliteal vessels (*arrow* **c**)

17.5 Scan Preparation:

- Creatinine obtained, 18–20 gauge IV in or near the antecubital fossa, obtain history of contrast allergy or prior surgery and/or intervention

    Scan Plan (16- to 64-row MDCTA): Scan field from the diaphragm to the mid-thigh (short scan; **Fig. 17.10a**).

Scan goal:

- ○ Assess mesenteric vessels, renovascular disease, aortoiliac and pelvic stenoses as well as aneurysms, and follow-up AAA stent grafts

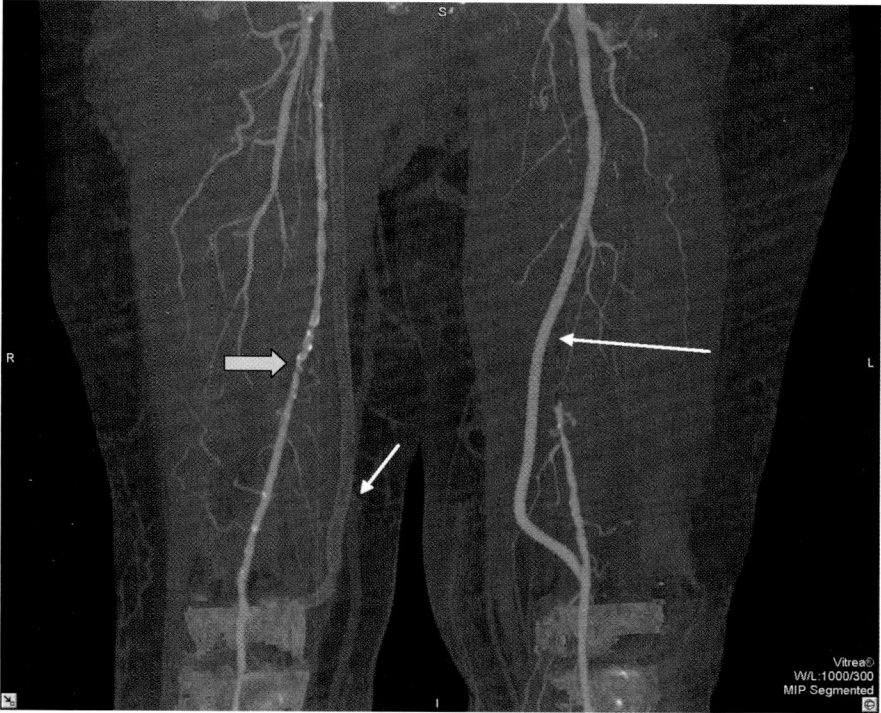

Fig. 17.9 New R-sided claudication. This image shows the femoral to popliteal region in a coronal view. A thick MIP provides an anatomic overview. Serrations are noted in a patent (*long arrow*) L fem-pop prosthetic (PTFE) above the knee graft and an occluded R fem-pop PTFE graft (*short arrow*). A significant residual mid-SFA lesion is present (*thick blue arrow*)

- Contrast type and injection protocol (see **Table 17.1**)
  - ○ Short scan field involves a shorter scan time. One must allow enough contrast to fill the vasculature before the scanner starts (This represents either starting at a high Hounsfield unit [HU] for bolus tracking or increasing an empiric scan delay with a timing bolus).
  - ○ Scan initiation by bolus tracking
    - ▪ Region of interest (ROI) in the aorta at the diaphragm
    - ▪ HU threshold for the scan at 200 HU allows the attenuation to be adequate in the area of interest.
  - ○ Scan initiation after timing bolus
    - ▪ 15–20 ml dose set for the initial rapid contrast delivery rate (e.g., 5 ml/s). Measure the time to arrival of contrast in the aorta at the diaphragm plus an empiric correction factor or scanning delay (e.g., 4–5 s).

(a)   (b)

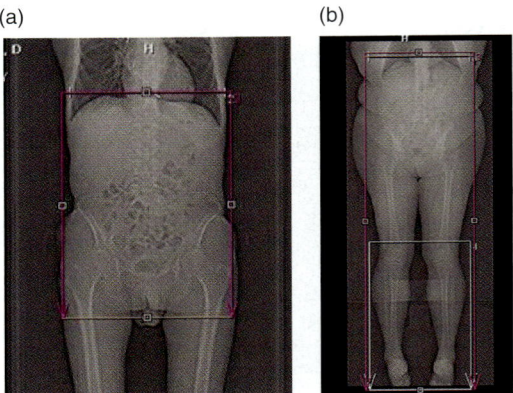

Fig. 17.10 The short scan field (**a**) for renal, mesenteric, abdominal aortic aneurysm, and AAA stent graft follow-up requires less contrast and can be imaged with a fast rotation time and table feed (however, slow table feed is recommended). The scan field of an abdominal aorta with runoffs (**b**) includes the diaphragm through the feet (*purple rectangle*). A second scan is set up from the suprapopliteal region through the feet (*white rectangle*) to follow immediately after the longer scan. This is to ensure that the infrapopliteal vessels are imaged

Table 17.1 Scan Protocols 16- through 64-row scanners

Scan Field: Diaphragm to Thigh	*#Contrast Rate and Volume	Bolus Tracking
(**Post-stent graft: see below)	4–5 ml/s for 120 ml, then saline 5 ml/s for 40 ml	HU threshold = 200
Table feed <30 mm/s; 0.5 s/rotation; scan time <40 s or Table feed >30 mm/s; <0.5 s/rotation; scan time <40 s		ROI at diaphragm
Scan Field: Diaphragm to Toes	*#Contrast Rate and Volume*	*Bolus Tracking*
(^Set up a second scan: popliteal to toes)	5 ml/s for 80 ml and then 3.5 ml/s for 60 ml, then saline at 3.5 ml/s for 40 ml	HU threshold = 150
Table feed <30 mm/s; 0.5 s/rotation; scan time >40 s		ROI at diaphragm

*Increase rate of injection for wt > 90 kg and decrease for wt < 60 kg.
Post-stent graft: initial non-contrast scan reconstructed at 3–5 mm. May follow with a 90 second post-contrast scan reconstructed at 3–5 mm (Fig. 17.11**).
^Second scan will automatically initiate unless stopped by the technician (**Fig. 10b**).
#Use non-ionic contrast with iodine content from 300 to 370 mg/dl (Vascular attenuation = iodine flux = rate of injection (ml/s) × iodine content (mg/dl)).

○ Protocol (see **Table 17.1**; the slow scan with table feed of <30 mm/s; 0.5 s/ rotation is recommended)

   Scan Plan: (16- to 64-row MDCTA): Scan field from the diaphragm through the toes (long scan; **Fig. 17.10b**).

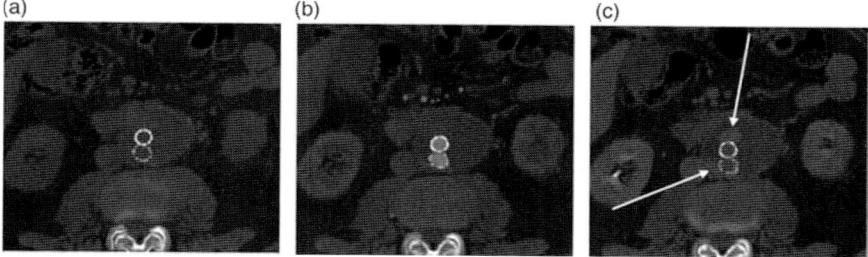

Fig. 17.11 Abdominal aortic stent graft follow-up after 1 year. Non-contrast (**a**), contrast (**b**), and 5 min post-contrast scan (**c**) performed. These axial slices are at the same position using a 3 mm thickness. HU (80–117) within the aneurysm sac shows a small contrast leak seen on the delayed scan (**c**) superiorly at 12 and 7 o'clock (*long arrows*). A lumbar a. branch connects to the region at 7 o'clock (not shown). This type II leak is small and the aneurysm size will be followed by serial scans

Scan goal

○ Evaluate the entire abdominal aorta through the infrapopliteal arteries

- Recommend slowing the table feed to <30 mm/s (0.5 s rotation time) to minimize the potential of "outrunning the contrast bolus" (**Fig. 17.11**)
- Despite the slower gantry rotation time and table feed, pre-plan a second scan (**Fig. 17.10b**) to start immediately following the first scan (e.g., a technician can elect to cancel the second scan if the initial infrapopliteal arterial contrast levels are adequate).
- The longer the scan time, the greater the distal peripheral vascular attenuation with a constant injection rate [18] (e.g., SFA vessels become brighter than the more proximal abdominal aorta).
- Injection protocol (see **Table 17.1**)

○ Scan initiation by bolus tracking

- ROI in the aorta at the diaphragm
- HU threshold of 150 for the scan initiation

○ Scan initiation after timing bolus

- 15–20 ml dose set for the initial rapid contrast delivery rate (e.g., 5 ml/s). Measure the time to arrival of contrast in the aorta at the diaphragm plus an empiric correction factor or scanning delay (e.g., 4 5 s).

17.6 Image interpretation

Clinical Pearls):

- Abdominal aorta or branch artery aneurysm assessment (**Figs. 17.3–17.5**)

○ Identify where the aneurysm starts (e.g., infrarenal) and ends (e.g., just proximal to the distal common iliac bifurcation).

o Measure aneurysm size including the outer edge to the outer edge that includes both the largest area of contrast and the intramural thrombus. Measure in the axial orientation with both AP and right-to-left dimensions, and provide the slice number at the site with the largest dimension for comparison using serial studies. Obtain a centerline measurement to give a major and minor axis dimension that identifies the largest pathophysiologic dimension (e.g., tortuous vessels may be obliquely cut in arbitrary views such as an axial orientation).

o Pre-stent graft planning includes a diameter of the aneurysm neck just beneath the lowest renal artery, the length from the start of the neck to the beginning of the aneurysm, degree of tortuosity of the neck, length starting 15 mm distal to the start of the neck through the extent of the aneurysm (often including the distance up to the external and internal iliac bifurcation).

• Celiac axis

o Identify the major branches and possible anatomic variants (e.g., combined celiac and SMA origin or separate gastric or common hepatic artery off the aorta). Check for aneurysms (e.g., splenic artery aneurysms are often silent and found incidentally).

o The median arcuate ligament can compress the celiac trunk with inspiration and be the cause of arterial narrowing in the absence of atherosclerotic disease

• Superior mesenteric artery (SMA)

o Combined ostium with the celiac artery may falsely suggest an SMA occlusion.

o May be a source of collaterals to the celiac or inferior mesenteric artery (IMA) or receive collaterals from the IMA (e.g., arc of Riolan) (**Fig. 17.1**).

o Abdominal angina usually requires at least a severe stenosis in two of the three mesenteric vessels (**Fig. 17.1**).

• Inferior mesenteric artery

o Often occluded or stenotic in the presence of an infrarenal abdominal aortic aneurysm

o Common source of collaterals to the SMA (**Fig. 17.1**)

• Renal arteries

o Multiple ostia may branch from the abdominal aorta for each kidney. The arteries may rarely originate from the common iliac arteries.

o Atherosclerotic disease often involves the ostia or proximal vessel, and fibromuscular dysplasia occurs in the distal arterial segments.

o Fibromuscular dysplasia may be present at any age but should be suspected in those with hypertension starting at age <30 years. Use the smallest voxel (0.4 mm or 0.6–0.75 mm slice width) to evaluate vascular beading because the spatial resolution of the thicker slices may be inadequate to see the beading (**Fig. 17.2**).

○ Report kidney size (longest length from pole to pole) in the setting of renal artery stenoses.

• Common and external iliac artery occlusions are often collateralized by vessels communicating with an internal mammary artery along the chest wall and then to the common femoral artery (**Fig. 17.7**).

• Internal iliac stenoses may be isolated and create buttock claudication with normal ABIs.

• Femoral, external, and common iliac artery size and severity of tortuosity should be mentioned for each possible stent graft candidate.

• Superficial femoral artery lesions (**Fig. 17.6**) are a common cause of calf claudication and often present as a collateralized total occlusion.

○ Measure the total length of an occlusion. Technical factors that negatively influence long-term post-PTA patency include an occlusion >10 cm, multiple lesions, <2 infrapopliteal unobstructed run-off vessels.

• Popliteal artery aneurysms are bilateral in 50–70%, and 30–50% have AAAs [16]. They are often asymptomatic but may present with an acute occlusion or distal embolization (**Fig. 17.3**).

• Critical limb ischemia can be improved by correcting inflow problems. If this is not adequate alone, revascularization (e.g., fem-tibial graft) of an infrapopliteal vessel that provides continuous flow to the foot can eliminate resting ischemia and prevent amputation.

17.7 Dataset Reconstruction

• In order to create a manageable number of images, we initially reconstruct a dataset with 1 mm slices and no overlapping intervals. If there is unclear stenosis severity or a heavily calcified segment, we create the thinnest slice compatible with an acceptable level of noise (e.g., 0.6 mm without overlap).

17.8 Software Techniques for Interpretation

• The volume-rendered (VR) technique and/or thick maximal intensity projection (MIP) images [19] provide an important overview of the vascular pathology but are insufficient for a precise diagnosis (**Figs. 17.2, 17.4, 17.5, 17.7**).

○ This is particularly useful in viewing the course of vascular grafts, assessing collaterals, and transmitting information about complex anatomy.

• Axial images are reviewed and measurements made to help for comparison with future studies.

- Thin (1–5 mm) MIP images are useful for review in any orientation.
- Vascular stenoses

  ○ The smaller the vessel or greater the level of calcium, the thinner the slice width (smaller voxel) required to accurately measure a stenosis (**Fig. 17.8**).
  ○ Multiple orientations are useful, including a vessel cross-section to assess the severity of an eccentric stenosis. The centerline technique is useful with a multipurpose reconstruction (MPR) to help evaluate the vessel wall adjacent to an area of calcification (**Fig. 17.8**).
  ○ "Blooming" of calcium can be reduced or the assessment of in-stent restenosis improved by widening the window and/or by using a sharper reconstruction kernel (**Fig. 17.8**).

References

1. Rubin GD, S. A., Logan L, et al. (2001). "Muti-detector row CT angiography of the lower extremity arterial inflow and runoff: initial experience." Radiology **221**: 146–158.
2. Adriaensen M, K. M., Stijnen T, et al. (2004). "Peripheral arterial disease: Therapeutic confidence of CT versus digital subtraction angiography and effects on additional imaging recommendations." Radiology **233**: 385–391.
3. Catalano C, F. F., Laghi A, et al. (2004). "Infrarenal aortic and lower-extremity arterial disease: Diagnostic performance of multi-detector row CT angiography." Radiology **231**: 555–563.
4. Ota H, T. K., Igarashi K, et al. (2004). "MDCT compared with digital subtraction angiography for assessment of lower extremity arterial occlusive disease: Importance of reviewing cross-sectional images." American Journal of Roentenology **182**: 201–209.
5. Sun, Z. (2006). "Diagnostic accuracy of multislice CT angiography in peripheral arterial disease." J Vasc Interv Radiol **17**: 1915–1921.
6. Kohl, G. (2005). "The evolution and state-of-the-art principles of multi-slice computed tomography." Proc Am Thorac Soc **2**: 470–476.
7. Schertler T, W. S., Alkadhi H, et al. (2005). "Sixteeen-detector row CT angiography for lower-leg arterial occlusive disease: analysis of section width." Radiology **237**: 649–656.
8. Ouwendijk R, K. M., van Dijk L , et al. (2006). "Vessel wall calcifications at multi-detector row CT angiography in patients with peripheral vascular disease: Effect on clinical utility and clinical predictors." Radiology **241**: 603–608.
9. Willmann JK, W. S., Pfammatter T, et al. (2003). "Aortoiliac and renal arteries: Prospective intraindividual comparison of contrast-enhanced three-dimensional MR angiography and multi-detector row CT angiography." Radiology **226**: 798–811.
10. Ouwendijk R, d. V. M., Pattynama P, et al. (2005). "Imaging peripheral arterial disease:a randomized controlled trial comparing contrast-enhanced three-dimensional MR angiography and multi-detector row CT angiography." Radiology **236**: 1094–1103.
11. Chernyak V, R. A., Patlas M, et al. (2006). "Type II endoleak after endograft implantation: Diagnosis with helical CT arteriography." Radiology **240**: 885–893.
12. Cademartiri F, R. R., Kuiper JW, et al. (2004). "Multi-detector row CT angiography in patients with abdominal angina." Radiographics **24**: 969–984.
13. Elizabeth A. Sadowski, Lindsey K. Bennett, Micah R. Chan, Andrew L. Wentland, Andrea L. Garrett, Robert W. Garrett, and Arjang Djamali (2007). "Nephrogenic Systemic Fibrosis: Risk Factors and Incidence Estimation." Radiology **243**: 148–157.

14. Willmann JK, B. B., Schertler T et al. (2005). "Aortoiliac and lower extremity arteries assessed with 16-detector row CT angiography: Prospective comparison with digital subtraction angiography." Radiology **236**: 1083–1093.
15. Hirsch AT, Z. Z., Hertzer NR, et al. (2006). "ACC/AHA Guidelines for the management of patients with peripheral arterial disease (lower extremity, renal, mesenteric, and abdominal aortic)." J Am Coll Cardiol **47**: 1239–1312.
16. Wright LB, M. W., Cruz CP, et al. (2004). "Popliteal artery disease: Diagnosis and treatment." Radiographics **24**: 467–479.
17. Stavropoulos SW, C. T., Carpenter JP, et al. (2005). "Use of CT angiography to classify endoleaks after endovascular repair of abdominal aortic aneurysms." J Vasc Interv Radiol **16**: 663–667.
18. Fleischmann D, R. G. (2005). "Quantification if intraveneously administered contrast medium transit through the peripheral arteries: Implications for CT angiography." Radiology **236**: 1076–1082.
19. Fishman EK, N. D., Heath DG, et al. (2006). "Volume rendering versus maximum intensity projection in CT angiography: What works best, when, and why." Radiographics **26**: 905–922.
20. Fleischmann D, H. R., Rubin GD (2006). "CT angiography of peripheral arterial disease." J Vasc Interv Radiol **17**: 3–26.

Chapter 18
Imaging Decisions: Cardiovascular CT Versus Cardiovascular MR

Jerold S. Shinbane, Jabi Shriki, and Patrick M. Colletti

The decision to perform cardiovascular computed tomography (CCT) versus cardiovascular magnetic resonance (CMR) imaging for the characterization of cardiovascular substrates requires knowledge of the individual strengths and limitations of these imaging techniques, the specific details of a patient's medical history, and the clinical question that needs to be addressed. In many clinical scenarios, cardiac echo is performed as an initial study to assess cardiovascular substrates, with CCT or CMR performed when further cardiovascular characterization is necessary and a noninvasive approach is preferable. Given the rapid evolution of these technologies, appropriateness criteria are being developed for specific cardiovascular indications [1].

18.1 Patient Selection and Preparation

While there is considerable effort focused on reducing the radiation exposure with CT techniques, the lack of ionizing radiation is an important strength of CMR. This issue is especially important in young patients, who may be at increased long-term risk of malignancy [2]. As opposed to iodinated contrast agents used in CT, which enhance vascular structures by increasing CT Hounsfield units, gadolinium-based contrast agents are paramagnetic and change the magnetic properties of water in close proximity to the contrast agent. The relative safety of gadolinium-based MR contrast agents is a significant strength of MR. Iodinated contrast agents are associated with a significant incidence of acute side effects including hypotension with tachycardia, hypotension with bradycardia, bronchospasm, and pulmonary edema along with acute and chronic nephropathy. Recently, gadolinium-based contrast agents though have been associated with both worsening renal function and nephrogenic systemic fibrosis in patients with moderate-to-severe renal dysfunction, particularly for patients on dialysis [3, 4].

J.S. Shinbane
Division of Cardiovascular Medicine, USC Keck School of Medicine, Los Angeles, CA, USA
e-mail: shinbane@usc.edu

M.J. Budoff, J.S. Shinbane (eds.), *Handbook of Cardiovascular CT*,
DOI: 10.1007/978-1-84800-091-9_18, © Springer-Verlag London Limited 2008

Patient size and body habitus are also important in deciding which imaging modality to employ. Image quality can be compromised in patients with an increased body mass index with CT and may require increased radiation exposure for adequate imaging [5]. This limitation is less significant with MR, although there are limitations in MR access due to extreme patient size related to magnet bore diameter and table weight limits.

Prior to scheduling CMR, patients require a complete history for ferromagnetic prosthetic implants, devices, or depositions. These may have relative or absolute contraindications to magnetic resonance imaging (MRI). It is important to ensure that patients with susceptible devices are not exposed to the MR environment [6]. Cardiac devices such as pacemakers and defibrillators are almost always considered absolute contraindications for MRI, although there is some controversy regarding the MRI of patients with these devices, with some preliminary data suggesting that MRI may not be absolutely contraindicated in this setting [7, 8]. Detailed knowledge of patient, device, scanner, scanning protocol, alternative imaging techniques, and importance of the clinical question are important factors in determination of individualized risk versus benefit of performance of an MR study [9].

Although study times for CMR have decreased due to advances in technology as well as efficiency of labs in performing protocols, studies are still significantly longer than those achieved with CCT with scanning times in the order of 6–10 s. The patient's ability to lie still and comply with breath-hold commands is important to both technologies, but can be more easily achieved with CCT, given the short study times. Claustrophobia is a common consideration in imaging some patients, although with appropriate premedication, this is seldom a cause for premature termination of an examination [10].

Special attention needs to be focused on electrocardiographic recording for monitoring and gating, as the MR environment can interfere with sensing of the QRS complex. Attention to skin prep, lead placement, and ECG vector can improve the ability to perform ECG gating and is especially important when stress imaging is being considered [11, 12]. Due to acoustic noise associated with scanning, auditory protection with earplugs is necessary.

18.2 Characterization of Cardiovascular Substrates

The ability of CMR and CCT to provide comprehensive assessment of cardiovascular structure and function, as well as extracardiac thoracic structures, makes these techniques useful in the diagnosis, facilitation of percutaneous and surgical procedures, and follow-up of patients with congenital heart disease, electrophysiologic disease, and disease processes affecting the thoracic and peripheral vasculature [13, 14, 15]. Both CMR and CCT can characterize cardiac structures and function by reproducibly assessing right and left ventricular volumes, ejection fractions, wall thickness, and wall motion [16, 17, 18]. In order to ensure visualization of the right ventricle, CCT requires attention to the timing of contrast agent injection.

Although CMR is useful in defining anomalous coronary arteries, currently CCT provides practical coronary angiography as a routinely clinically useful study [1, 5, 19, 20, 21]. Both CCT and CMR can assess tissue characteristics of coronary artery plaque, but identification of vulnerable plaques requires further study [22]. The performance of rest and stress first-pass imaging as well as delayed enhancement imaging are practical strengths of CMR over CCT. This is important to characterize ischemia and myocardial infarction. With CMR, the first-pass study during gadolinium injection at rest or with adenosine or dobutamine pharmacologic stress can be used to assess myocardial perfusion (**Fig. 18.1**). This correlates with invasive fractional flow reserve and offers prognostic information important to risk stratification [23, 24].

With delayed enhancement images, obtained 10 min after gadolinium-based contrast administration, gadolinium clears from normal myocardium, but enhances areas of fibrosis or inflammation [25]. Delayed enhancement imaging using iodinated contrast agent with CTA is also able to image fibrosis associated with myocardial infarction, but is currently less well established and limited by the overall radiation exposure required to perform the additional delayed imaging [26]. Interpretation of gadolinium delayed contrast enhancement has become more complex as it has been recognized to occur in a variety of cardiovascular disease processes associated with fibrosis or inflammation. Interpretation of delayed enhancement requires correlation of the individual patient's medical history and the posed clinical question with the pattern of delayed enhancement. The sensitivity and specificity of delayed enhancement patterns for particular disease processes requires greater investigation.

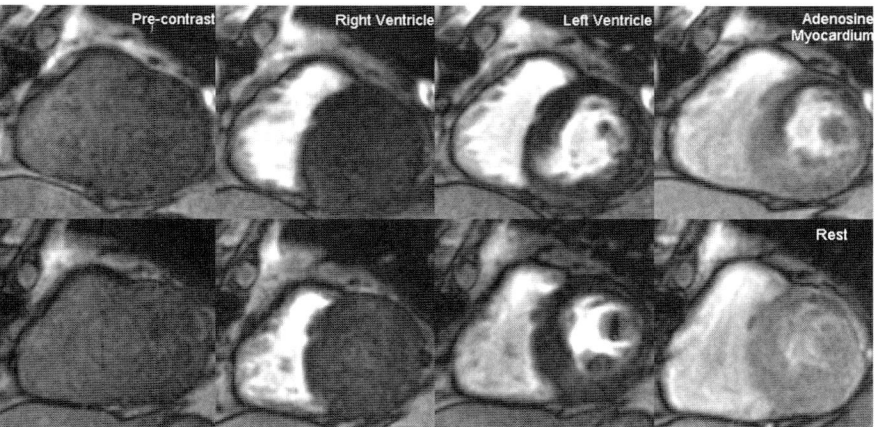

Fig. 18.1 First-pass perfusion imaging demonstrating resting normal perfusion (*lower panels*) and adenosine perfusion imaging with evidence of ischemia. Note that resting images (*bottom row*) demonstrate normal perfusion throughout the left ventricle. After administration of adenosine (*top row*), an area of slightly decreased signal intensity is demonstrated in a subendocardial distribution involving much of the anterior wall. This is consistent with an area of ischemia in the distribution of the left anterior descending coronary artery

Delayed gadolinium enhancement may be useful in assessing a variety of cardio-myopathic processes. Infarct-related delayed contrast enhancement typically occurs in the anatomic distribution of coronary arteries. There is typically subendocardial delayed enhancement with increasing degrees of transmural extension depending on the extent of infarct (**Fig.18.2**) [27]. There may be areas of peri-infarct tissue

(a)

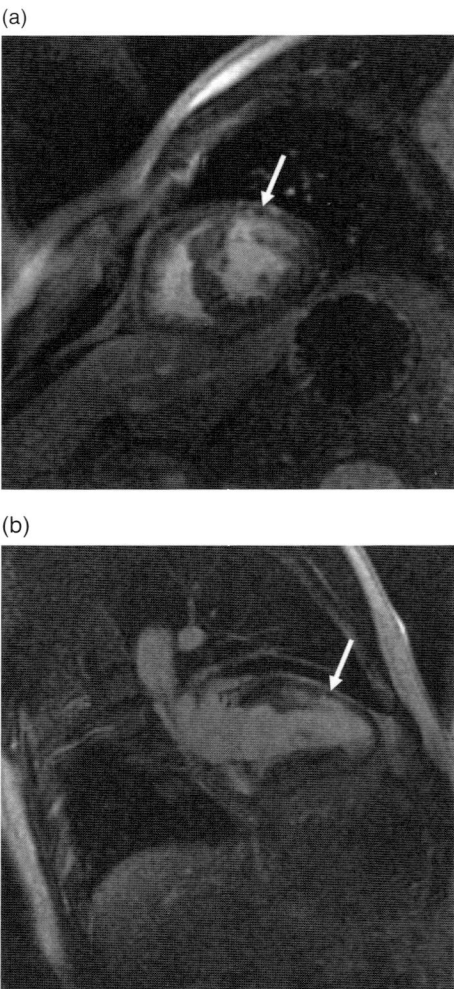

(b)

Fig. 18.2 This image demonstrates a small, mostly subendocardial infarction in the LAD territory on short axis (**a**) and two chamber, vertical long axis (**b**) views. The delayed image demonstrates hyperenhancement in the wall of the left ventricle involving the LAD territory (*arrow*), consistent with an infarction. Note that portions of the infarct are transmural, although most of the distribution is subendocardial, confirming that ischemic cardiomyopathy is the likely etiology. The presence of delayed enhancement indicates nonviability

heterogeneity, representing areas of viable myocardium and fibrosis. These hetero-geneous areas may increase the propensity for the development of ventricular tachy-cardia [28]. Delayed contrast enhancement may be useful in differentiating ischemic dilated cardiomyopathy from non-ischemic one. A delayed enhancement subendo-cardial and transmural infarct pattern is consistent with ischemic cardiomyopathy, while other patterns are not consistent with infarct, including subepicardial and mid-wall fibrosis [27]. Mid-wall fibrosis in dilated cardiomyopathy has been associated with worse prognosis and ventricular arrhythmias [29].

Delayed enhancement imaging is also useful in the characterization of other cardiomyopathic processes. In the setting of hypertrophic cardiomyopathy, delayed contrast enhancement has potential prognostic significance related to ventricular arrhythmias. In comparison to non-ischemic dilated cardiomyopathy, the dilated phase of hypertrophic cardiomyopathy has a greater extent of delayed enhancement predominantly in the septal and anterior walls [30]. In the setting of arrhythmo-genic right ventricular cardiomyopathy, delayed contrast enhancement of the right ventricle may be identified, in addition to right ventricular intramyocardial fat, increased trabeculation, abnormal ventricular size or shape, and asynergy [31].

A variety of infiltrative and of inflammatory processes can also be associ-ated with delayed contrast enhancement. In cardiac amyloid, the typical delayed enhancement pattern is a patchy subendocardial pattern (**Fig. 18.3**) [32].

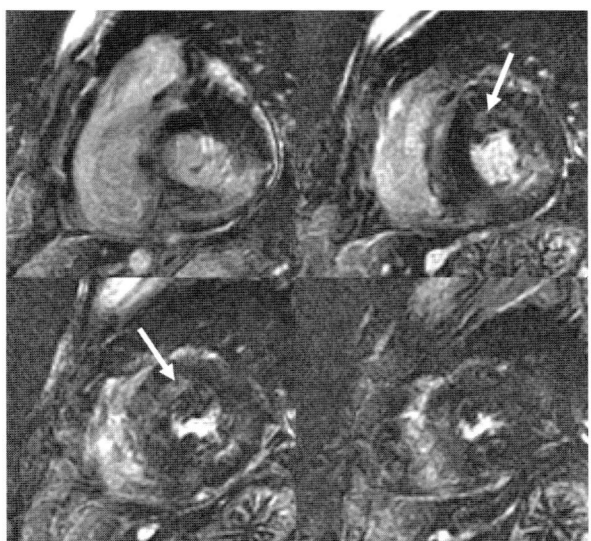

Fig. 18.3 Short-axis delayed contrast enhancement images show thickening of the left ventricle, whereas the usual pattern of coronary artery disease tends to attenuate the left ventricular wall. There are several patchy areas of delayed enhancement that do not conform well to the subendocardial distribution typically found in ischemic cardiomyopathy. Instead, there are also areas of subepicardial and mid-wall enhancement (*arrows*). In conjunction with thickening of the left ventricle, this pattern is suggestive of an infiltrative cardiomyopathy such as sarcoidosis or amyloidosis

In sarcoid, mid-wall delayed enhancement often involves the basal septum, especially the right ventricular side of the basal septum [33]. Transmural enhancement correlates with wall motion abnormalities, which may represent fibrogranulomatous tissue involvement [34]. In Chagas disease, the extent of myocardial fibrosis correlates with disease severity, and delayed enhancement imaging can detect involvement in the early asymptomatic phase of disease [35]. Delayed gadolinium enhancement can be seen in acute and chronic myocarditis and can help differentiate acute myocardial infarction from acute myocarditis, with delayed enhancement imaging pattern demonstrating a non-subendocardial distribution (**Fig. 18.4**) [36, 37].

CCT and CMR can detect cardiac masses, and assess involvement of surrounding cardiac and thoracic structures (**Fig. 18.5**). With the use of multiple pulse sequences with emphasis on T1 and T2 weighting, proton density, and perfusion imaging, CMR is especially useful in assessment of tissue characteristics of masses [38]. Mass location, tissue characteristics, and presence of pericardial or pleural

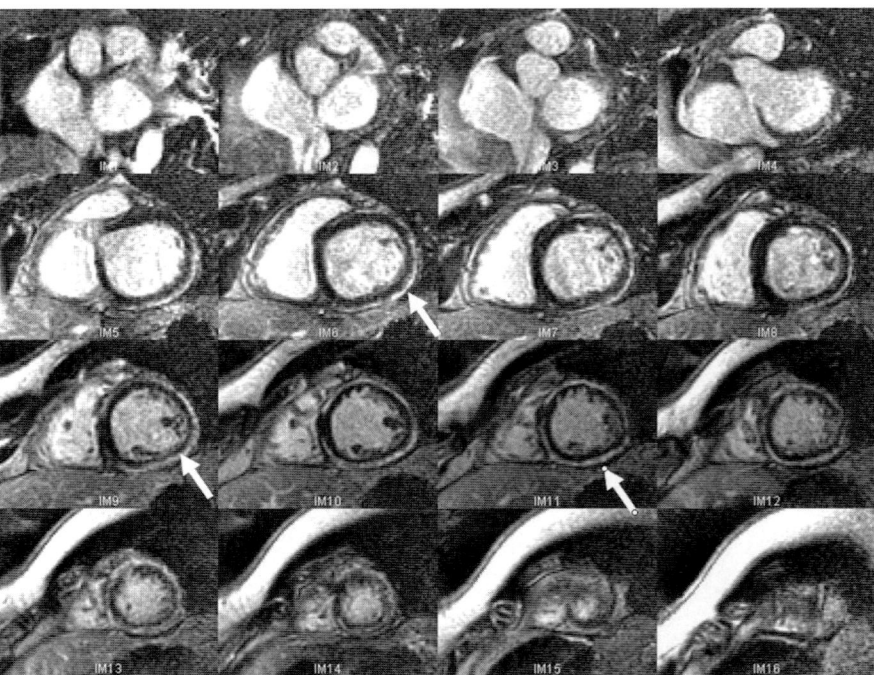

Fig. 18.4 Short-axis delayed contrast enhancement images demonstrate a large area of subepicardial enhancement (*arrows*) consistent with myocarditis. In contradistinction to **Fig. 18.2**, there is a large, band-like area of delayed enhancement mostly involving the lateral wall. Note that in this case, the enhancement involves the subepicardial portion of the wall of the left ventricle. This should raise the possibility of an alternative diagnosis rather than ischemic cardiac disease. In this case, the clinical history was consistent with viral myocarditis, and catheterization showed no significant coronary disease

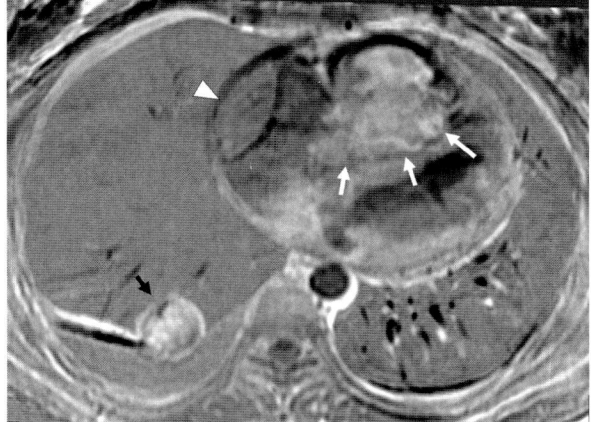

Fig. 18.5 In this case, a large, broad-based mass is present, arising from the right ventricle (*white arrows*). There is also an enhancing mass in the right atrium (*arrowhead*) with an elliptical border with the right atrial lumen. It is important to not overlook extracardiac findings. A right lower lobe enhancing mass is present (*black arrow*), likely representing a metastasis. A right pleural effusion is also present

(a)   (b)   (c)

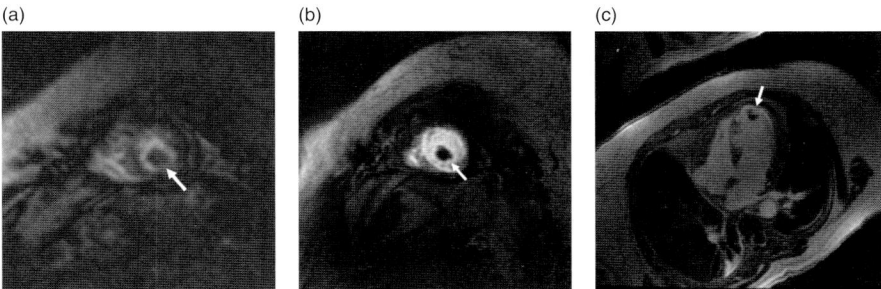

Fig. 18.6 A large ventricular infarction with apical thrombus (*arrows*) is shown. CMR is useful for demonstrating infarctions and also findings associated with infarctions including a thrombus, demonstrated on this image. Thrombi are frequently well seen on first-pass perfusion images as a non-enhancing structure within an enhancing, contrast-filled ventricle (**a**). The thrombus is also well demonstrated here on the short axis (**b**), and four-chamber (**c**) views. They frequently demonstrate low signal on all sequences and are seen adjacent to areas of infarction

involvement are important factors for evaluating and staging benign or malignant cardiac neoplasms [39]. CCT and CMR can demonstrate intracardiac thrombi. CMR is excellent for assessment of left ventricular thrombus compared to echo [40] (**Fig. 18.6**), but transesophageal echo may still be the study of choice to assess for left atrial thrombi [41, 42]. CMR also provides excellent imaging of ventricular structures such as trabeculae and is helpful in the diagnosis of ventricular non-compaction (**Fig. 18.7**) [43]. A ratio of non-compacted to compacted myocardium of greater than 2.3 by echocardiography, CMR, or CCT is useful in

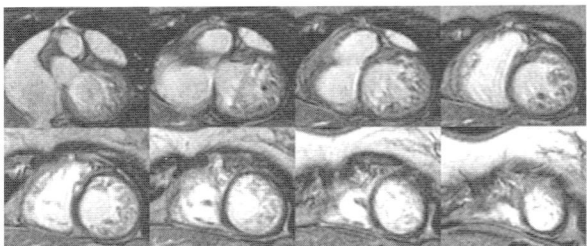

Fig. 18.7 Short-axis delayed enhancement views show deep trabeculation. Delayed enhancement images were obtained with an inversion time chosen to null myocardial signal, which would normally suppress or darken myocardium. In this case, there is bright signal from contrast in the blood pool interdigitating into the bands of non-compacted myocardium

differentiating ventricular non-compaction from other conditions including hypertrophic cardiomyopathy, dilated cardiomyopathy, hypertensive heart disease, and aortic stenosis.

Both CCT and CMR are robust imaging modalities for characterization of cardiovascular substrates. An understanding of the strengths of each modality as well as the specific clinical question, specific patient history, and imaging expertise of an individual center can help in guiding imaging decisions. Advances are rapidly occurring with newer technology and require continued updates on new applications for each individual technology.

18.3 Imaging Pearls

- Decisions related to performing CMR versus CCT require information including patient age, allergy history, clinical stability to be in the MR environment for the amount of time necessary for study given the limitations to patient monitoring, history of claustrophobia, history of ferromagnetic devices, implant or deposits, devices, renal function, cardiac rhythm and rate, strengths and limitations of other imaging modalities, and the posed clinical question.
- Contrast agents for both CT and MR are problematic in the setting of renal insufficiency, although in mild-to-moderate degrees of renal dysfunction, MR contrast agents generally carry lower risks.
- Iodinated contrast agents commonly are causally related to increasing renal dysfunction. The osmotic load of iodinated contrast agents may be high, with increased potential for both renal failure and pulmonary edema, particularly in the setting of CCT followed by catheter angiography–guided intervention.
- Gadolinium-based CMR contrast agents have been associated with nephrogenic systemic fibrosis in patients with moderate-to-severe renal dysfunction and in patients on dialysis, and are problematic to use in this setting.
- As opposed to data acquisition with CCT as one axial imaging sequence, CMR requires multiple views and MRI sequences. This requires a detailed

understanding of the cardiovascular anatomy and imaging sequences necessary to answer a particular clinical question.

- When gadolinium-based contrast agents are used in a study, a decision needs to be made whether to use the initial gadolinium injection for first-pass perfusion or to provide an MR angiogram (MRA) with the bolus timed to image a particular cardiac or vascular structure. Alternatively, a second bolus may be used if both perfusion and MRA are required.

- First-pass perfusion images of the heart, obtained just after injection of gadolinium, can be performed with CMR due to the superior temporal resolution compared with CCT. This may be helpful in evaluating for perfusion abnormalities at rest and during administration of adenosine.

- Interpretation of gadolinium delayed contrast enhancement images requires the integration of the patient's medical history, the clinical question being addressed, and the common patterns of gadolinium delayed enhancement associated with different pathologic disease states.

- Although it may be frequently difficult to discern whether an area or areas of gadolinium enhancement are related to myocardial infarctions or other causes of cardiomyopathy (HOCM, amyloidosis, sarcoidosis, etc.), subendocardial involvement with variable degrees of transmurality are more suggestive of infarctions, especially when in the expected vascular distribution of a coronary artery. Mid-wall, subepicardial, or nodular enhancement patterns should raise suspicion that other processes may be causing the abnormality.

- In the setting of ischemic heart disease, the presence of delayed enhancement suggests that the enhancing area of the myocardium is nonviable. Conversely, if a focal wall motion abnormality is identified without delayed enhancement, this may represent an area of viable myocardium, which may be chronically ischemic or stunned.

- Characterization of ancillary findings associated with infarcts, including areas of microvascular obstruction, thrombus, and aneurysms is probably better achieved with CMR compared to CCT. Microvascular obstruction is usually depicted as a subendocardial area, which is completely surrounded by delayed enhancement, but which does not itself demonstrate delayed enhancement. Thrombi are typically shown as intraluminal masses that do not enhance and are low in signal on all sequences, and occur in the regions of infarctions.

- Although there have been limited applications of CMR to evaluate the coronary arteries, CCT is currently the modality of choice for most routine clinical applications to evaluate the coronary arteries due to the inherently better temporal resolution of CCT than CMR.

- CCT has the advantage of imaging calcifications, which are less conspicuous on CMR, especially in the coronary arteries. In addition to imaging coronary calcifications, CCT may also demonstrate calcifications in valves, and in other cardiac structures, such as the left atrium in rheumatic heart disease.

- Infarctions may be demonstrated on CT, and are frequently seen as areas of low attenuation on CT, with attenuation values approaching that of fat.

- Because ionizing radiation is not needed to perform CMR, other sequences can be frequently obtained, including dynamic imaging of the left ventricle and delayed contrast-enhanced sequences, whereas these additional imaging protocols would require more radiation with CT.

- MR techniques are preferable for evaluating dynamic processes in general. Valvular pathology is better demonstrated by CMR, since regurgitant and stenotic lesions can be depicted by loss of signal. Wall motion is also better imaged with CMR.
- In employing either cardiac CCT or cardiac CMR, care should be taken to search for extracardiac pathology, which may be contributing to symptoms of cardiac disease.

References

1. Hendel RC, Patel MR, Kramer CM, et al. ACCF/ACR/SCCT/SCMR/ASNC/NASCI/SCAI/SIR 2006 appropriateness criteria for cardiac computed tomography and cardiac magnetic resonance imaging: a report of the American College of Cardiology Foundation Quality Strategic Directions Committee Appropriateness Criteria Working Group, American College of Radiology, Society of Cardiovascular Computed Tomography, Society for Cardiovascular Magnetic Resonance, American Society of Nuclear Cardiology, North American Society for Cardiac Imaging, Society for Cardiovascular Angiography and Interventions, and Society of Interventional Radiology. J Am Coll Cardiol 2006, 48(7): 1475–97.
2. Einstein AJ, Henzlova MJ, Rajagopalan S. Estimating risk of cancer associated with radiation exposure from 64-slice computed tomography coronary angiography. Jama 2007, 298(3): 317–23.
3. Ergun I, Keven K, Uruc I, et al. The safety of gadolinium in patients with stage 3 and 4 renal failure. Nephrol Dial Transplant 2006, 21(3): 697–700.
4. Sadowski EA, Bennett LK, Chan MR, et al. Nephrogenic systemic fibrosis: risk factors and incidence estimation. Radiology 2007, 243(1): 148–57.
5. Raff GL, Gallagher MJ, O'Neill WW, Goldstein JA. Diagnostic accuracy of noninvasive coronary angiography using 64-slice spiral computed tomography. J Am Coll Cardiol 2005, 46(3): 552–7.
6. Shellock FG. Reference Manual for Magnetic Resonance Safety, Implants, and Devices: 2006 Edition. Los Angeles: Biomedical Research Publishing Group; 2006.
7. Martin ET, Coman JA, Shellock FG, Pulling CC, Fair R, Jenkins K. Magnetic resonance imaging and cardiac pacemaker safety at 1.5-Tesla. J Am Coll Cardiol 2004, 43(7): 1315–24.
8. Gimbel JR, Kanal E, Schwartz KM, Wilkoff BL. Outcome of magnetic resonance imaging (MRI) in selected patients with implantable cardioverter defibrillators (ICDs). Pacing Clin Electrophysiol 2005, 28(4): 270–3.
9. Shinbane JS, Colletti PM, Shellock FG. MR in patients with pacemakers and ICDs: Defining the issues. J Cardiovasc Magn Reson 2007, 9(1): 5–13.
10. Eshed I, Althoff CE, Hamm B, Hermann KG. Claustrophobia and premature termination of magnetic resonance imaging examinations. J Magn Reson Imaging 2007, 26(2): 401–4.
11. Chia JM, Fischer SE, Wickline SA, Lorenz CH. Performance of QRS detection for cardiac magnetic resonance imaging with a novel vectorcardiographic triggering method. J Magn Reson Imaging 2000, 12(5): 678–88.
12. Wahl A, Paetsch I, Gollesch A, et al. Safety and feasibility of high-dose dobutamine-atropine stress cardiovascular magnetic resonance for diagnosis of myocardial ischaemia: experience in 1000 consecutive cases. Eur Heart J 2004, 25(14): 1230–6.
13. Valente AM, Powell AJ. Clinical applications of cardiovascular magnetic resonance in congenital heart disease. Cardiol Clin 2007, 25(1): 97–110, vi.
14. Dong J, Dickfeld T, Dalal D, et al. Initial experience in the use of integrated electroanatomic mapping with three-dimensional MR/CT images to guide catheter ablation of atrial fibrillation. J Cardiovasc Electrophysiol 2006, 17(5): 459–66.

15. Shiga T, Wajima Z, Apfel CC, Inoue T, Ohe Y. Diagnostic accuracy of transesophageal echocardiography, helical computed tomography, and magnetic resonance imaging for suspected thoracic aortic dissection: systematic review and meta-analysis. Arch Intern Med 2006, 166(13): 1350–6.

16. Belge B, Coche E, Pasquet A, Vanoverschelde JL, Gerber BL. Accurate estimation of global and regional cardiac function by retrospectively gated multidetector row computed tomography: comparison with cine magnetic resonance imaging. Eur Radiol 2006, 16(7): 1424–33.

17. Raman SV, Shah M, McCarthy B, Garcia A, Ferketich AK. Multi-detector row cardiac computed tomography accurately quantifies right and left ventricular size and function compared with cardiac magnetic resonance. Am Heart J 2006, 151(3): 736–44.

18. Dewey M, Muller M, Eddicks S, et al. Evaluation of global and regional left ventricular function with 16-slice computed tomography, biplane cineventriculography, and two-dimensional transthoracic echocardiography: comparison with magnetic resonance imaging. J Am Coll Cardiol 2006, 48(10): 2034–44.

19. Ropers D, Pohle FK, Kuettner A, et al. Diagnostic accuracy of noninvasive coronary angiography in patients after bypass surgery using 64-slice spiral computed tomography with 330-ms gantry rotation. Circulation 2006, 114(22): 2334–41; quiz

20. Shabestari AA, Abdi S, Akhlaghpoor S, et al. Diagnostic performance of 64-channel multi-slice computed tomography in assessment of significant coronary artery disease in symptomatic subjects. Am J Cardiol 2007, 99(12): 1656–61.

21. Ehara M, Kawai M, Surmely JF, et al. Diagnostic accuracy of coronary in-stent restenosis using 64-slice computed tomography: comparison with invasive coronary angiography. J Am Coll Cardiol 2007, 49(9): 951–9.

22. Yeon SB, Sabir A, Clouse M, et al. Delayed-enhancement cardiovascular magnetic resonance coronary artery wall imaging: comparison with multislice computed tomography and quantitative coronary angiography. J Am Coll Cardiol 2007, 50(5): 441–7.

23. Costa MA, Shoemaker S, Futamatsu H, et al. Quantitative magnetic resonance perfusion imaging detects anatomic and physiologic coronary artery disease as measured by coronary angiography and fractional flow reserve. J Am Coll Cardiol 2007, 50(6): 514–22.

24. Jahnke C, Nagel E, Gebker R, et al. Prognostic value of cardiac magnetic resonance stress tests: adenosine stress perfusion and dobutamine stress wall motion imaging. Circulation 2007, 115(13): 1769–76.

25. Kim RJ, Fieno DS, Parrish TB, et al. Relationship of MRI delayed contrast enhancement to irreversible injury, infarct age, and contractile function. Circulation 1999, 100(19): 1992–2002.

26. Gerber BL, Belge B, Legros GJ, et al. Characterization of acute and chronic myocardial infarcts by multidetector computed tomography: comparison with contrast-enhanced magnetic resonance. Circulation 2006, 113(6): 823–33.

27. McCrohon JA, Moon JC, Prasad SK, et al. Differentiation of heart failure related to dilated cardiomyopathy and coronary artery disease using gadolinium-enhanced cardiovascular magnetic resonance. Circulation 2003, 108(1): 54–9.

28. Schmidt A, Azevedo CF, Cheng A, et al. Infarct tissue heterogeneity by magnetic resonance imaging identifies enhanced cardiac arrhythmia susceptibility in patients with left ventricular dysfunction. Circulation 2007, 115(15): 2006–14.

29. Assomull RG, Prasad SK, Lyne J, et al. Cardiovascular magnetic resonance, fibrosis, and prognosis in dilated cardiomyopathy. J Am Coll Cardiol 2006, 48(10): 1977–85.

30. Matoh F, Satoh H, Shiraki K, et al. Usefulness of delayed enhancement magnetic resonance imaging to differentiate dilated phase of hypertrophic cardiomyopathy and dilated cardiomyopathy. J Card Fail 2007, 13(5): 372–9.

31. Casolo G, Di Cesare E, Molinari G, et al. Diagnostic work up of arrhythmogenic right ventricular cardiomyopathy by cardiovascular magnetic resonance (CMR). Consensus statement. Radiol Med (Torino) 2004, 108(1–2): 39–55.

32. Maceira AM, Joshi J, Prasad SK, et al. Cardiovascular magnetic resonance in cardiac amyloidosis. Circulation 2005, 111(2): 186–93.
33. Smedema JP, Snoep G, van Kroonenburgh MP, et al. Evaluation of the accuracy of gadolinium-enhanced cardiovascular magnetic resonance in the diagnosis of cardiac sarcoidosis. J Am Coll Cardiol 2005, 45(10): 1683–90.
34. Tadamura E, Yamamuro M, Kubo S, et al. Effectiveness of delayed enhanced MRI for identification of cardiac sarcoidosis: comparison with radionuclide imaging. AJR Am J Roentgenol 2005, 185(1): 110–5.
35. Rochitte CE, Oliveira PF, Andrade JM, et al. Myocardial delayed enhancement by magnetic resonance imaging in patients with Chagas' disease: a marker of disease severity. J Am Coll Cardiol 2005, 46(8): 1553–8.
36. De Cobelli F, Pieroni M, Esposito A, et al. Delayed gadolinium-enhanced cardiac magnetic resonance in patients with chronic myocarditis presenting with heart failure or recurrent arrhythmias. J Am Coll Cardiol 2006, 47(8): 1649–54.
37. Laissy JP, Hyafil F, Feldman LJ, et al. Differentiating acute myocardial infarction from myocarditis: diagnostic value of early- and delayed-perfusion cardiac MR imaging. Radiology 2005, 237(1): 75–82.
38. Grizzard JD, Ang GB. Magnetic resonance imaging of pericardial disease and cardiac masses. Cardiol Clin 2007, 25(1): 111–40, vi.
39. Hoffmann U, Globits S, Schima W, et al. Usefulness of magnetic resonance imaging of cardiac and paracardiac masses. Am J Cardiol 2003, 92(7): 890–5.
40. Srichai MB, Junor C, Rodriguez LL, et al. Clinical, imaging, and pathological characteristics of left ventricular thrombus: a comparison of contrast-enhanced magnetic resonance imaging, transthoracic echocardiography, and transesophageal echocardiography with surgical or pathological validation. Am Heart J 2006, 152(1): 75–84.
41. Achenbach S, Sacher D, Ropers D, et al. Electron beam computed tomography for the detection of left atrial thrombi in patients with atrial fibrillation. Heart 2004, 90(12): 1477–8.
42. Mohrs OK, Nowak B, Petersen SE, et al. Thrombus detection in the left atrial appendage using contrast-enhanced MRI: a pilot study. AJR Am J Roentgenol 2006, 186(1): 198–205.
43. Petersen SE, Selvanayagam JB, Wiesmann F, et al. Left ventricular non-compaction: insights from cardiovascular magnetic resonance imaging. J Am Coll Cardiol 2005, 46(1): 101–5.

Chapter 19
Radiation Safety: Radiation Dosimetry and CT Dose Reduction Techniques

Kai H. Lee

19.1 Introduction

With the advent of 64-slice systems having high temporal and spatial resolution, the utilization of CT for cardiac studies is rapidly expanding. However, we must be aware that CT is a high-dose application of x-rays and be cognizant of the associated radiation risks to the patients. It is incumbent upon the practitioners of CT to apply the lowest dose consistent with the clinical study. Based on our current knowledge of radiation biology, the deleterious effect of radiation is cumulative and medical radiation is increasingly a significant contributor to the amount of radiation accumulated in a person's lifetime [1, 2, 3]. The risk of cancer from radiation exposure is especially worrisome to children and young women who may receive multiple CT examinations early in their life. For example, studies found that one CT examination of the female chest gives as much radiation as 10 mammograms to each breast [4].

One of the difficulties confronting the cardiologists when dealing with radiation safety of CT is the plethora of terms used to quantify the radiation dose. Thus, this chapter sets out on two aims. The first aim is to explain the fundamental concepts of radiation dosimetry relevant to cardiac CT examinations. The second aim is to describe the techniques available to the cardiologists to control radiation exposure to their patients.

19.2 Fundamentals of Radiation Dosimetry

19.2.1 Absorbed Dose

The international unit (SI units) of radiation dose measurement is the *Gray* (Gy) [5]. Because one Gray is a relatively large quantity of radiation when dealing with

K.H. Lee
Department of Radiology, Los Angeles County and University of Southern California Medical Center, Los Angeles, CA, USA
e-mail: Kailee@usc.edu

M.J. Budoff, J.S. Shinbane (eds.), *Handbook of Cardiovascular CT*,
DOI: 10.1007/978-1-84800-091-9_19, © Springer-Verlag London Limited 2008

radiation safety purposes, two smaller divisions of the Gray are frequently used. These are the milliGray (mGy) and centiGray (cGy).

$$1 \text{ mGy} = 10^{-3} \text{Gy}$$

$$1 \text{ mGy} = 10^{-2} \text{Gy}$$

In the United States the SI units are used in the literature, but the traditional unit *rad* is still widely quoted in routine radiation safety procedures [6]. The unit *rad* is the acronym for *r*adiation *a*bsorbed *d*ose. The conversion between the radiation doses measurements of the two systems is simple. 1 Gy = 100 rad. It follows that 1 cGy = 1 rad.

19.2.2 Equivalent Dose

The severity of biological damage depends not only on the *amount* of radiation absorbed, but also on the *type* of radiation absorbed. For example, 1 Gy of neutron radiation is 10 times more damaging than 1 Gy of x-rays [7]. We therefore need a biological equivalent unit to quantify radiation damage, taking into account the effectiveness of different types of the radiation in producing biological damages. The biological equivalent unit used in radiation protection is the Sievert (Sv), and the traditional unit is the rem (acronym for radiation equivalent man). The biological equivalent dose commonly symbolized by the letter H is equal to the radiation absorbed dose, D, measured in Gy multiplied by the radiation weighting factor W_r; that is

$$H \text{ (Sv)} = D(\text{Gy}) \times W_r,$$

When using the traditional units, the biological equivalent dose in rem is equal to the absorbed dose in rad multiplied by the quality factor Q; that is

$$H \text{ (rem)} = D(\text{rad}) \times Q$$

where the quality factor Q serves the same function as W_r to account for the relative effectiveness of different types of radiation in producing biological damage. The numerical values of Q and W_r are, in fact, identical for the same type of radiation. Some typical radiation weight factors are given in **Table 19.1**.

The values of W_r or Q are proportional to the density of ionization created by the incident radiation along its path of travel in tissue. For x-rays, gamma rays, beta particles, and electrons from radioactive materials, the density of ionization created in tissue is relatively low. The weighting factor W_r equals to 1. Thus, when working with x-rays from CT, the equivalent dose and absorbed dose are numerically equal;

Table 19.1 Radiation-weighting factors

Type of radiation	Weighting factor
x- and gamma rays, electrons, positrons	1
Neutrons	10
Protons	2
Alpha particles	20

that is 1 Sv = 1 Gy, and 1 rem = 1 rad. For neutrons, the weighting factor W_r is equal to 10. The equivalent dose for 1 Gy of neutron absorbed dose equals to

$$H(\text{Sv}) = 1(\text{Gy}) \times 10$$
$$= 10\,\text{Sv}$$

The above example shows that neutrons are 10 times more damaging to the human body than x-rays for the same absorbed dose. In other words, 1 Gy of neutron produces 10 times greater risk than 1 Gy of x-ray.

For radiation protection purposes, sub-units of Sievert and rem are used. Sub-units of Sievert and rem are the milliSievert (mSv) and millirem (mrem), respectively. Since both the traditional and SI units are used in the United States [6], it should be noted that 1 mSv = 100 mrem. A convenient method to convert an equivalent dose given in SI unit to the traditional unit is by multiplying the SI values by 100 and changing the unit name from Sv to rem, but leave the numeric prefix unchanged.

In summary, *absorbed dose* is the amount of radiation energy deposited in tissue. The *equivalent dose* is a measure of biological damage equal to the absorbed dose modified by a weighting factor according to the relative effectiveness of the incident radiation to produce tissue damage.

Now that we have a metrics to quantify radiation; **Table 19.2** lists the average equivalent dose received annually to the total body by workers in various occupations [8, 3, 9]. The table also gives the natural background radiation and the regulatory limits on radiation exposure as reference to occupational exposures. It is interesting to note that the airline flight crews who are not classified as occupational radiation workers receive annual equivalent dose from the cosmic rays nearly twice as much as the nuclear medicine technologists who routinely handle radioactive materials on the job.

Table 19.2 Typical annual whole body radiation dose

	mSv	mrem
Nuclear medicine technologists	1.2	120
Airline flight crews	2.2	220
Nuclear power plant workers	5.5	550
Intervention radiologists	18	1,800
Cardiologists (catheterization)	16	1,600
Natural background radiation	2.5	250
Regulatory limit on the occupational workers	50	5,000
Regulatory limit on the general public	5	500

19.2.3 Effective Dose

Unlike the absorbed dose and the equivalent dose, the effective dose is not a physically measurable quantity. It is an imaginary total body dose calculated from the absorbed dose given to any part or parts of the body. The purpose of the effective dose is to translate a partial body exposure such as a CT scan to an equivalent uniform total body dose to assess the risk of carcinogenesis and genetic defects.

One way to explain why we want to calculate the effective dose is that our current knowledge of the risk of radiation-induced carcinogenesis and genetic defects is based on data collected from the total body exposed uniformly to certain doses of radiation. If we wish to estimate the risk resulting from CT of the chest for example, we must translate the partial body irradiation to an equivalent whole body dose in order to utilize the database for risk estimates. To do so, a mathematical model is used to compute the secondary doses to all other organs resulting from CT of the chest. These computed organ doses are additionally multiplied by a weighting factor according to the sensitivity of each organ to radiation. Summation of the product of these computed organ doses and their associated risk-weighting factor is called the effective dose. That is, the effective dose E is computed using the equation

$$E = \sum H_i w_i$$

where E is the effective dose

H_i is the dose equivalent to a given organ
w_i is the risk-weighting factor for that organ.

The effective dose is thus a weighted sum of the computed doses to all organs in the body. A table of weighting factors for different body organs is given in a report by the International Commission on Radiation Protection [7, 10].

One may interpret the effective dose as a calculated equivalent dose of radiation given to the entire body that would be required to produce the same risk as a dose of radiation delivered to a localized region of the body as in a CT examination. In other words, the risk from a part of the body exposed to a given dose of radiation is the same as the total body uniformly receiving the effective dose. Thus, the effective dose is an extrapolated whole body dose from a partial body dose. As such, the effective dose is a computed value rather than a physically measurable quantity. The purpose of the effective dose is to serve as a common scale for comparison of risk between different medical or non-medical procedures involving the use of radiation.

Now that we understand the concept of the absorbed dose, equivalent dose, and effective dose, the next step is to learn the methodology to calculate the risk of radiation received from CT examinations.

19.2.4 CT Dosimetry

Special dosimetric techniques have to be developed for measuring CT doses because the geometry of the x-ray field employed in CT scans is very different from the conditions of conventional radiographic exposures [11]. The fundamental parameter developed for CT dosimetry is the computed tomography dose index (CTDI). From the CTDI, the dose-length product (DLP) is calculated, and then used to derive the effective dose (E) for risk comparison.

19.2.5 CTDI

The CTDI, or specifically the $CTDI_{100}$, is measured using a dosimeter 100 mm long in a cylindrical acrylic phantom of 16- or 32-cm diameter to simulate a head or body [**Fig.19.1**]. Four measurements are made in the periphery and one in the center of the phantom. The average of the four peripheral measurements and the central measurement is used to compute the weighted average of the $CTDI_{100}$ in the phantom, as follows:

$$CTDI_w = 0.87 \times [2/3\, CTDI_{100}(periphery) + 1/3\, CTDI_{100}(center)]$$

where $CTDI_w$ is the weighted average of $CTDI_{100}$ in the phantom.

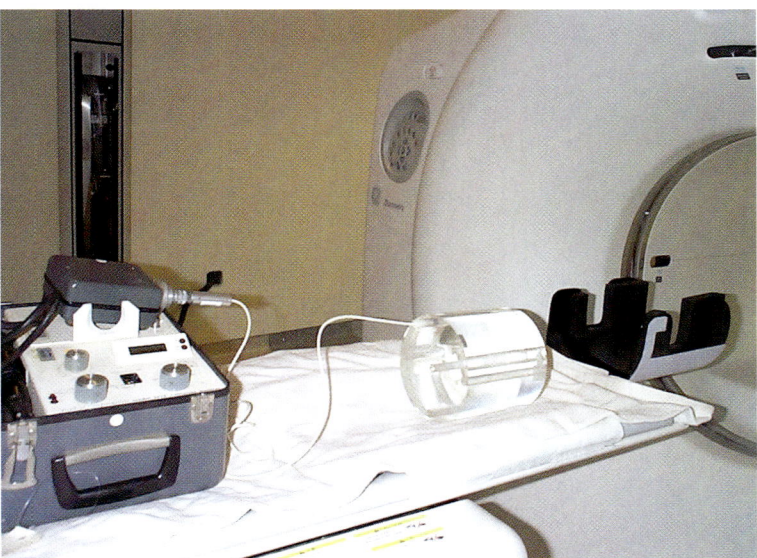

Fig. 19.1 A typical setup of the dosimeter, ionization chamber, and 16-cm diameter acrylic phantom for measuring the CTDI of the head. There are four holes 1 cm from the surface and one hole in the center of the phantom for insertion of the ionization chamber for dose measurements

The factor 0.87 is a conversion factor to relate dose measured in air to dose in soft tissues. The $CTDI_w$ can be considered as the average absorbed dose in the cross section of the patient from one axial scan.

For helical scans using a multi-slice CT, the average dose may be greater than or less than the dose from an axial scan. If in a helical scan the table moves the patient slowly through the gantry, the average absorbed dose in a transverse section of the patient may be greater than that in a non-helical scan due to the x-ray beam overlapping on the patient in successive rotation of the x-ray tube. Conversely, if the table moves at a high speed, the x-ray beam passes through the patient in a non-overlapping helical path as shown in **Fig. 19.2**. There would be less radiation delivered to the scan volume because of the gap between tracks of the x-ray beam.

The $CTDI_{vol}$ was developed to compute the average absorbed dose in the scan volume to take into account the variable overlaps in the spiral path of the x-ray beam. The $CTDI_{vol}$ is calculated using the following equation:

$$CTDI_{vol} = CTDI_w/pitch$$

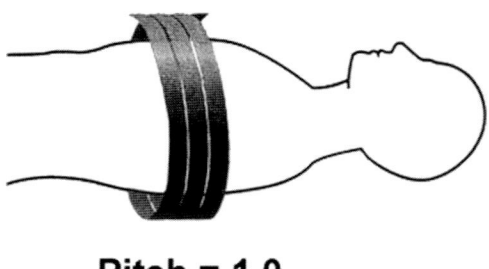

Pitch = 1.0

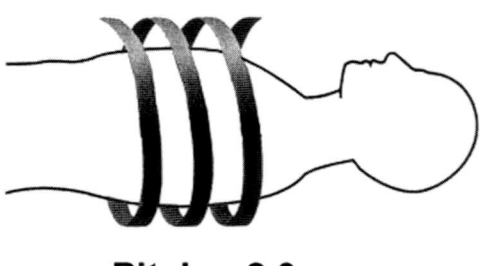

Pitch = 2.0

Fig. 19.2 The amount of overlap of the helical path of the x-ray beam becomes less as the pitch is increased. When the pitch is greater than 1, gap develops between passes of the x-ray beam

Pitch is a dimensionless unit equal to the distance the table traveled during one complete rotation of the x-ray tube divided by the width of the x-ray beam at the axis of rotation. For a multi-slice CT, the pitch is defined as follows:

$$\text{Pitch} = D/nT$$

where D is the distance the patient table moved in one rotation of the x-ray tube

   n is the number of slices produced in one tube rotation
   T is the thickness of each slice measured at the axis of rotation.

The product nT represents the width of the x-ray beam at the axis of rotation of the x-ray tube.

19.2.6 Dose-Length Product

One final dosimetric parameter for CT is the DLP. The DLP is proportional to the total amount of x-ray energy deposit in the scan volume, and is defined as follows:

$$\text{DLP} = \text{CTDI}_{vol} \times \text{scan length}$$

Since the cross-sectional area of the patient is implicitly included in CTDI_{vol}, by multiplying the CTDI_{vol} by the scan length, DLP describes the volume of tissues irradiated and the total amount of x-ray energy deposited in that volume. DLP is an important risk indicator because the severity of biological damage from radiation depends not only on the quantity and type of radiation given, but also on the volume of tissue irradiated as well. For example, a radiation oncologist could deliver 7000 cGy of x-rays to a small region surrounding the prostate gland to cure a patient with prostate cancer. If 7000 cGy was delivered over the entire body, the person will most certainly die from the radiation exposure. Thus, the risk of radiation increases with the volume of tissue irradiated. The two descriptors of CT dosimetry, CTDI_{vol} and DLP, serve to quantify the amount of x-ray energy absorbed per unit mass of tissue, the volume of tissue exposed to radiation, and the total amount of energy deposited in the scan volume. Because CTDI_{vol} and DLP are such important indicators of the risk from a CT procedure, the values of CTDI_{vol} and DLP are displayed on the control console in all MSCT systems manufactured in the last several years.

19.2.7 The Effective Dose from CT

A simple formalism was developed by the ICRP to compute the effective dose from the DLP [12]. The effective dose is conveniently calculated by multiplying the DLP by the corresponding conversion factor shown in **Table 19.3**, that is

$$E(\text{mSv}) = \text{DLP} \times \text{CF}$$

Table 19.3 CT effective dose conversion factors

Region of body	Conversion factor
Head	0.0023
Neck	0.0054
Chest	0.017
Abdomen	0.015
Pelvis	0.019

Table 19.4 Typical effective doses of radiological examinations

Radiologic examination	Typical effective dose (mSv)
Head/neck CT	2–5
Chest CT	5–7
Abdomen/pelvis CT	8–11
Coronary CT angiogram	5–15
Coronary bi-plane angiogram	3–10
PET cardiac viability per 370 MBq	4–7
MIBI cardiac stress/rest per 1.3 GBq	10.6
PA chest x-ray	0.02
Skull x-ray	0.07
Lumbar spine	1.3
I. urogram	2.5
Upper GI	3.0
Barium enema	7.0

where CF is the conversion factor for the corresponding CT procedure.

By using the $CTDI_{vol}$, DLP, and conversion factors in **Table 19.3**, some typical values of the effective dose from different CT procedures and other radiologic examinations are also shown in **Table 19.4** for comparison [13, 14, 15].

19.2.8 CT Dose Reduction Techniques

It can be seen in **Table 19.4** that CT is a high-dose procedure compared with other x-ray examinations. Studies found that CT examinations consisted of 12% of all diagnostic examinations, but contributed to 45% of the medical radiation to the population [16, 17, 18, 19]. The contribution of CT dose to the population is expected to continue to rise, given the ever-expanding use of CT. It is therefore imperative for the practitioners of CT to utilize low-dose techniques to obtain the desired diagnostic information.

The CT manufacturers responded by building into their equipment a variety of dose reduction options. The various CT dose reduction techniques are actually different implementations of automatic exposure control (AEC) that have been in use for decades in fluoroscopy and radiography. In a nutshell, the AEC controls dose to the patient by modulating the x-ray beam intensity according to the patient's anatomy to produce the desired image quality. A convenient way to vary the intensity of the x-ray beam is to adjust the milliamperage of electron current (mA) across the x-ray tube. By modulating the tube current according to the amount of x-ray attenuation presented by the patient, the desired image quality can be maintained without imparting unnecessary radiation to the patient.

There are three conditions under which the AEC can be called upon to modulate the tube current (mA) to produce the desired image quality, and in the process, reduce the unnecessary radiation to the patient. First, the AEC could be programmed to adjust the mA along the long axis of the patient so that the mA is reduced when the x-ray beam passes through large volume of air in the thorax, and is raised when the beam goes through the more attenuating soft tissues in the abdomen and pelvis. Second, the mA is adjusted in the transverse plane of the patient according to the tube angle during its rotation around the patient. That is, the mA is reduced when the x-ray beam is passing through the patient in the thinner anterior-posterior and posterior-anterior directions, and increased in the thicker lateral directions. Third, the overall tube current is adjusted according to the patient's size such that a lower mA would be used on pediatric patients rather than on adult patients, and on thinner patients rather than on heavy-set patients. All multi-slice CT systems on the market today provide AEC controls that utilize combinations of the above methods to optimize the radiation dose and image quality. The debates on the merit of each AEC control focus not so much on the efficacy of the mechanisms to modulate the x-ray intensity, but on the objective of the algorithm to optimize the radiation dose and image quality.

19.2.9 Dose Optimization Objectives

Modulating the tube current according to the patient attenuation in real time is technologically relatively simple. The difficulty lies in deciding the trade-offs between the patient dose and image quality. When we reduce the intensity of the x-ray beam passing through the patient, we reduce the patient dose, but we reduce the quality of the images as well. The question becomes one of deciding the minimum dose to the patient that would still produce an acceptable image quality. Answer to this question obviously depends on the comfort level of the interpreting physician, and this subjectivity varies from physician to physician. There are three general methods used by the manufacturers to set the AEC [20, 19, 21], each with their advantages and disadvantages.

19.2.10 AEC Guided by Image Noise

The image noise can be described qualitatively as the graininess of the image. Low noise images appear smooth with continuous shade of gray from the darkest to the lightest portions of the image. High noise images show the characteristic salt and pepper grains interspersed throughout the image. Resolution of low contrast objects can be greatly impaired by image noise. Image noise is influenced by a number of factors, but is ultimately determined by the number of x-ray photons that contribute to the image. A simple way to quantify noise in an image is to calculate the percentage standard deviation. The standard deviation of an image is the square root of the total number of counts or dots that make up the image. The resulting standard deviation is then divided by the total counts in the image to arrive at the percentage standard deviation. The standard deviation of the number of counts in an image is an expression of the fraction of noise in an image. The percentage standard deviation as computed by the ratio of the standard deviation to the total number of counts in the image indicates what fraction of the image is occupied by noise.

The number of counts in a given CT image is directly proportional to the number of x-ray photons available for image formation, which in turn depends on the intensity of the x-ray beam striking the detectors and the length of time the x-ray beam is on. As discussed, the AEC modulates the beam intensity by varying the tube current. The exposure time is determined by the speed of the x-ray tube to make one rotation around the patient. The product of the tube current in mA and the rotation time in seconds is commonly called the *mAs*. The mAs set for a CT scan determines the number of x-ray photons striking the patient. Higher the mAs, greater is the number of photons available to pass through the patient to reach the detectors, and lower is the noise in the reconstructed images. When all the other technical factors are held constant, the image noise is inversely proportional to the square root of the mAs, that is

$$\text{Noise} \sim 1/\sqrt{\text{mAs}}$$

During CT scans, the tube rotation time is fixed. The image noise–guided AEC continually adjusts the mAs by varying the mA to maintain the same number of photons reaching the detectors, and hence keeping the image noise at a pre-selected level. For example, the AEC can reduce the mA when the beam is passing through in the thinner anterior-posterior direction of the patient, and increases the mA when passing through laterally.

The CT user has great flexibility in patient dose optimization by providing the AEC with a target image noise appropriate for the particular CT procedure. The disadvantage is that the target noise level selected by the user may be lower than necessary for obtaining the diagnostic information, and results in giving unnecessary dose to the patient. A simple rule to remember is that reducing the image noise by a factor of 2 increases the mAs and hence the patient dose by a factor of 4.

19.2.11 AEC Guided by Reference Image

This method of AEC is an extension of the constant image noise algorithm. Here, the target image noise is set on the AEC using a clinical image that is selected by the reader as of adequate quality for the given CT procedure. During scan, the mA at each tube position is adjusted by the AEC to yield an image noise approximating the noise in the reference image. The advantage of the reference image approach is that the target image noise is derived from a database of clinical images rather than some abstract percentage standard deviation. The major disadvantage of the reference image approach is the user inclination to select the prettier image as the reference image even though a less attractive image will do. This results in the patient receiving a more radiation dose than necessary.

19.2.12 AEC Guided by Reference mAs

This approach uses the mAs of a reference patient as a guide to modulate the mA for the actual patient. For a given CT procedure, a certain mAs that was found to produce images of acceptable quality on a reference patient is used as the standard of reference. From the attenuation profiles measured on a scout view of the actual patient, the AEC adjusts the tube current at each tube position to compensate for the difference in attenuation between the actual and reference patients. The image noise is not maintained for different patient sizes. The technique, however, relies on the experience of the user to select the proper degree of tube current modulation for a given patient and CT procedure.

19.2.13 Computed Tomography of the Heart

One of the methods implemented by the manufacturers to reduce patient dose for cardiac CT studies is called prospective gating [22, 23]. Prospective gating is based on the finding that least motion artifacts were found in the images reconstructed from data in the ventricular diastolic phase. Therefore, the x-ray beam needs to turn on only during diastole to acquire the data for image reconstruction, and to be turned off during the other phases of the cardiac cycle. Having the x-ray beam turned on only when is needed would result in substantial reduction of radiation dose to the patient.

To implement this prospective gating technique, the tube current is modulated by the ECG tracings to synchronize with the patient's cardiac cycle. Signals from the ECG monitor trigger the x-ray beam to turn on for data acquisition during diastole, and turn off when not taking data during the systolic and early diastolic phases. The heart is thus scanned in a sequential step-and-shoot fashion as shown in **Fig. 19.3**. Immediately before the scan, a sample of the ECG traces is taken to measure the average R–R time interval. When the CT is set to scan, the AEC sets the clock to zero upon receiving an R-wave from the ECG monitor. The tube current is turned off until 70% of the cardiac cycle has elapsed. After this initial delay, the tube current is turned on to the maximum, and it maintains the maximum output for the next 10% of the cardiac cycle, corresponding to the time during which the heart is in the diastolic phase. The AEC then turns off the tube current at the 80% mark that approximates the end of the diastolic phase to stop data acquisition. The time marker is reset to zero upon receiving the next R-wave. While the x-ray beam is off, the table moves

Prospective Gating Technique

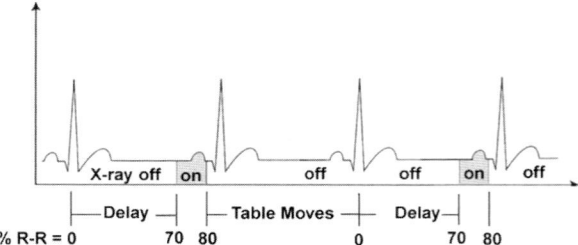

Fig. 19.3 In prospective gating, the x-ray beam is turned on only for a short duration in the R–R interval

the patient to the next scanning position. By turning the x-ray beam on only during 10% of the cardiac cycle for data acquisition, the patient dose was reported to reduce by 50–70% in comparison with the retrospective gating that requires the x-ray beam on continuously throughout the scan [24].

Rapid advances in MSCT technology also bring changes to cardiovascular imaging techniques and radiation dose to the patient in a fast pace. Of particular interest to cardiologists are the introduction of 256-slice and dual-source MSCT. Preliminary studies [25] using the 256-slice CT found that image data for the entire heart volume could be acquired in a single rotation, thus avoiding helical scans and bed indexing to acquire data over several cardiac cycles. When combined with prospective gating and elimination of scan overlap of the x-ray helical path, 50–80% dose reduction was realized in pilot studies. On the other hand, the dual-source CT by use of a special cardiac bow-tie filter and the ECG to modulate the tube current and pitch was able to reduce the patient dose up to a factor of 2 according to one study [26]. However, more studies need to be done to confirm the dose reduction factors in these initial studies.

19.3 Conclusion

Multi-slice CT with its high temporal and spatial resolution is increasingly applied for a wide spectrum of cardiac studies. Because of the high radiation dose associated with cardiac CT examinations, it is necessary for the clinicians to become familiar with the dosimetric principles, and to adopt dose reduction techniques in their clinical practice. Although brief, this chapter reviewed the basic dosimetry parameters necessary to understand the terms and concepts invariably brought up in any discussion of radiation dose optimization methods. The abstract concept of effect dose should be well understood in order to explain to the patients the relative risks of different medical procedures that involve the use of radiation, for example the comparative risks of coronary CT angiography, chest x-rays, and radionuclide perfusion studies.

It is not within the scope of this chapter to explore the influence on patient dose from the interacting CT scan parameters such as the kilovoltage, pitch, tube current, rotation time, slice width, and image noise. However, several of the key parameters pertinent to patient dose reduction are discussed in the AEC systems implemented in commercial CT systems. The trade names of CT dose reduction techniques are confusing. However, the guiding principle of all techniques involves seeking the minimum dose necessary to produce acceptable quality of image for interpretation.

Modulating the x-ray tube current according to attenuation by the patient's anatomy is the methodology adopted by CT manufacturers for dose reduction. The option controllable by the user for patient dose reduction is the tube current–time product, or mAs. Regardless of the different definitions of the mAs in the manufacturer's literature, selecting a lower mAs with other variables held constant always results in lowering the dose given to the patient. The trade-off for lowering the mAs is increasing graininess of the reconstructed images. The clinician then has to decide the minimum mAs they could use to produce the quality of images that they confidently could draw diagnostic information from.

References

1. NCRP Report #93, "Ionizing Radiation Exposure of the Population of the United States" (1987).
2. United Nations Scientific Committee on the Effects of Atomic Radiation. Sources and effects of atomic radiation: ionizing radiation. Publication n. E.00.IX4. New York, NY: United Nations, 2000.
3. NCRP Report #101, "Exposure of the U.S. Population From Occupational Radiation", 1989
4. Parker, MS, Hui, FK, Camacho, MA, et al NN. Female Breast Radiation Exposure During CT Pulmonary Angiography. Am J Roentgenol. 2005; 185(5): 1228–1233.
5. Huda, W. Medical Radiation Dosimetry. In From Invisible to Visible – The Science and Practice of X-ray Imaging and Radiation Dose Optimization. 2006 Categorical Course Syllabus, Radiologicqal Society of North America.
6. NCRP Report #82. SI Units in Radiation Protection and Measurements (1985)
7. ICRP. *ICRP Publication 92: Relative Biological Effectiveness (RBE), Quality Factor (Q), and Radiation Weighting Factor (wR)*. Elsevier Science Ltd, Oxford, UK. November 2003. ISBN 0-08-044311-7.
8. Feng YJ et al. Estimated cosmic radiation doses for flight personnel. Space Med Med Eng 2002, 15(4): 265–9.
9. 1997 Report on Occupational Radiation Exposures in Canada. Radiation Protection Bureau, Ottawa, Ontario K1A 1C1. http://dsp-psd.pwgsc.gc.ca/Collection/H46-2-97-213E.pdf
10. ICRP. *ICRP Publication 60: 1990 Recommendations of the International Commission on Radiological Protection*. Elsevier Science Pub Co (April 1, 1991). ISBN 0-08-041144-4.
11. International Electrotechnical Eommission. Medical Electrical Equipment. Part 2-44: Particular Requirements for the Safety of X-ray Equipment for Computed Tomography. IEC publication No. 60601-2-44. International Electrotechnical Commission (IEC) Central Office: Geneva, Switzerland, 2002.
12. European Commission study group. European guidelines on quality criteria for computed tomography. Publication no. EUR 16262 EN. Brussels, Belgium: Office for Official Publications of European Communities, 2000.
13. http://www.fda.gov/cdrh/ct/risks.html as of May 18, 2007.

14. Morin, RL, Gerber, MD, McCollough, CH. Radiation Dose in Computed Tomography of the Heart. Circulation, 2003, 107: 917–922.
15. Hausleiter, J, Meyer, T, Hadamitzky, M, et al. Radiation Dose Estimates From Cardiac Multi-slice Computed Tomography in Daily Practice, Impact of Different Scanning Protocols on Effective Dose Estimates. Circulation, 2006, 113: 1305-1310.
16. Mettler, FA, Wiest PW, Locken JA, et al. CT scanning: patterns of use and dose. Journal of Radiological Protection 2000 20: 353–359.
17. Kalender, WA. Computed Tomography – Fundamentals, System Technology, Image Qaulity, Application, Publicis Corporate Publishing, Erlanger, 2005.
18. Goodman, TR, Brink, JA. Adult CT: Controlling Dose and Image Quality. In From Invisible to Visible – The Science and Practice of X-ray Imaging and Radiation Dose Optimization. 2006 Categorical Course Syllabus, Radiologicqal Society of North America.
19. http://www.impactscan.org/slides/ecr2005/index.htm as of May 18, 2007.
20. McCollough, CH, Bruesewitz, MR, Kofler, JM. CT Dose Reduction and Dose Management Tools: Overview of Available Options. Radiographics 2006, 26: 503–512.
21. Prokop, M and Galanski, M [Ed]. Spiral and Multislice Computed Tomography of the Body. Thieme, 2003, 131–160.
22. Bae, KT, Hong, C, Whiting, BR. Radiation Dose in Multidetector Row Computed Tomography Cardiac Imaging. J Magn Reson Imaging. 2004 19: 859–863.
23. Abada HT, Larchez C, et al. MDCT of the Coronary Arteries: Feasibility of Low Dose CT with ECG-Pulsed Tube Current Modulation to Reduce Radiation Dose. Am J Roentgenol. 2006, 186: S387–90.
24. Mori, S, Endo, M, Nishizawa, K, et al. Comparison of Patient Doses in 256-Slice CT and 16-Slice CT Scanners. The Brit J Radiol. 2006, 56–61.
25. McCollough, CH, Primak, AN, et al. Dose Performance of a 64-Channel Dual-Source CT Scanner. Radiology. 2007, 243: 775–784.
26. Watson, SJ, Jones, AL, Oatway, WB, Hughes, JS. Ionizing Radiation Exposure of the UK Population: 2005 Review. Health Protection Agency, Report HPA-RPD-001, 2005.

Chapter 20
Competency, Appropriateness, and Quality in Cardiovascular CT

Allen J. Taylor, Lance E. Sullenberger, and Todd C. Villines

- Competency

  - For all levels of cardiac computed tomography (CCT) competence, clinicians must attend lectures and include a parallel self-study reading program on the basic concepts of CCT.
  - Level 1 training is the minimal introductory training for familiarity with CCT, but is not sufficient for independent interpretation of CCT images.
  - Level 2 training is the minimum training for a physician to independently perform and interpret CCT.
  - Level 3 trainees qualify to serve as a director of a CCT facility or training program, responsible for quality control and technologist and physician training.
  - The deadline to achieve experience-based competency in CCT is July 1, 2010. After this date, formal program-based training is required.

- Appropriateness

  - An appropriate imaging study is one in which the expected information gained, combined with clinical expertise, significantly exceeds expected negative consequences such that the procedure is generally considered acceptable for a specific indication.
  - "Appropriateness" is a work in progress, remaining flexible as data emerges on developing technologies such as CCT.
  - Appropriate indications for CCT currently include the evaluation of chest pain (among intermediate probability patients unable to exercise, with uninterpretable electrocardiograms, suspected coronary anomalies, acute chest pain with negative standard evaluations, and uninterpretable or equivocal stress

The opinions or assertions herein are the private views of the authors and are not to be construed as reflecting the views of the Department of the Army or the Department of Defense.

A.J. Taylor
Department of Cardiology, Walter Reed Army Medical Centre, Washington, DC 20307-5001, USA; The Uniformed Services University of the Health Sciences, Bethesda MD, USA.
e-mail: allen.taylor@na.amedd.army.mil

tests), new-onset heart failure, and evaluation of cardiac masses and other anatomical structures.

- A Clinical Expert Consensus Document of the American College of Cardiology has extended appropriateness to coronary calcium scanning in patients with an intermediate risk of coronary heart disease as a method to refine the coronary risk assessment and alter treatment paradigms [1].

- Quality in CCT

  - Quality imaging extends to all aspects of CCT including patient selection, image acquisition, image interpretation, and reporting/communication.
  - Provider certification and laboratory accreditation in CCT are external methods of ensuring quality standards in CCT.

The science and application of CCT is rapidly evolving and involves practitioners from different background disciplines. In an effort to ensure quality care and patient safety, the American College of Cardiology Foundation (ACCF)/American Heart Association (AHA) published in 2005 a statement addressing the knowledge, skills, and minimum specific training required to achieve and maintain clinical competence in CCT [2]. This document serves to guide clinicians seeking training in CCT and medical staff organizations responsible for granting clinical privileges.

All candidates must have completed a cardiovascular fellowship or a residency in general radiology or nuclear medicine. Additionally, there are cognitive skills inherent to CCT that clinicians must thoroughly understand (**Table 20.1**).

Table 20.1 Cognitive skils required for competence in CCT

General:
- Knowledge of the physics of CT and radiation generation and exposure
- Knowledge of scanning principles and scanning modes for non-contrast and contrast-enhanced cardiac imaging using multidetector and/or electron beam methods
- Knowledge of the principles of intravenous iodinated contrast administration for safe and optimal cardiac imaging
- Knowledge of recognition and treatment of adverse reactions to iodinated contrast
- Knowledge of the principles of image postprocessing and appropriate applications

Cardiac:
- Clinical knowledge of coronary heart disease and other cardiovascular diseases
- Knowledge of normal cardiac, coronary artery, and coronary venous anatomy, including associated pulmonary arterial and venous structures
- Knowledge of pathologic changes in cardiac and coronary artery anatomy due to acquired and congenital heart disease
- Basic knowledge in ECG to recognize artifacts and arrhythmias

Aorta:
- Knowledge of normal thoracic arterial anatomy
- Knowledge of pathologic changes in central arterial anatomy due to acquired and congenital vascular disease

Reproduced with permission of the ACCF/AHA

Achievement of specific levels of competence (Level 1, 2, or 3) is based on cumulative training duration, minimum number of mentored CCT examinations performed (physically present) and interpreted, and the amount of course/lecture exposure (**Table 20.2**). At least 25 (Level 2) to 50 cases (Level 3) should include evaluation of ventricular function, as well as simple congenital heart disease lesions (e.g., anomalies of the aorta or pulmonary veins). A portion of live cases may be obtained through videotaped cases. A portion of mentored case interpretations may include studies from established teaching files, previous cases, journals, textbooks, or electronic courses/CME. Proof of competence must be documented in the form of a letter from a training supervisor or a Level 2/3-trained CCT physician mentor. Accordingly, the Society of Cardiovascular Computed Tomography (SCCT) has initiated a training verification program based on the ACCF/AHA competence statement requirements (http://www.scct.org/credentialing/verification.cfm). The deadline for achieving experience-based competency is July 1, 2010.

Competence for CCT interpretation may be acquired within an accredited cardiovascular medicine fellowship as directed by the ACCF Update for Training in Adult Cardiovascular Medicine [3]. Cardiovascular fellows may reach three levels of expertise with CCT. Level 1 training is the minimum goal for all graduating cardiovascular medicine fellows and is comprised of at least 50 mentored cases in CCT interpretation during at least 1 month of dedicated CCT training. This level of training expects the graduating fellow will be familiar with indications, general capabilities, and limitations of CCT. Achieving Level 2 and 3 expects a cardiovascular medicine fellow to be familiar with all aspects of CCT including indications, use of contrast, data artifacts, CT acquisition, and post-processing. Level 2 training qualifies a graduating fellow for credentialing in CCT interpretation and, as such, seeks to have the fellow understand acquisition as well as interpretation of CCT examinations. This level requires at least 2 months of dedicated training, during which the cardiovascular medicine fellow is present for at least 35 CCT acquisitions in the presence of a mentor and at least 150 mentored examination interpretations.

Table 20.2 Requirements to achieve level 1, 2, and 3 clinical competence in cardiovascular CT

	Cumulative Duration of Training	Minimum Number of Mentored Examinations Performed	Minimum Number of Mentored Examinations Interpreted
Level 1	4 weeks*	–	50†
Level 2—non-contrast	4 weeks*	50	150†
Level 2—contrast	8 weeks*	50	150†
Level 3	6 months*	100	300†

* This represents cumulative time spent interpreting, performing, and learning about CCT, and need not be a consecutive block of time, but at least 50% of the time should represent supervised laboratory experience. In-lab training time is defined as a minimum of 35 h/week.

† The case load recommendations may include studies from an established teaching file, previous CCT cases, journals and/or textbooks, or electronic/on-line courses/CME.

	Level 2		Level 3
Initial Experience	• NON-CONTRAST REQUIREMENTS	• FULL CCT REQUIREMENTS	• Board certification or eligibility, valid medical license, and completion of 6 months (cumulative) of training in CCT,
	• Board certification or eligibility, valid medical license, and completion of 4 weeks of training (to include coursework, scientific meetings, and courses/on-line training)	• Board certification or eligibility, valid medical license, and completion of 8 weeks (cumulative) of training in CCT	• AND 300 contrast CCT examinations. For at least 100 of these cases, the candidate must be physically present, and be involved in the acquisition and interpretation of the case
	• AND 150 non-contrast CCT examinations (for at least 50 of these cases, the candidate must be physically present, and be involved in interpretation of the case)	• AND 150 contrast CCT examinations. For at least 50 of these cases, the candidate must be physically present, and be involved in the acquisition and interpretation of the case	• AND evaluation of 100 non-contrast studies
	• AND completion of 20 h of courses/lectures related to CT in general and/or CCT in particular	• AND evaluation of 50 non-contrast studies	• AND completion of 40 h of courses/lectures related to CT in general and/or CCT in particular
		• AND completion of 20 h/lectures related to CT in general and/or CCT in particular	
Continuing Experience	50 non-contrast CCT exams conducted and interpreted per year	50 contrast CCT exams conducted and interpreted per year	100 contrast CCT exams conducted and interpreted per year
Continuing Education	20 h Category I every 36 months of CCT		40 h Category I every 36 months of CCT

A graduating cardiovascular medicine fellow achieving level 3 certification in CCT angiography would be capable of serving as a director of a cardiac CT lab or facility. The fellow should spend at least 6 months of dedicated training in CCT imaging and be present for the acquisition of at least 100 CCT angiograms as well as the mentored interpretation of 300 cases.

20.1 Appropriateness and Quality

Along with the expanded options in noninvasive imaging, has come an increasing emphasis on appropriate use of imaging technology. To this end, a multi-society group undertook a process to determine the appropriateness of selected indications for cardiovascular CCT. As defined, an appropriate imaging study is one in which "the expected incremental information, combined with clinical judgment, exceeds the expected negative consequences by a sufficiently wide margin for specific indications that the procedure is generally considered acceptable care and a reasonable approach for the indication." Determined by expert opinion, a number of indications were considered appropriate in the use of CCT in the evaluation of chest pain (among intermediate probability patients unable to exercise, with uninterpretable electrocardiograms, suspected coronary anomalies, acute chest pain with negative standard evaluations, and uninterpretable or equivocal stress tests), new-onset heart failure, and evaluation of cardiac masses and other anatomical structures. More recently, a Clinical Expert Consensus Document of the American College of Cardiology has extended appropriateness to coronary calcium scanning in patients with an intermediate risk of coronary heart disease as a method to refine the coronary risk assessment and alter treatment paradigms [1].

Appropriately selected patients must still be examined within an environment of quality imaging standards. To this end, a "think tank" of the American College of Cardiology and Duke University has defined a pathway toward improved patient care outcomes through quality imaging [4]. Within this pathway of the imaging process are dimensions of patient selection, image acquisition, image interpretation, and reporting/communication. Many details remain to be determined; however, it is hoped that these theoretical discussions will pave the way for subsequent work toward continuous quality improvement.

20.2 Certification and Laboratory Accreditation

The certification of competency via a formal examination process is anticipated. The Certification Board of Cardiovascular Computed Tomography has been established with the first board examination anticipated in late 2008. More information on eligibility and the examination process can be found at www.cbcct.org. Similarly, assurance that quality standards in cardiovascular CT laboratory methods are met will be administrated via the Intersocietal Commission for the Accreditation of Cardiovascular CT Laboratories. This is also an area under development, and more information is available at www.icacctl.org.

References

1. Greenland P, Bonow RO, Brundage BH, Budoff MJ, Eisenberg MJ, Grundy SM, Lauer MS, Post WS, Raggi P, Redberg RF, Rodgers GP, Shaw LJ, Taylor AJ, Weintraub WS, Harrington RA, Abrams J, Anderson JL, Bates ER, Eisenberg MJ, Grines CL, Hlatky MA, Lichtenberg RC,

Lindner JR, Pohost GM, Schofield RS, Shubrooks SJ Jr, Stein JH, Tracy CM, Vogel RA, Wesley DJ. Coronary Artery Calcium Scoring: ACCF/AHA 2007 Clinical Expert Consensus Document on Coronary Artery Calcium Scoring By Computed Tomography in Global Cardiovascular Risk Assessment and in Evaluation of Patients With Chest Pain. J Am Coll Cardiol. 2007, 49: 378–402.

2. Budoff MJ, Cohen MC, Garcia MJ, Hodgson JM, Hundley WG, Lima JA et al. ACCF/AHA clinical competence statement on cardiac imaging with computed tomography and magnetic resonance: a report of the American College of Cardiology Foundation/American Heart Association/American College of Physicians Task Force on Clinical Competence and Training. J Am Coll Cardiol. 2005, 46: 383–402.

3. Budoff MJ, Achenbach S, Fayad Z, Berman DS, Poon M, Taylor AJ et al. Task Force 12: training in advanced cardiovascular imaging (computed tomography): endorsed by the American Society of Nuclear Cardiology, Society for Cardiovascular Angiography and Interventions, Society of Atherosclerosis Imaging and Prevention, and Society of Cardiovascular Computed Tomography. J Am Coll Cardiol. 2006, 47: 915–20.

4. Douglas P, Iskandrian AE, Krumholz HM, Gillam L, Hendel R, Jollis J et al. Achieving quality in cardiovascular imaging: proceedings from the American College of Cardiology-Duke University Medical Center Think Tank on Quality in Cardiovascular Imaging. J Am Coll Cardiol. 2006, 48: 2141–51.

Chapter 21
Cardiac Anatomy by Computed Tomographic Imaging

Ambarish Gopal

Cardiovascular CT (CCT) allows for the comprehensive analysis of a variety of cardiovascular diseases. The focus of this chapter is to orient the reader to the axial anatomy of the cardiovascular system through assessment of serial labeled axial images, as axial image analysis is essential to the interpretation of CCT.

- The word "tomography" is derived from Greek *tomos* (slice) and *graphein* (to write). The heart can be imagined as a loaf of bread, and the slices through the heart can be likened to the slices of the bread. The thinness of a slice enables the reader to further examine what may be contained in that slice with greater clarity and detail as opposed to using a thicker slice. Just as the slices can be stacked on top of one another in sequence to reconstitute the original loaf, the axial slices of the heart can be used in sequence to reconstruct the heart, using an advanced post-processing workstation.

- In many ways, reading CCT studies is more intuitive than reading invasive angiographic and echocardiographic studies. The axial anatomy is always in the same orientation (Image Explanation Figure). The images are acquired with the patient in the supine position; each axial slice is viewed from the foot of the supine patient. The reader should always "shake hands with the axial image," as the reader's left side will be the patient's right side. The "top" of the image is anterior for the patient and the "bottom" is posterior for the patient.

- The axial slices presented here are in sequence cranio-caudally and will help the reader to get easily oriented to the cardiovascular tomographic anatomy. The slices have a small sagittal navigator that will identify the axial slice in relation to the heart and thorax through the sagittal plane.

- The reader should never try to identify a structure just with one axial slice. Identification of a structure should be performed by assessing adjacent axial slices to establish anatomic continuity.

A. Gopal
Division of Cardiology, Los Angeles Biomedical Research Institute at Harbor -UCLA Medical Centre, Torrance, CA, USA
e-mail: ambarishgopal@hotmail.com

M.J. Budoff, J.S. Shinbane (eds.), *Handbook of Cardiovascular CT*,
DOI: 10.1007/978-1-84800-091-9_21, © Springer-Verlag London Limited 2008

- Using the axial slices, the workstations generate the other views used in CCT. These axial slices should always be used to verify, confirm, or exclude any potential lesions that might be seen with other reconstructions.
- Cardiac axial images are routinely acquired in a small field of view (FOV), allowing for an increase in the resolution of data analyzed for cardiac disease. However, all systems have multiple FOV settings to allow for imaging of the entire chest, not just the cardiac field. For an evaluation of the cardiac structures and the coronary arteries, a small FOV is recommended. CCT uses a 512×512 image matrix in the high-resolution mode. In a 512×512 matrix, each pixel represents a certain amount of data. The smaller FOV (i.e., 15 cm), each pixel represents more data (better spatial resolution). If the FOV is enlarged (i.e., 30 cm), this halves the resolution in each voxel, as 512 pixels are each divided into portions to constitute 30 cm. The small FOV focuses on the field of interest without degrading the image quality prior to transfer to the workstation, allowing the physician to zoom in on even smaller structures later (digital zoom).

Abbreviations

ACV	Anterior cardiac vein
Asc aorta	Ascending aorta
CS	Coronary sinus
CS os	Coronary sinus os
Desc aorta	Descending aorta
Diag	Diagonal branch
Eso	Esophagus
GCV	Great cardiac vein
IAS	Inter-atrial septum
IVC	Inferior vena cava
IVS	Inter-ventricular septum
LA	Left atrium
LAA	Left atrial appendage
LAD	Left anterior descending coronary artery
LV	Left ventricle
LCx	Left circumflex coronary artery
LIMA	Left internal mammary artery
LV	Left ventricle
LVOT	Left ventricular outflow tract
PA	Pulmonary artery
PDA	Posterior descending coronary artery
RSPV	Right superior pulmonary vein
RIPV	Right inferior pulmonary vein
LSPV	Left superior pulmonary vein
LIPV	Left inferior pulmonary vein
OM	Obtuse marginal branch
RA	Right atrium

RAA	Right atrial appendage
RCA	Right coronary artery
RIMA	Right internal mammary artery
RV	Right ventricle
RVOT	Right ventricular outflow tract
SVC	Superior vena cava

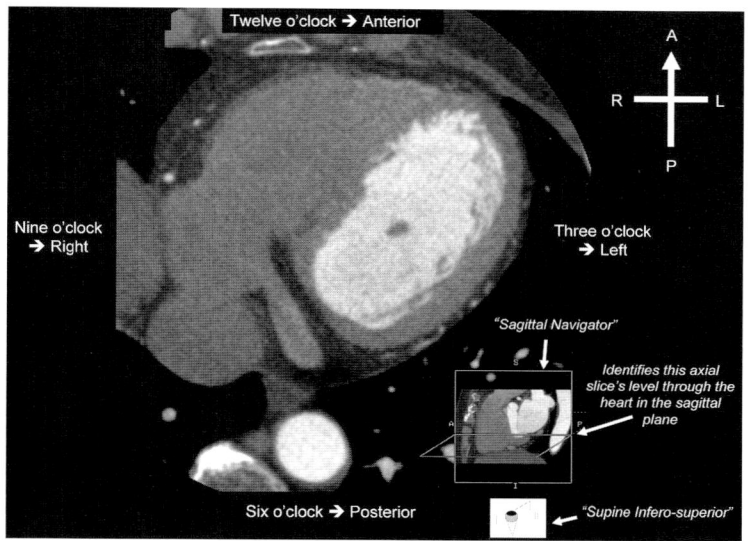

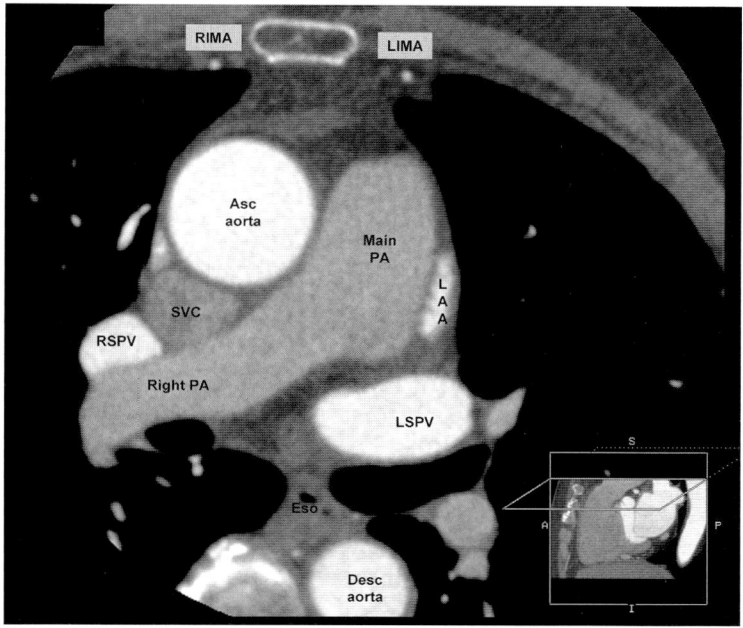

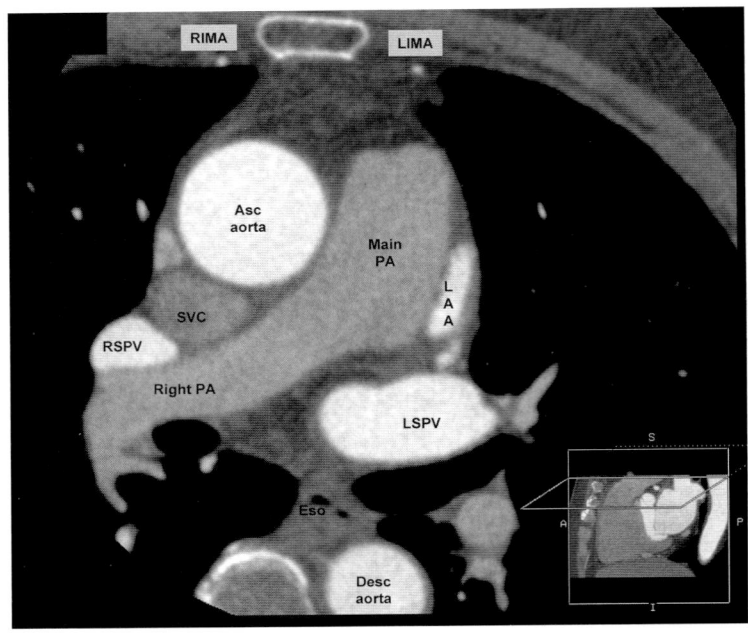

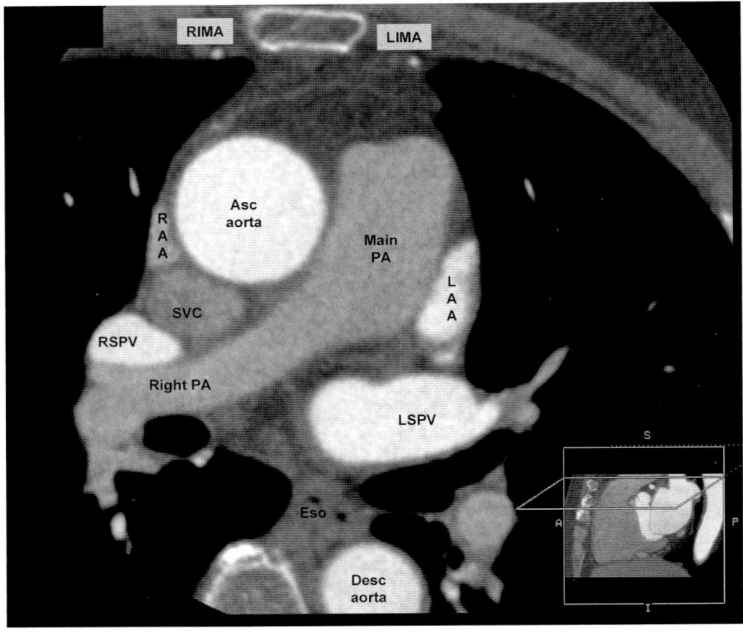

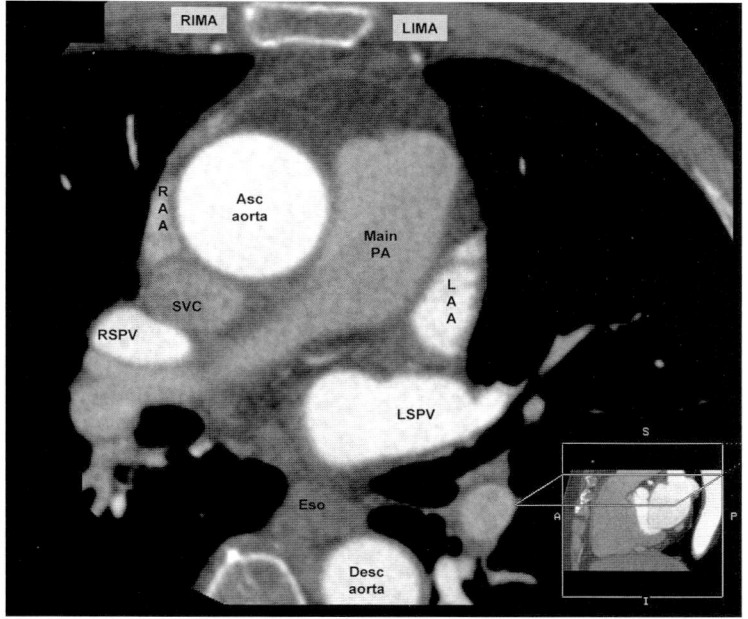

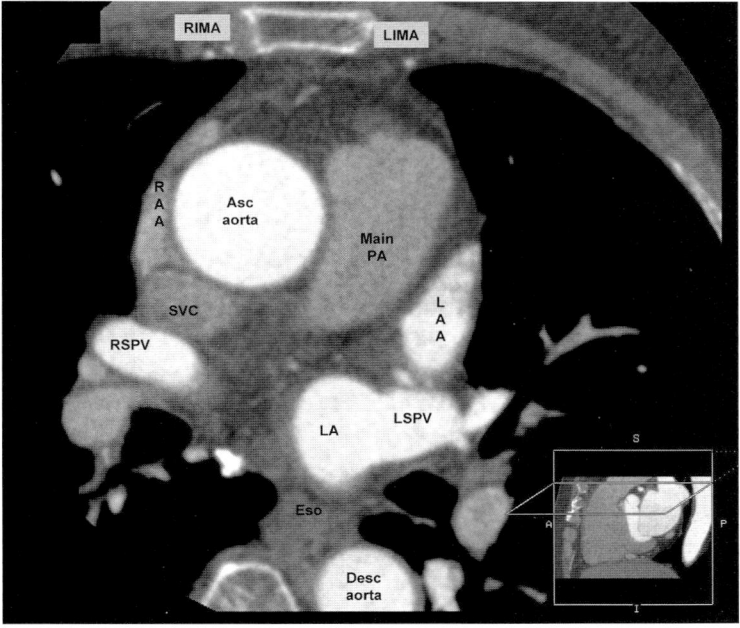

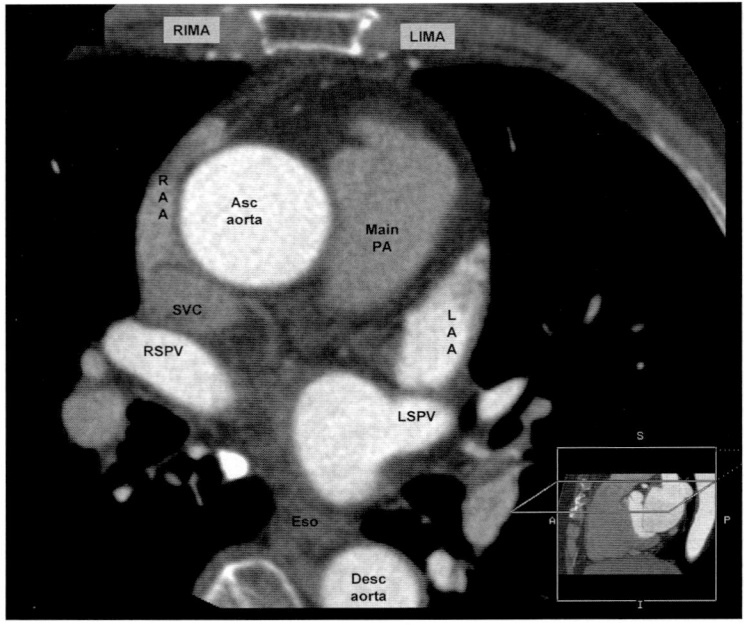

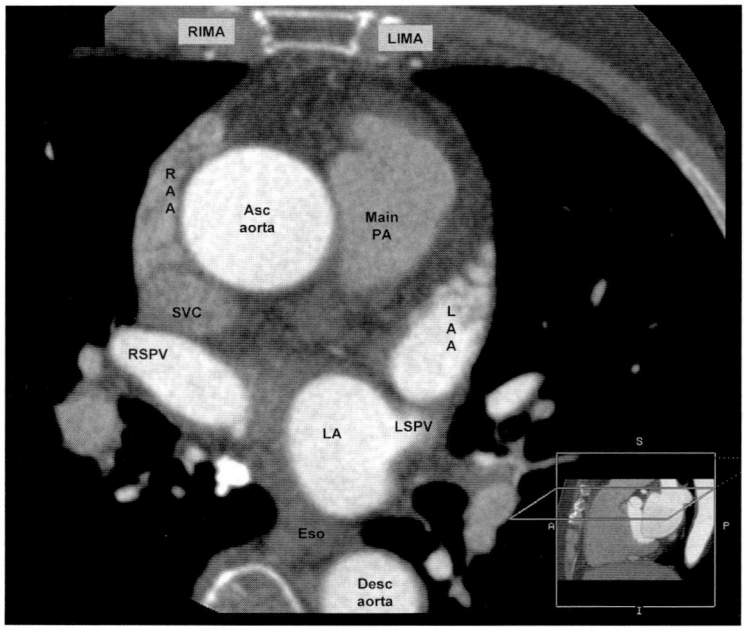

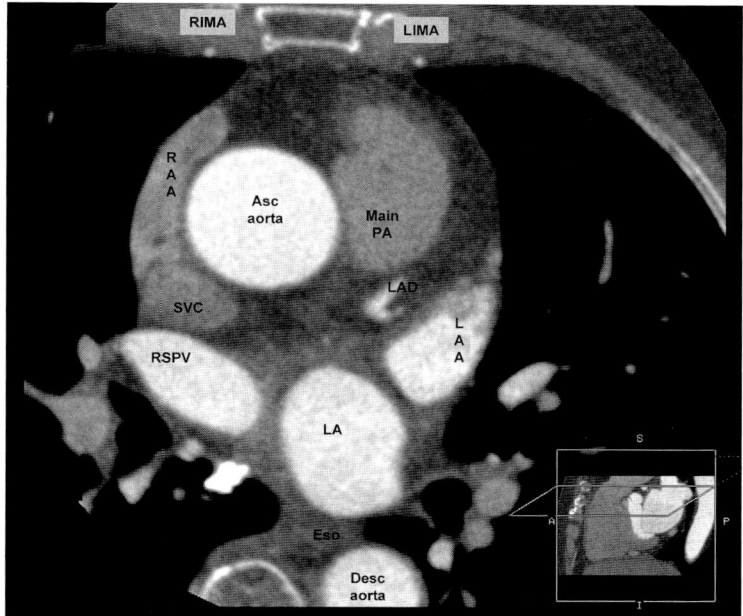

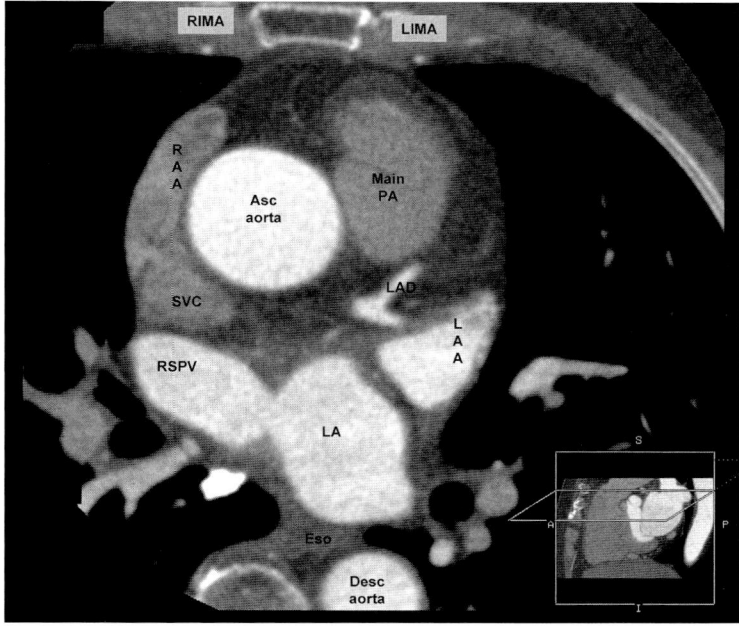

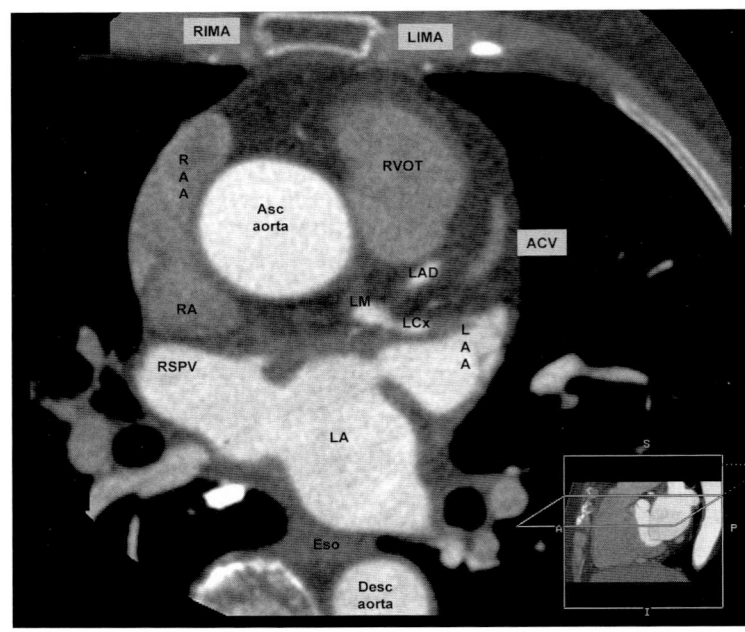

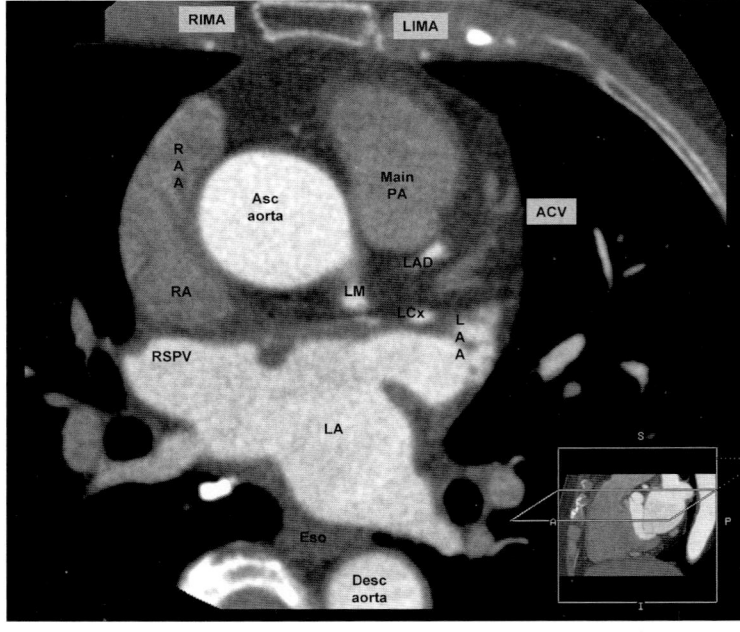

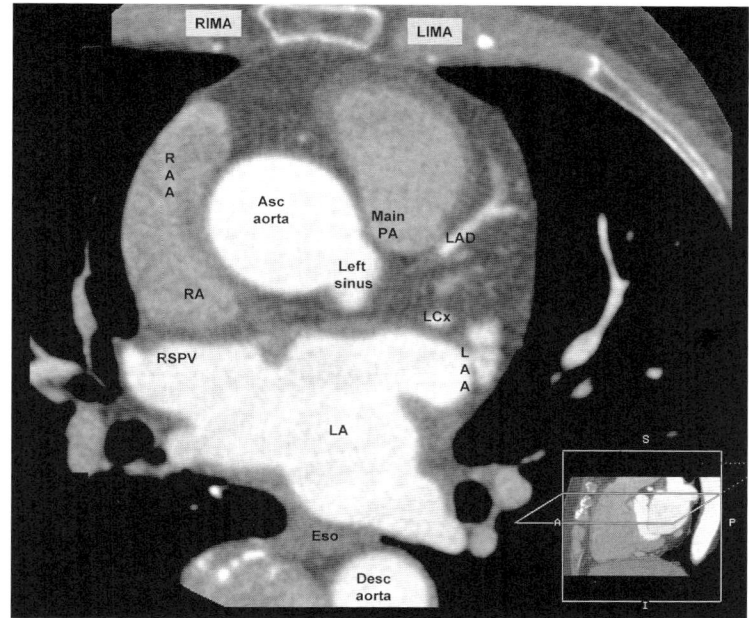

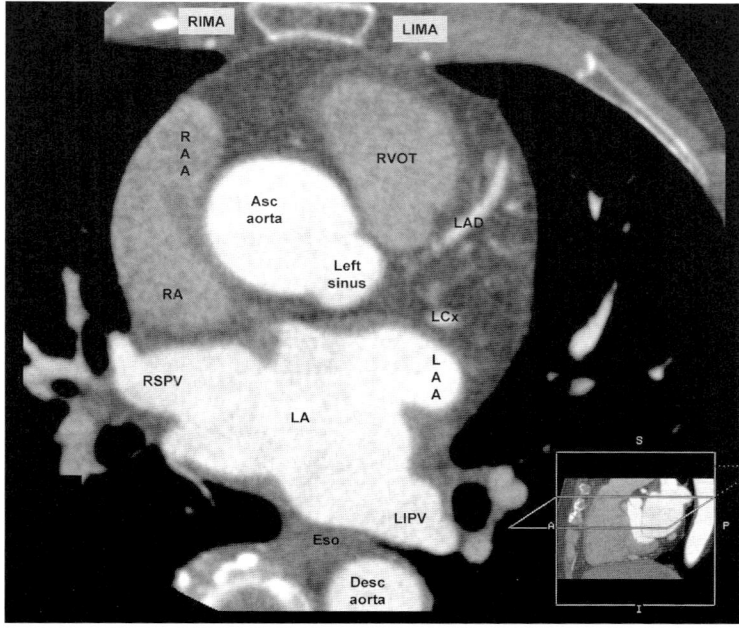

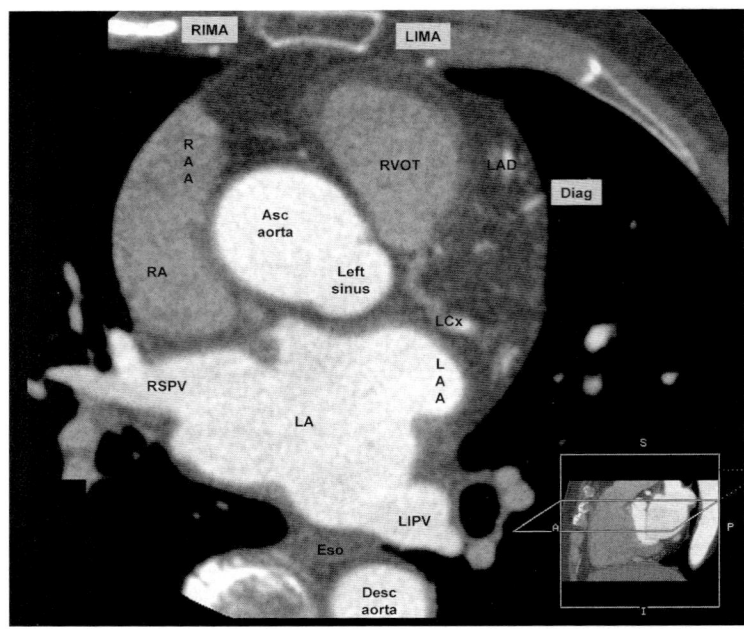

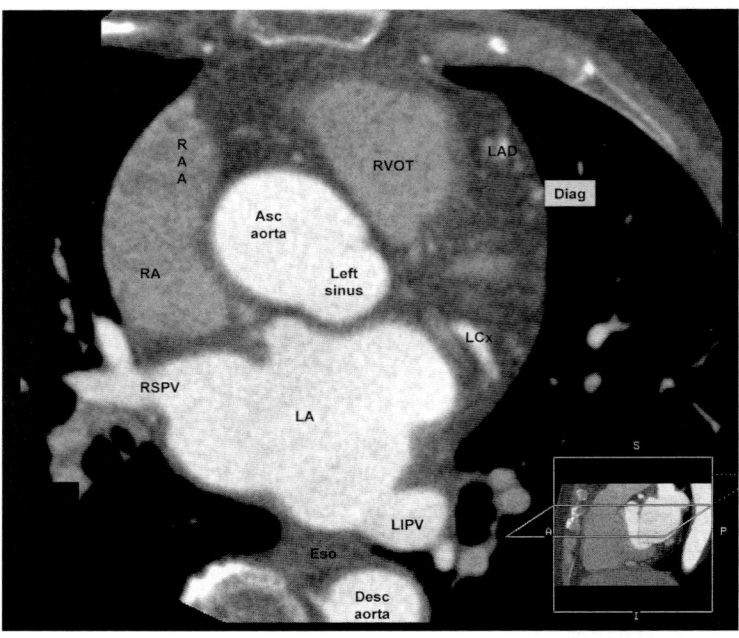

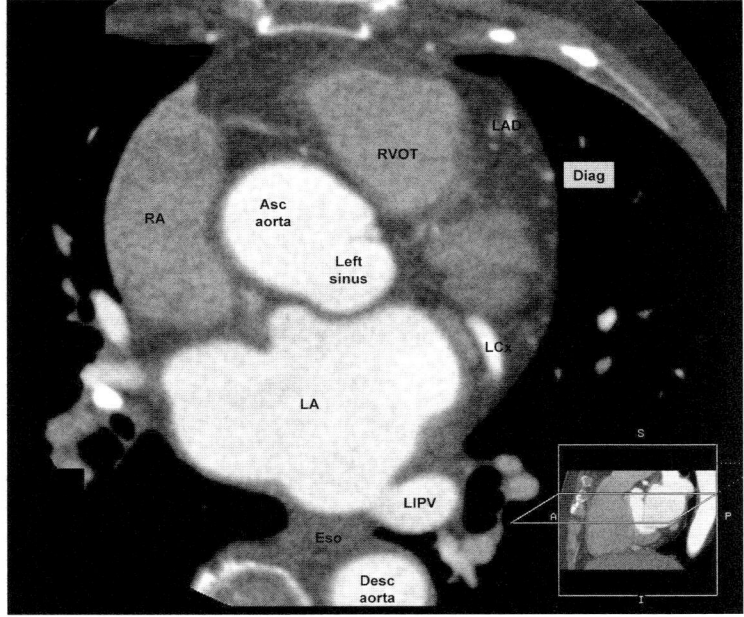

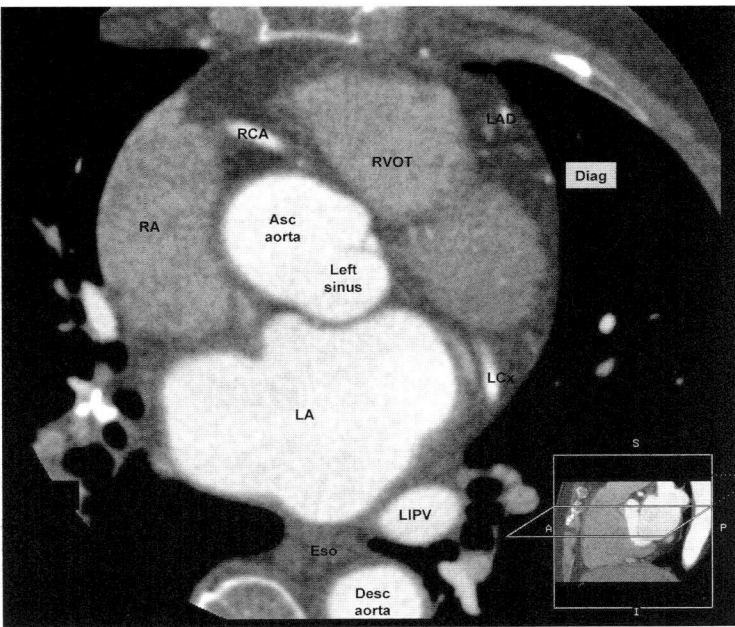

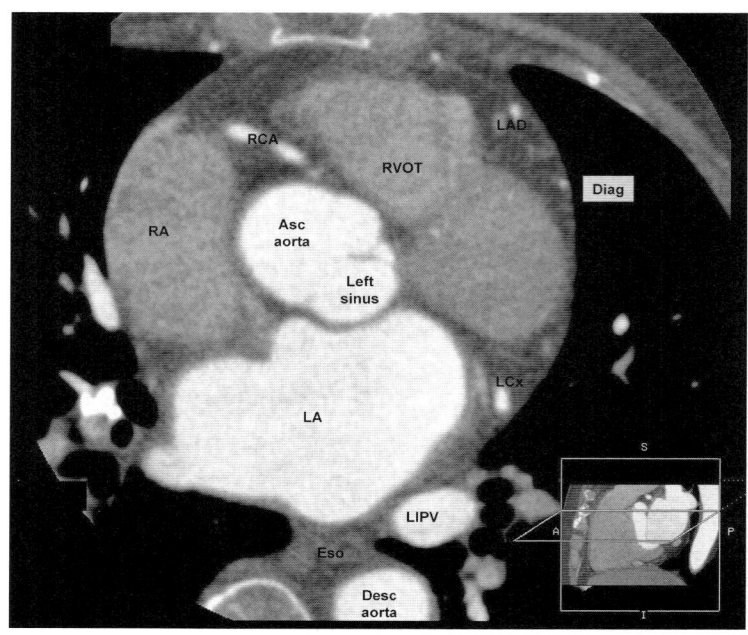

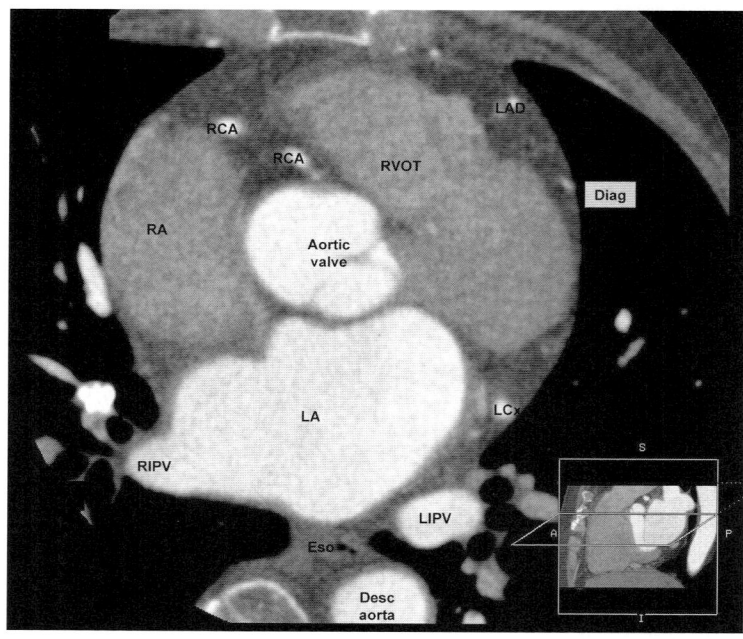

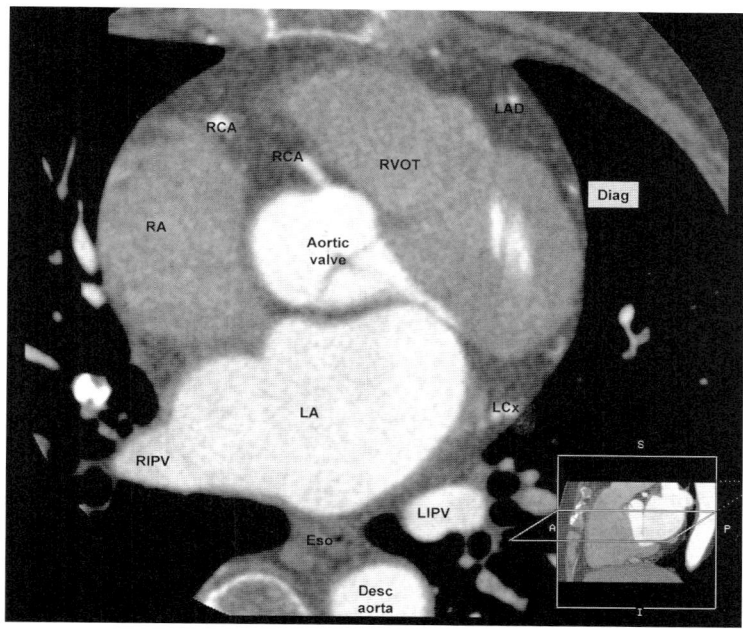

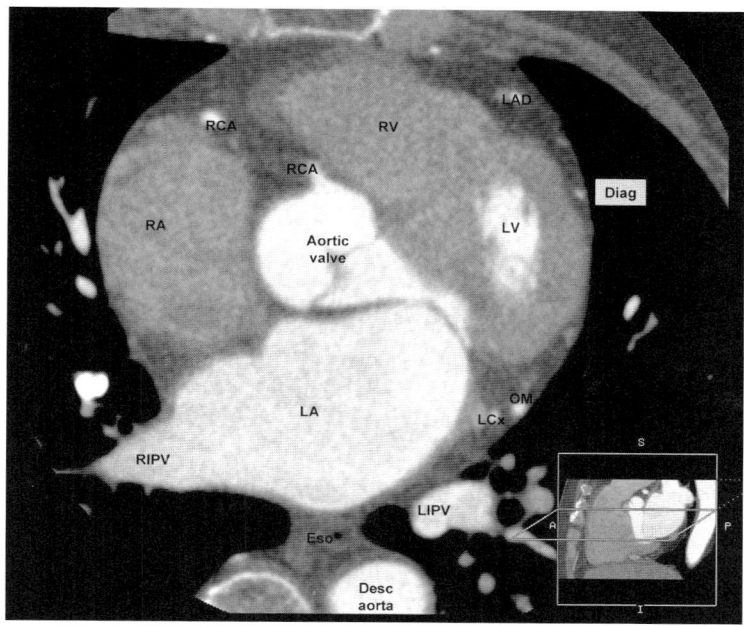

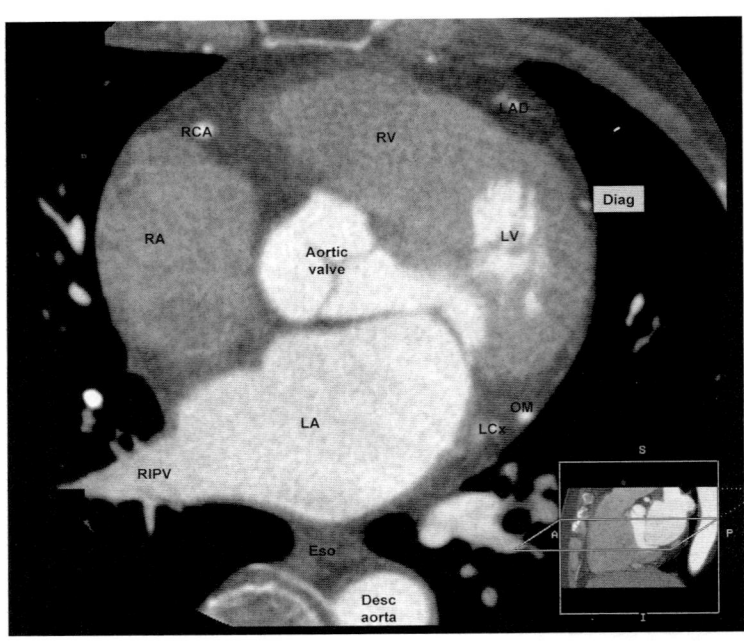

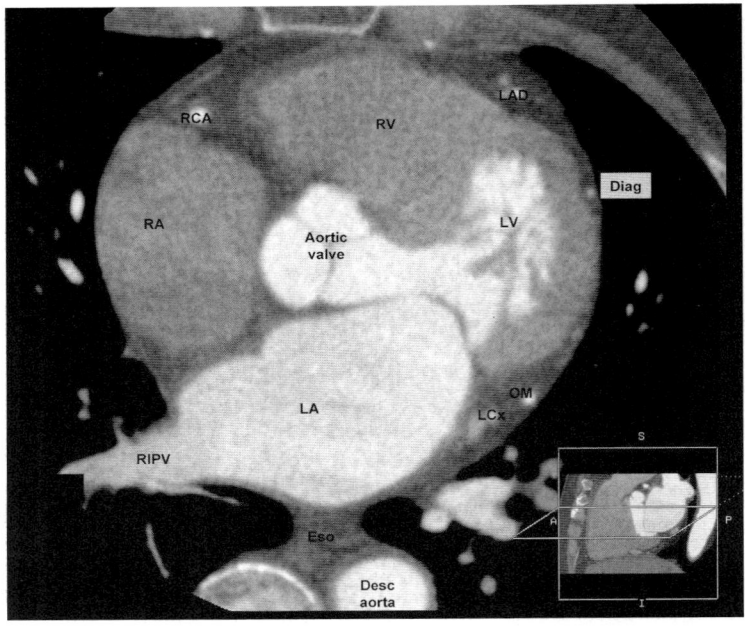

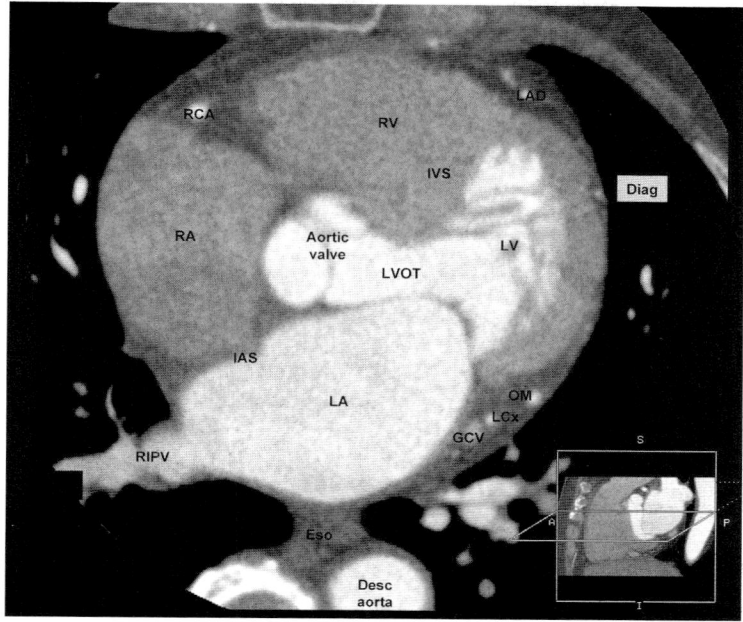

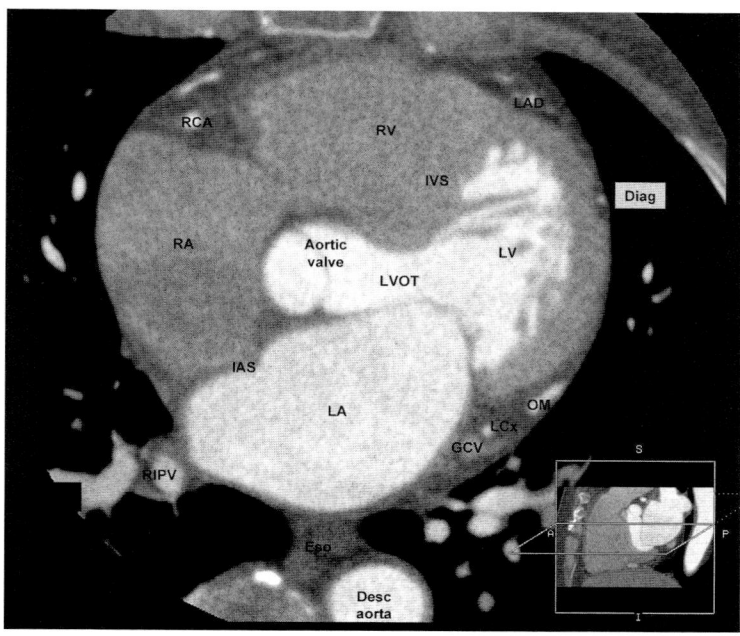

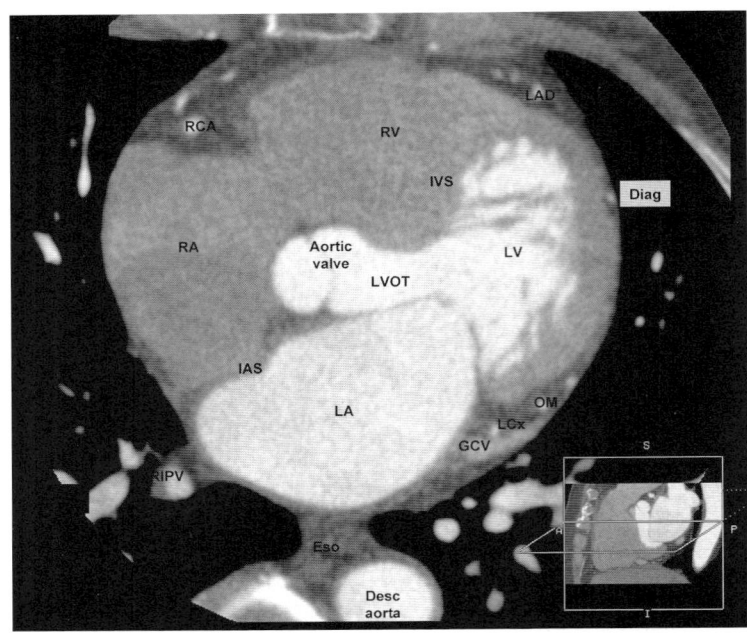

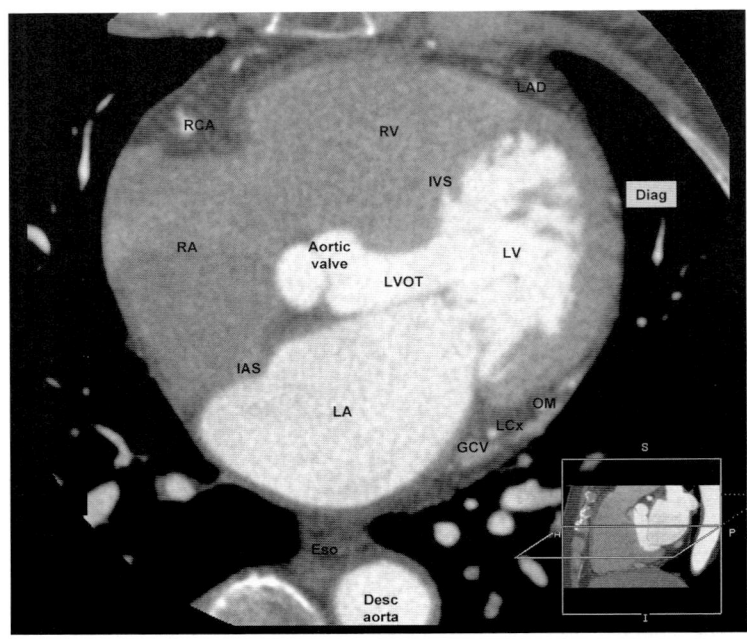

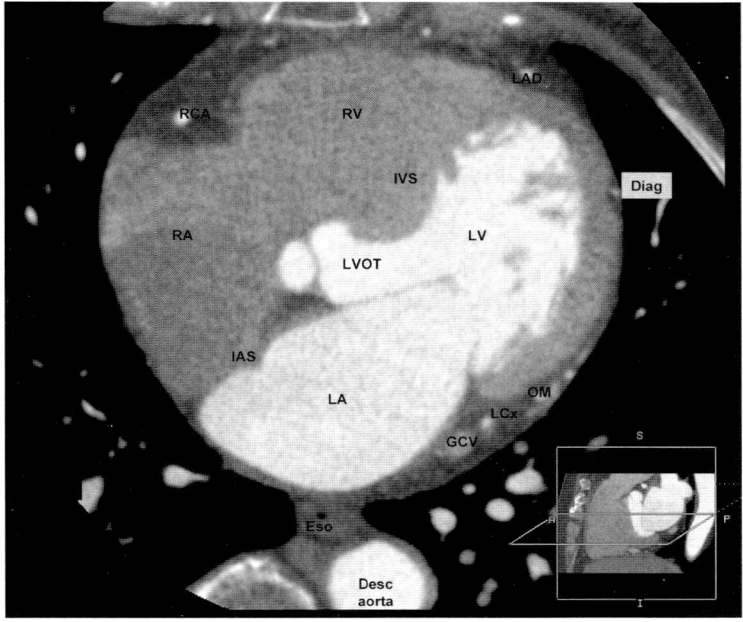

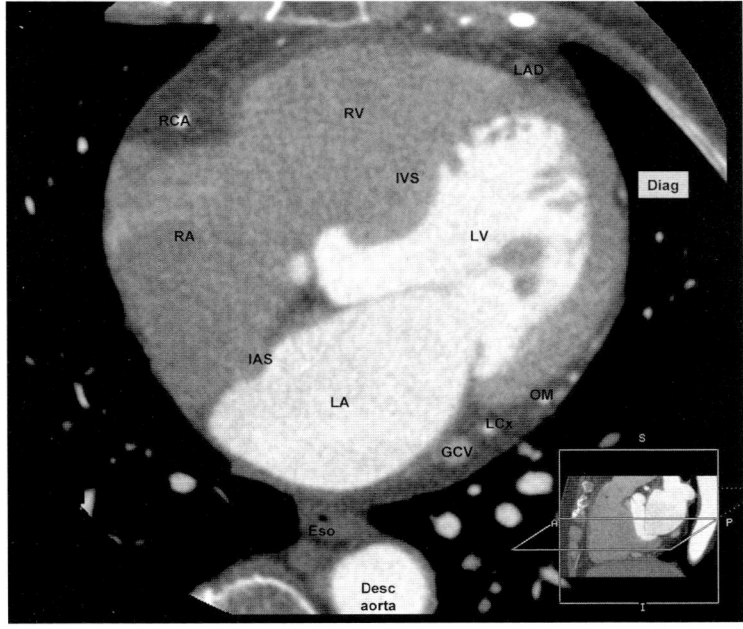

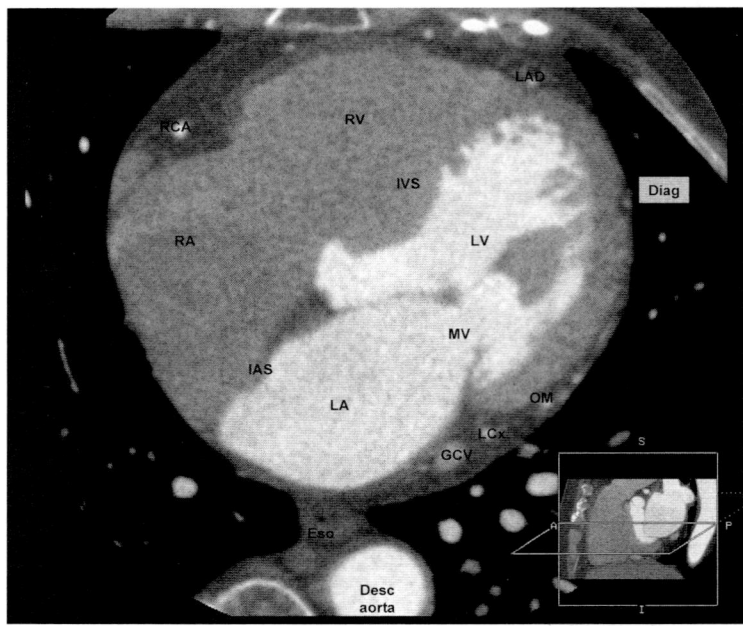

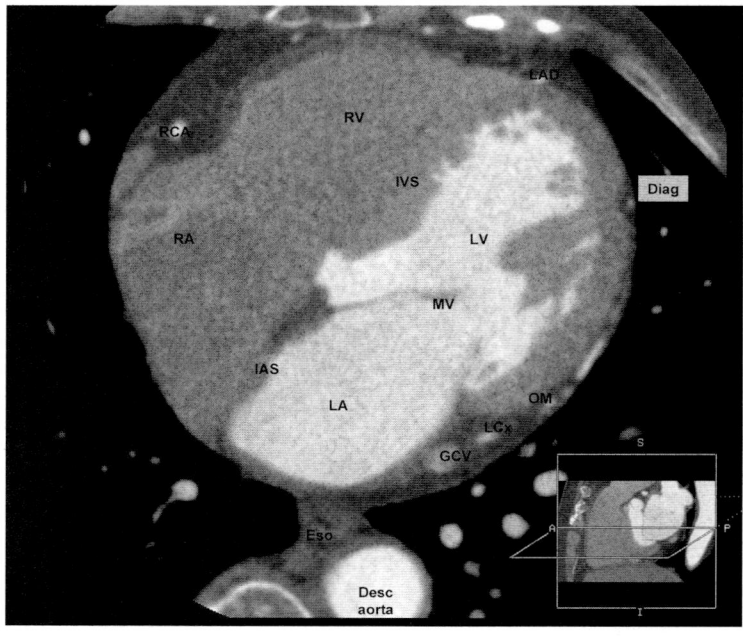

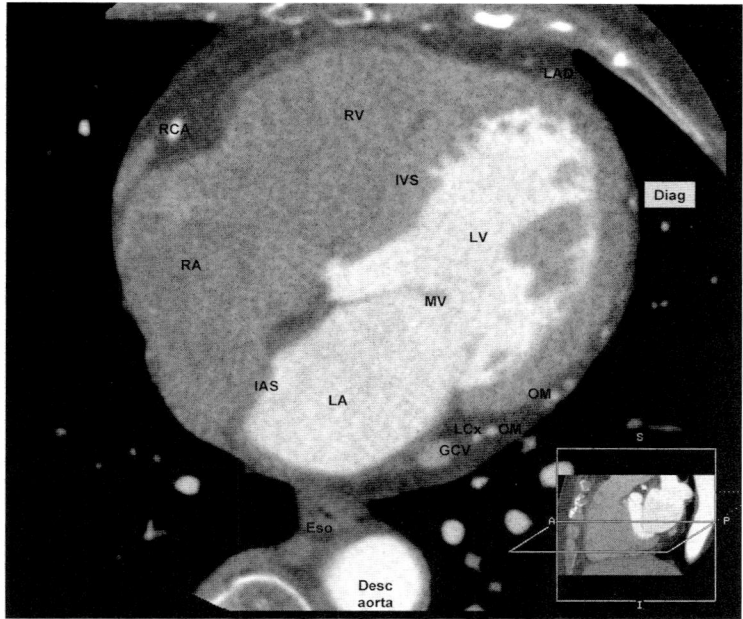

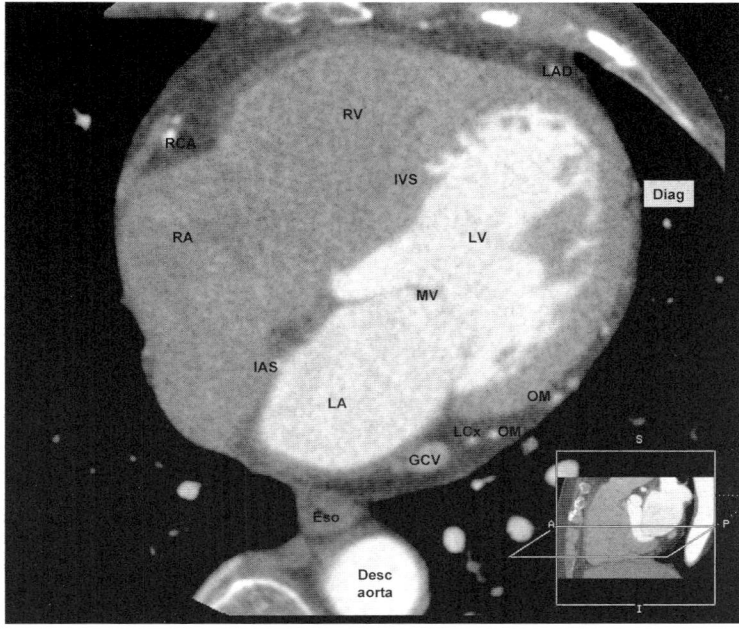

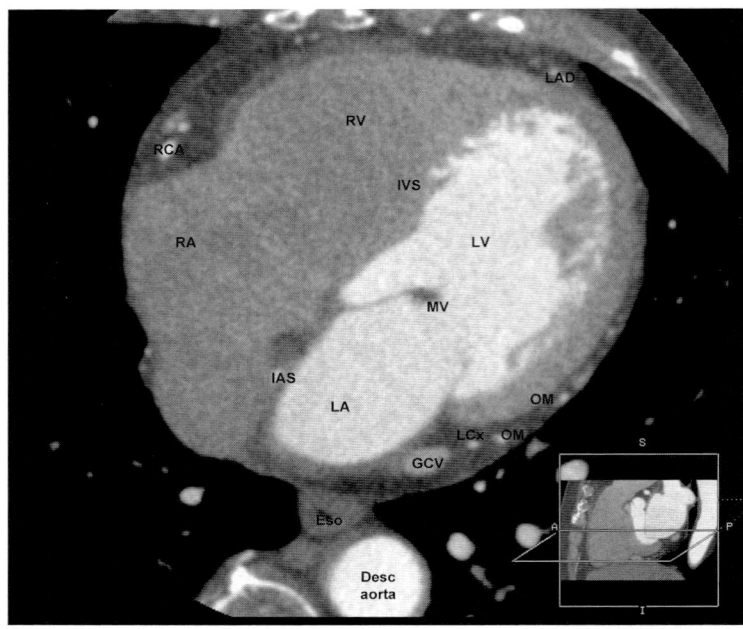

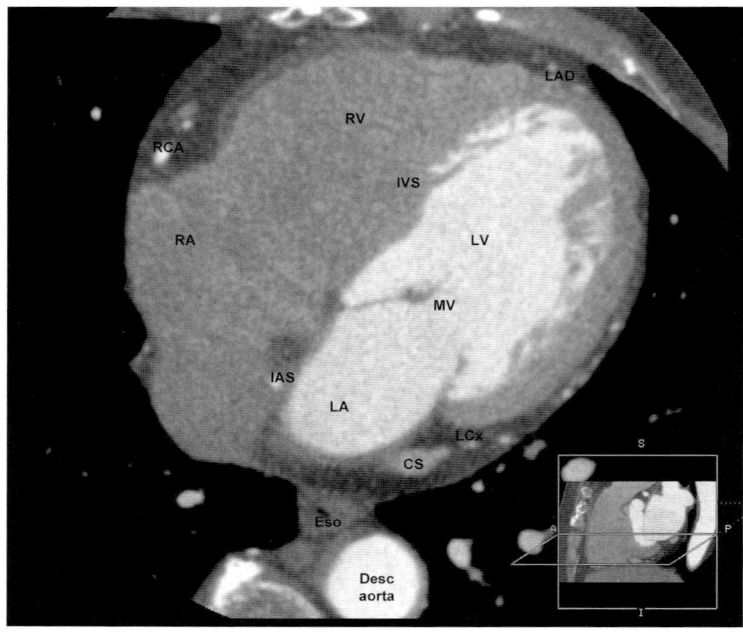

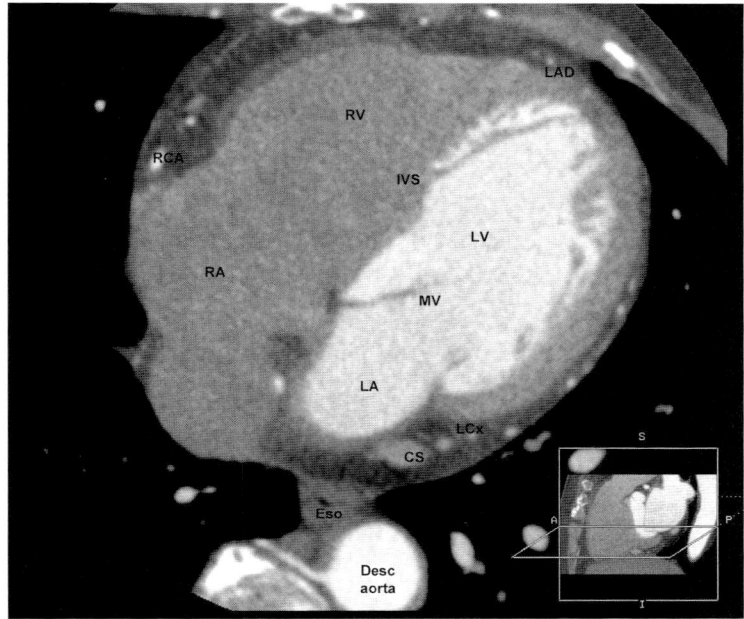

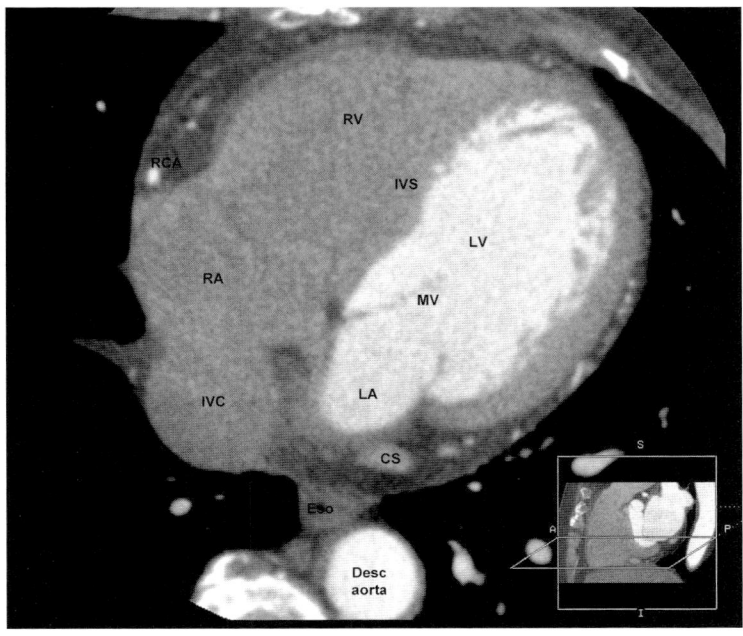

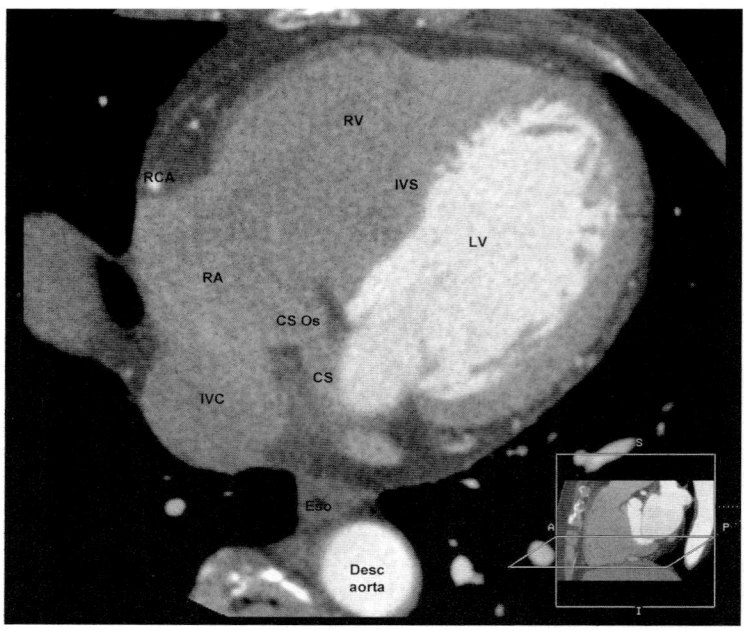

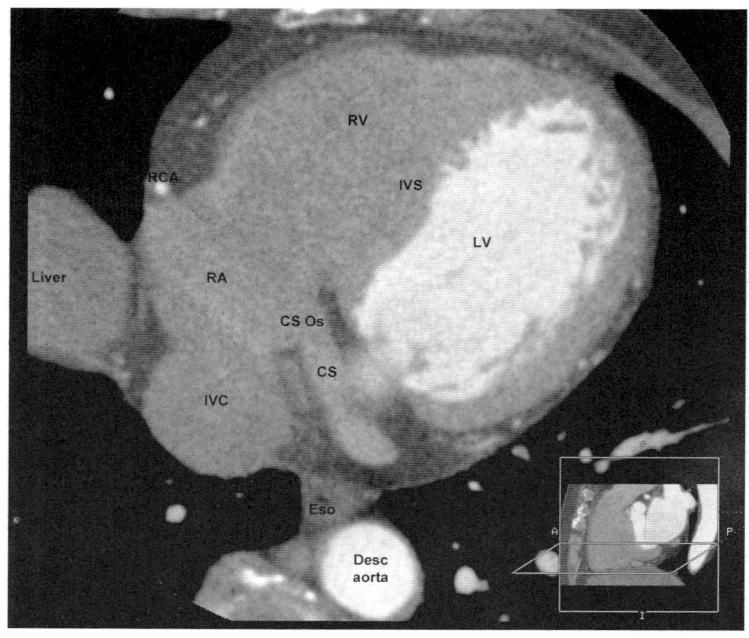

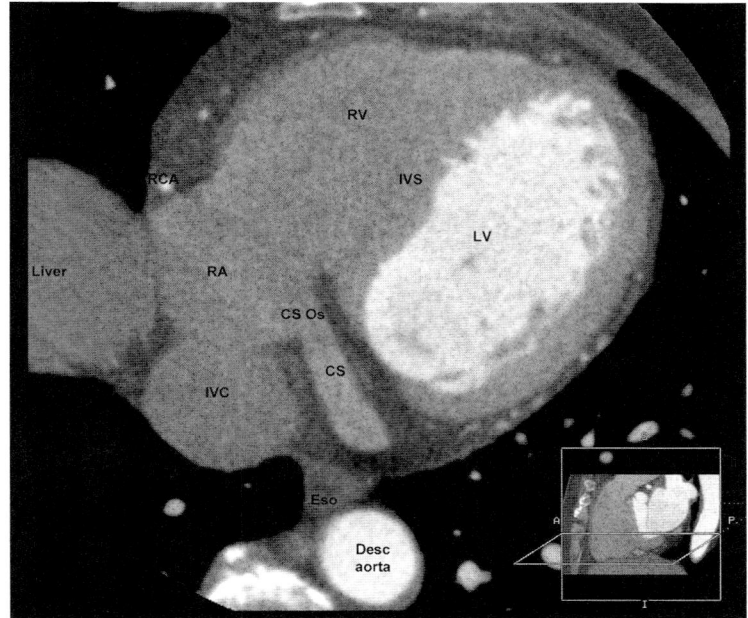

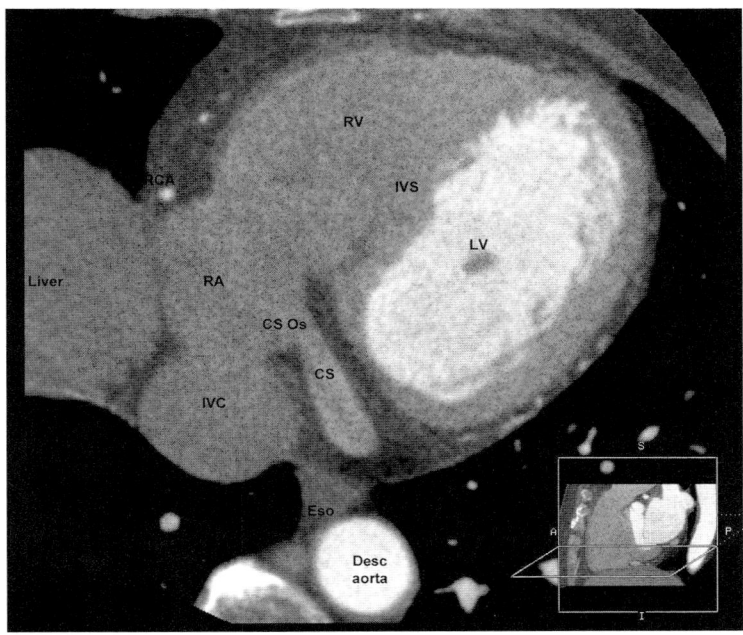

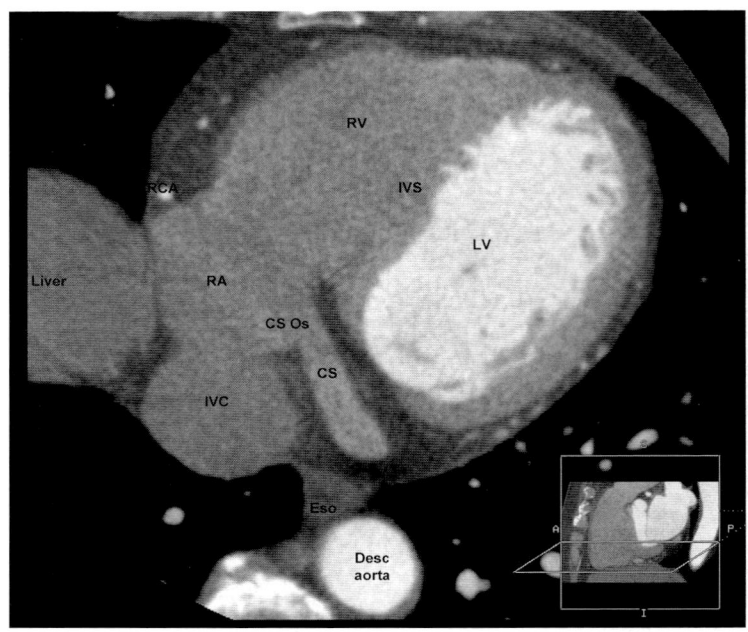

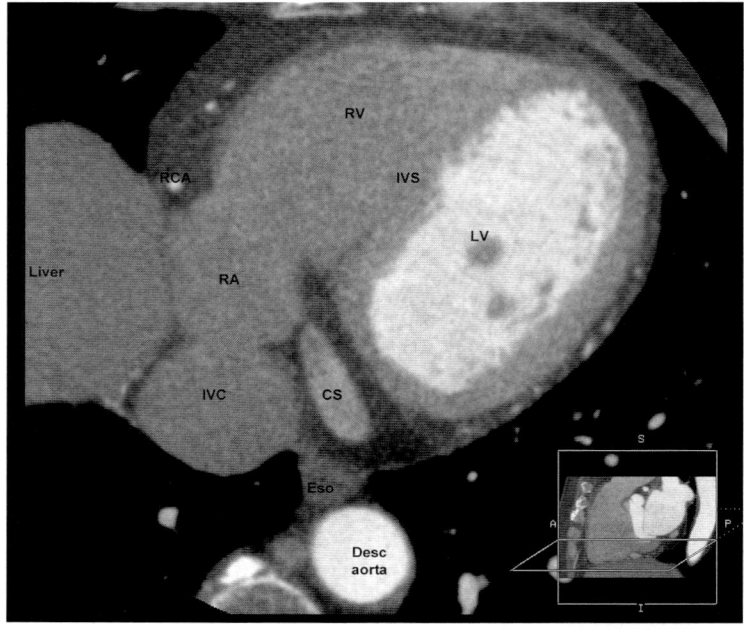

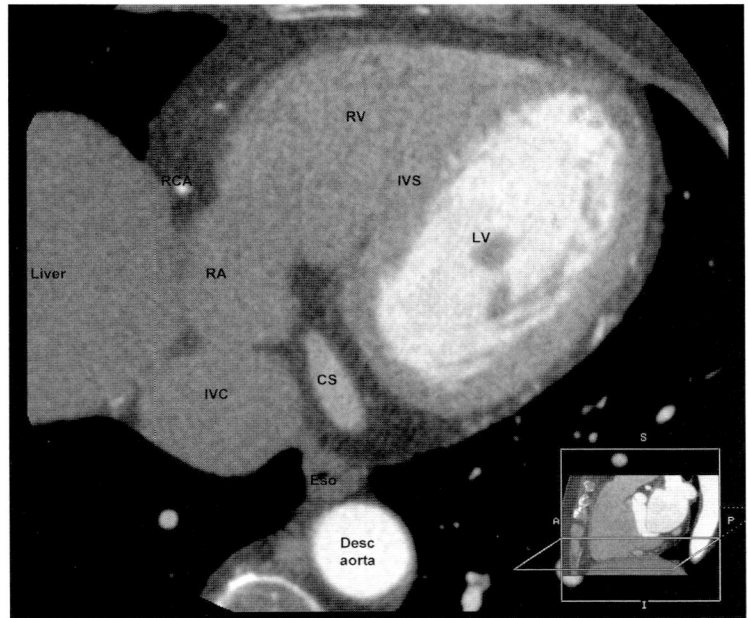

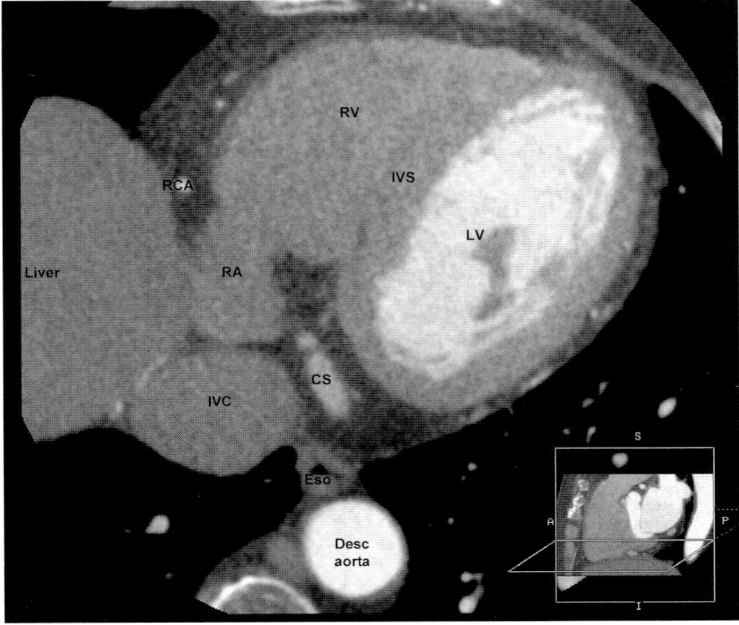

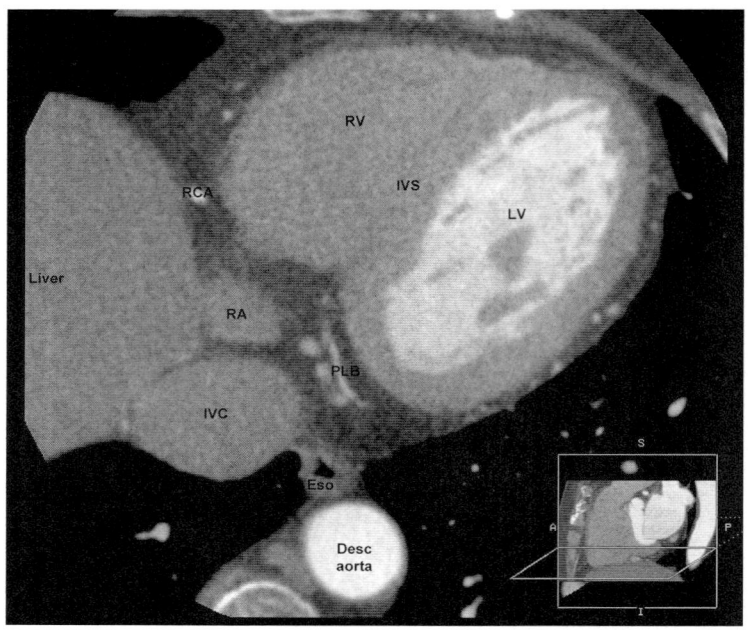

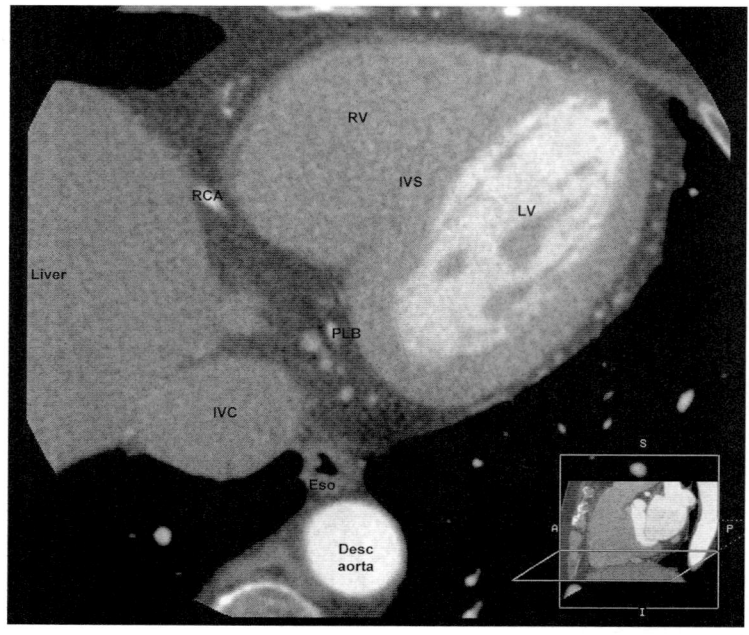

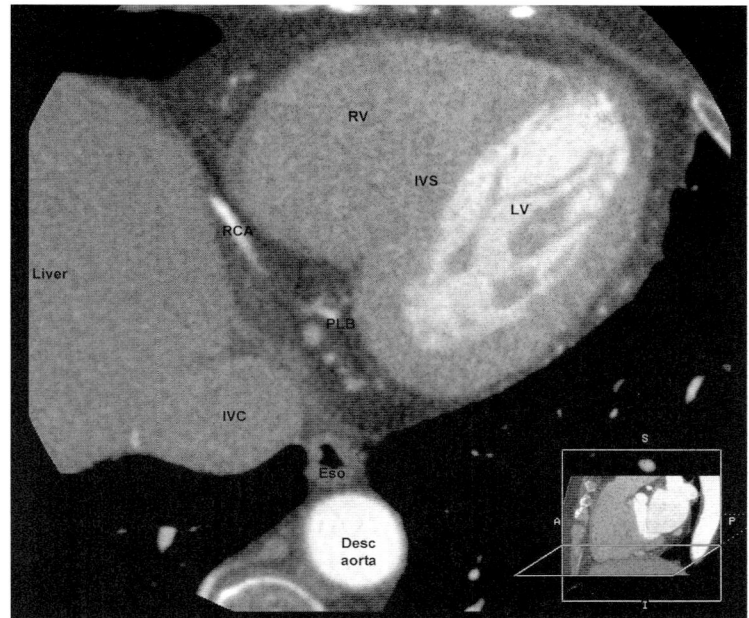

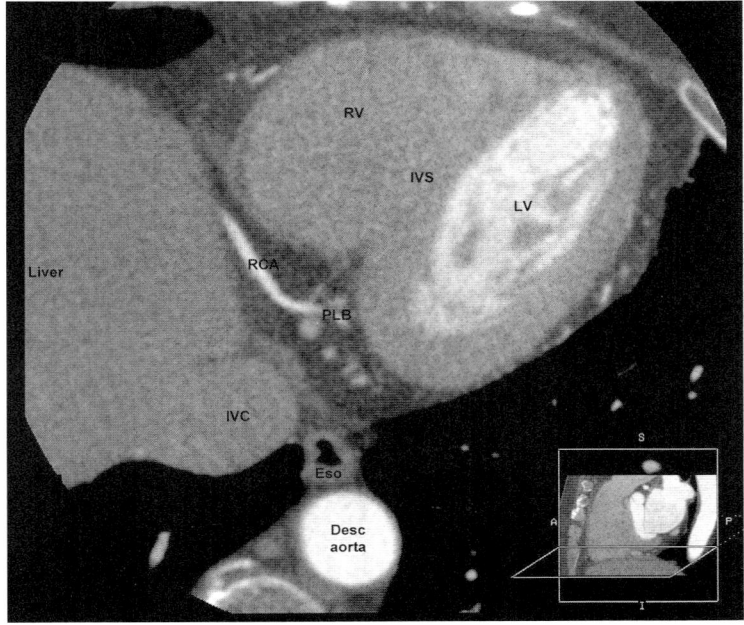

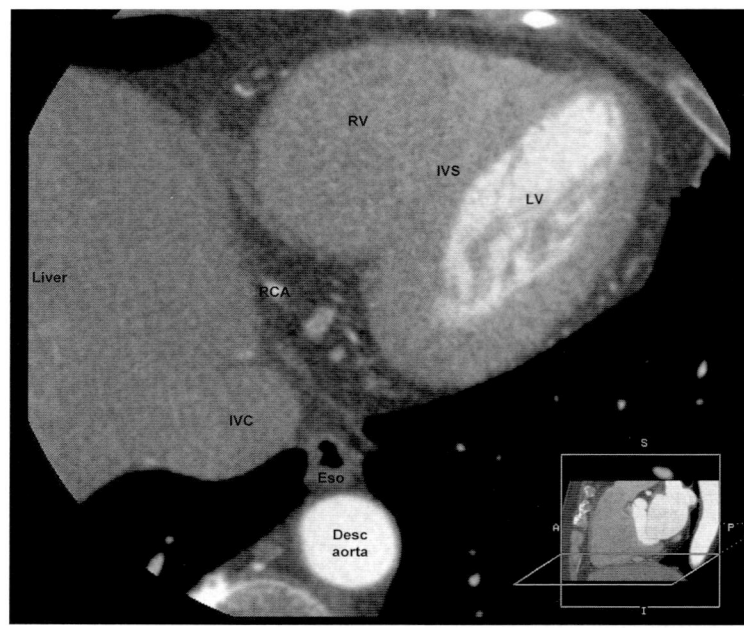

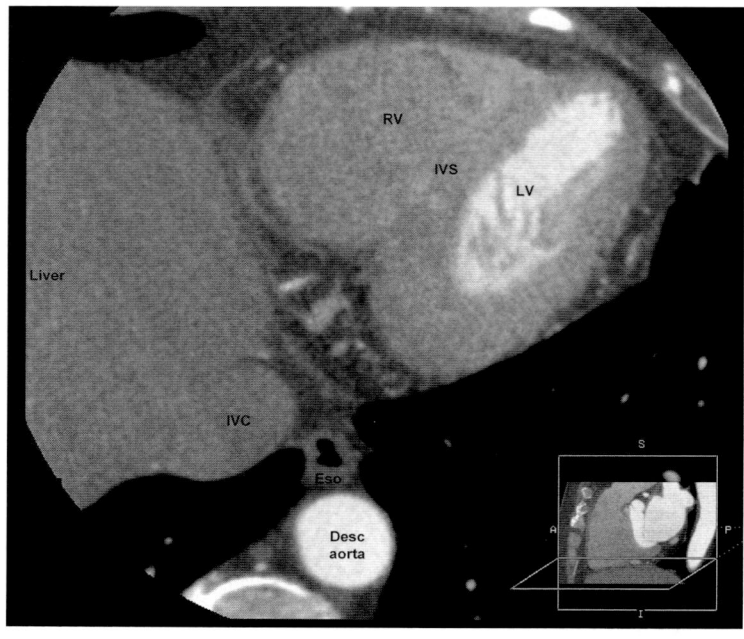

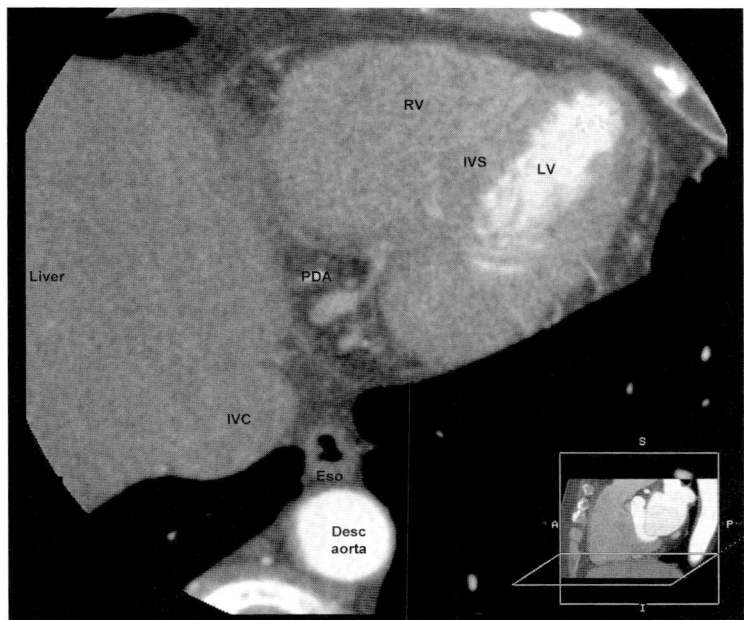

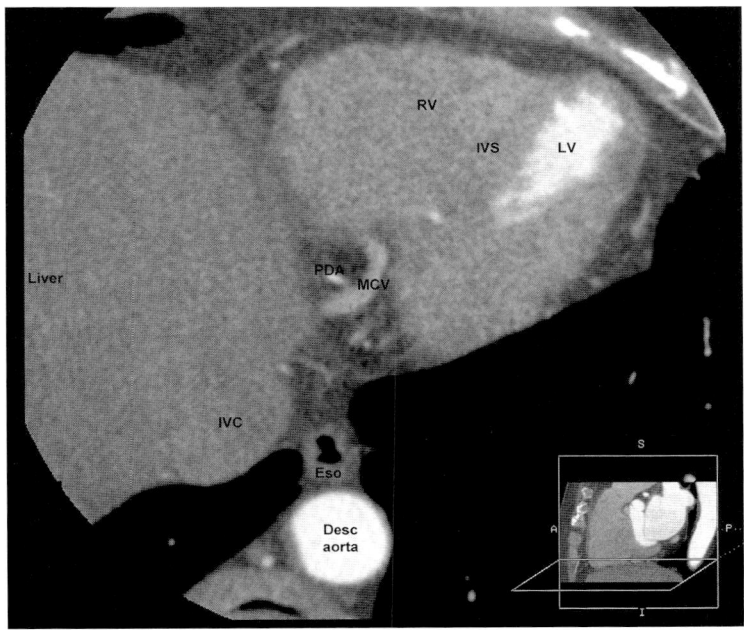

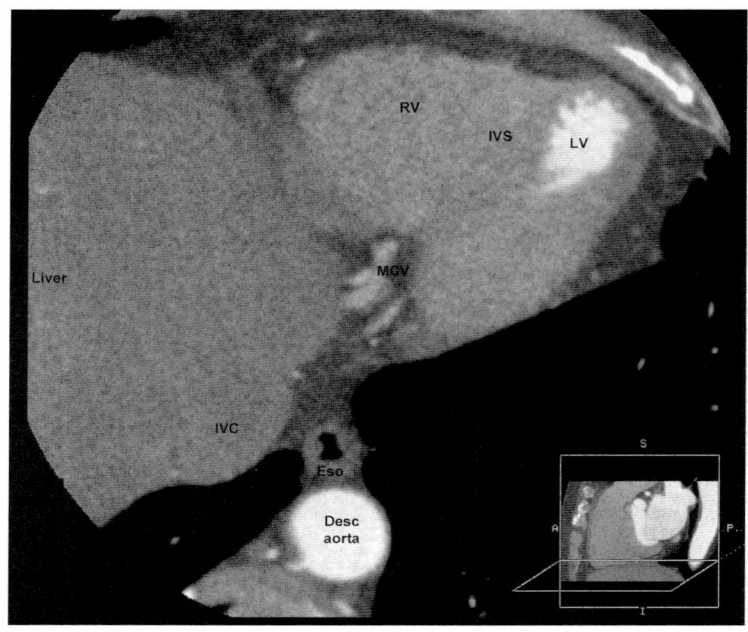

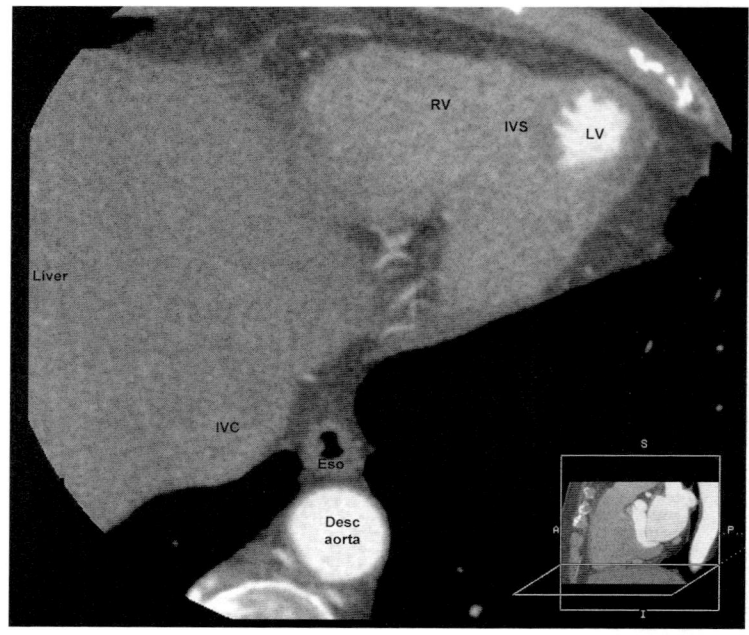

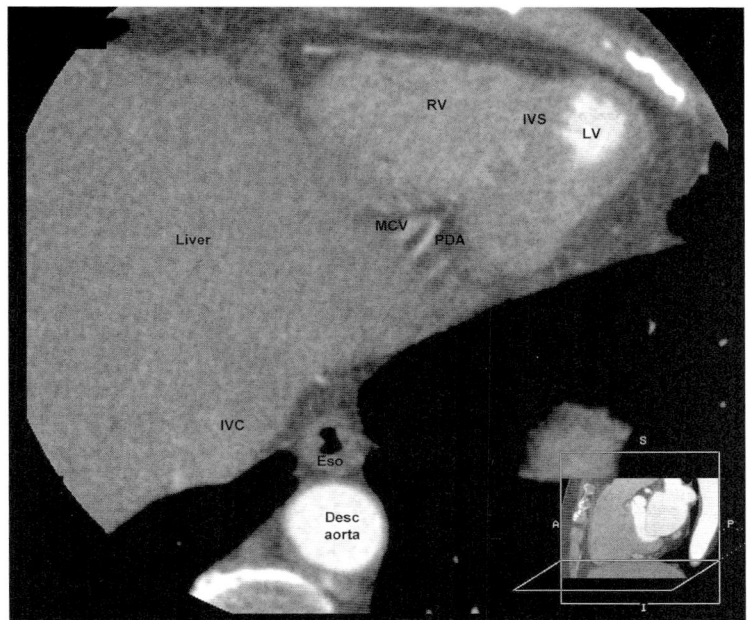

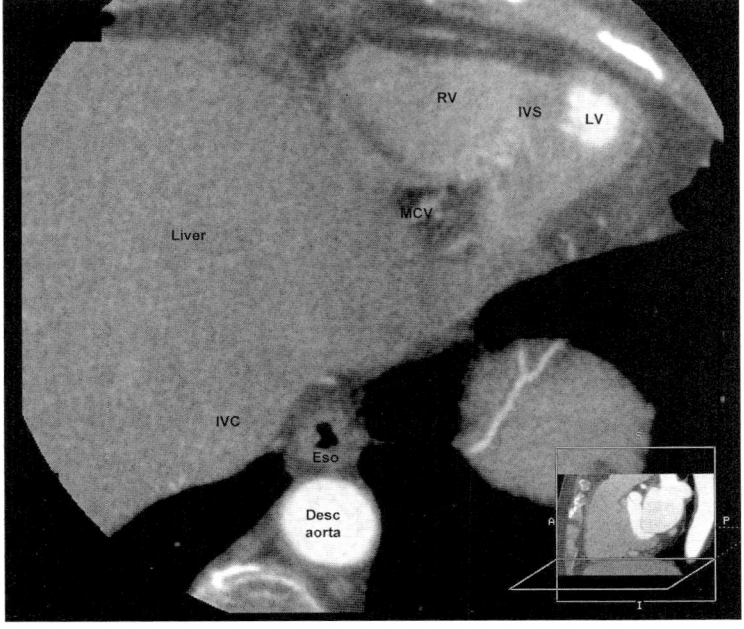

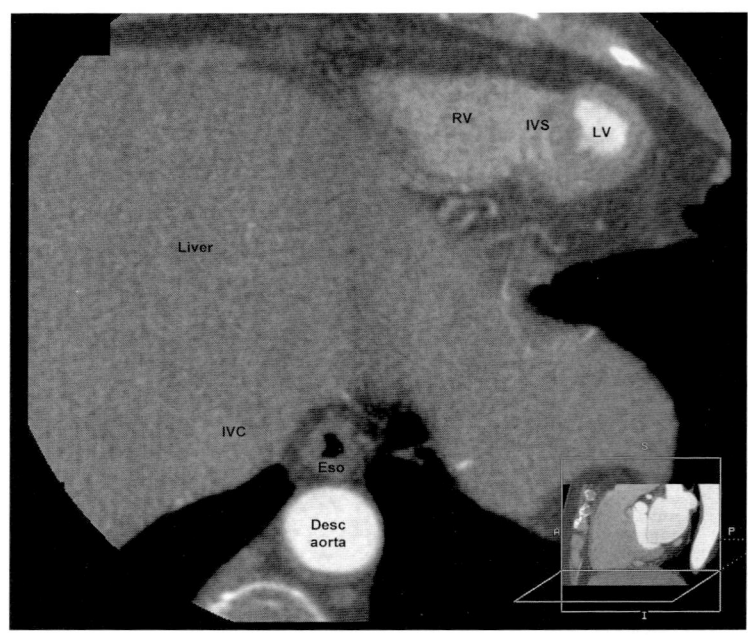

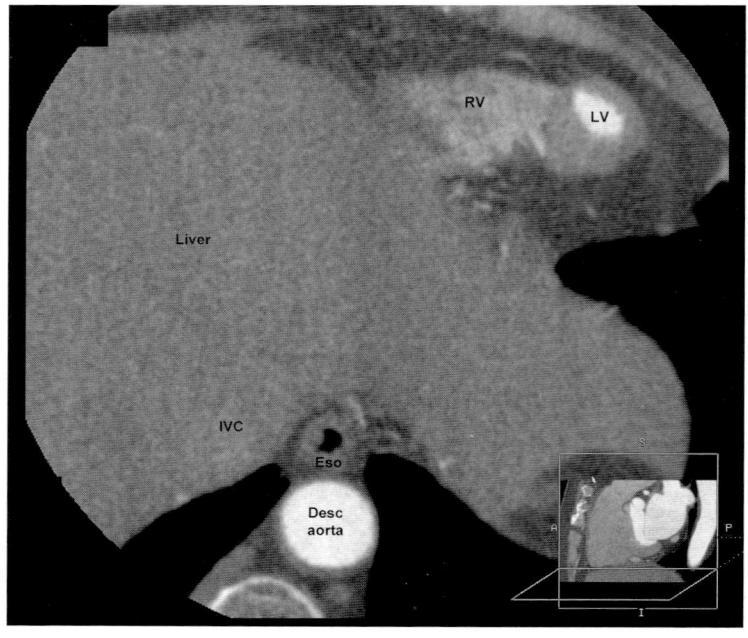

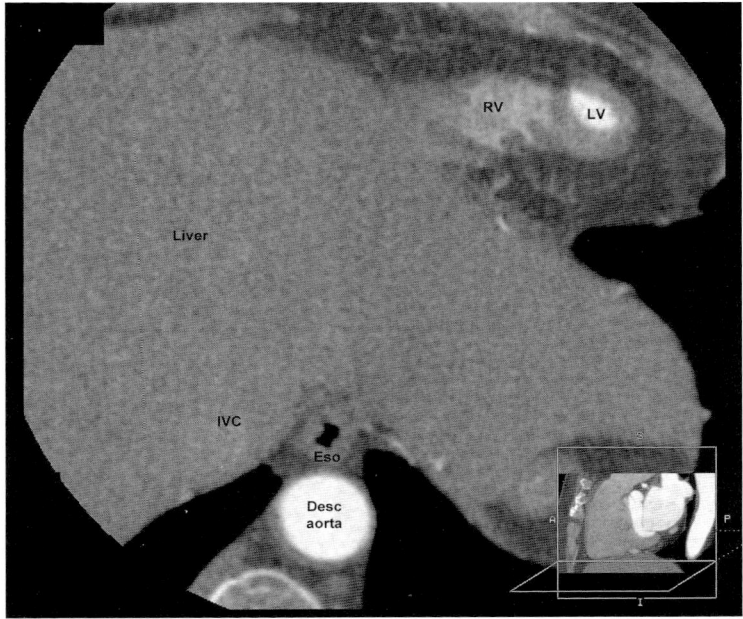

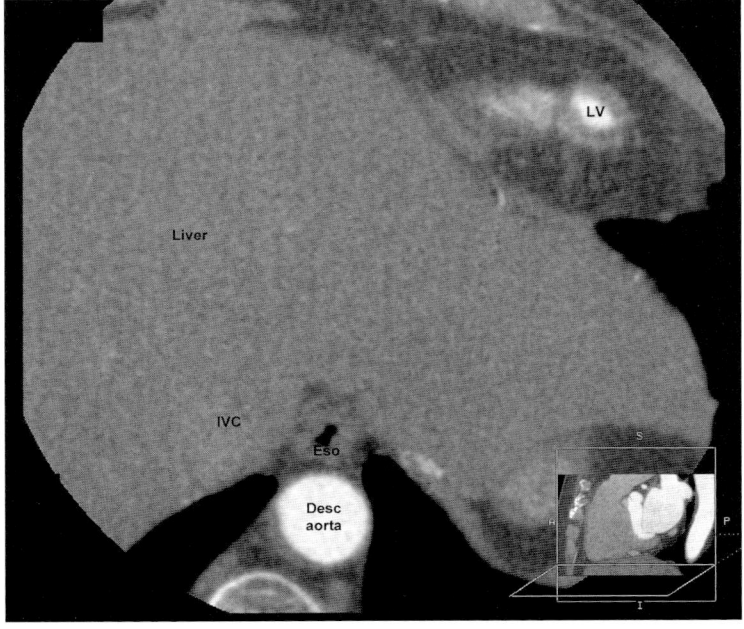

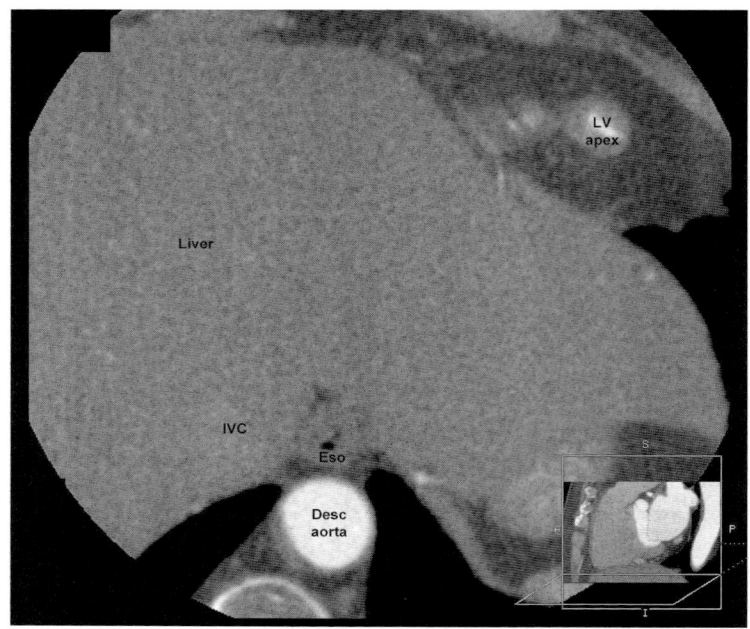

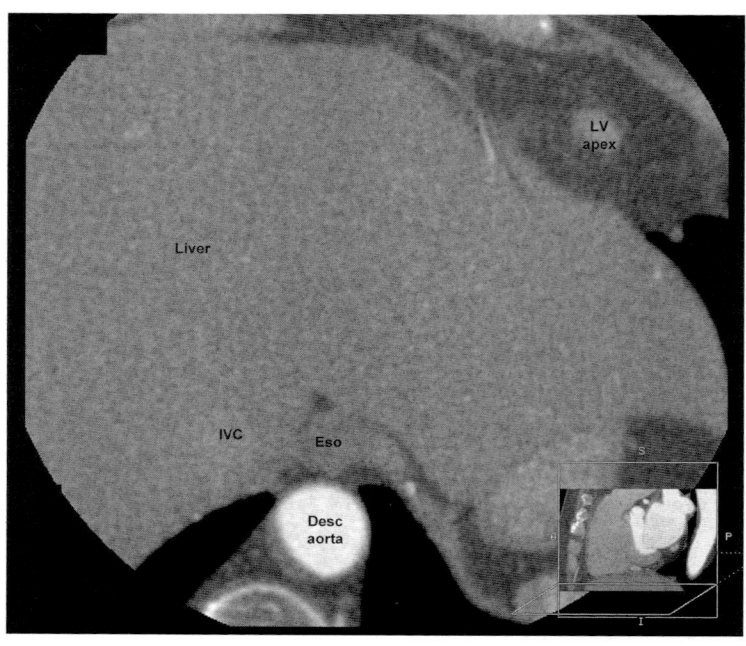

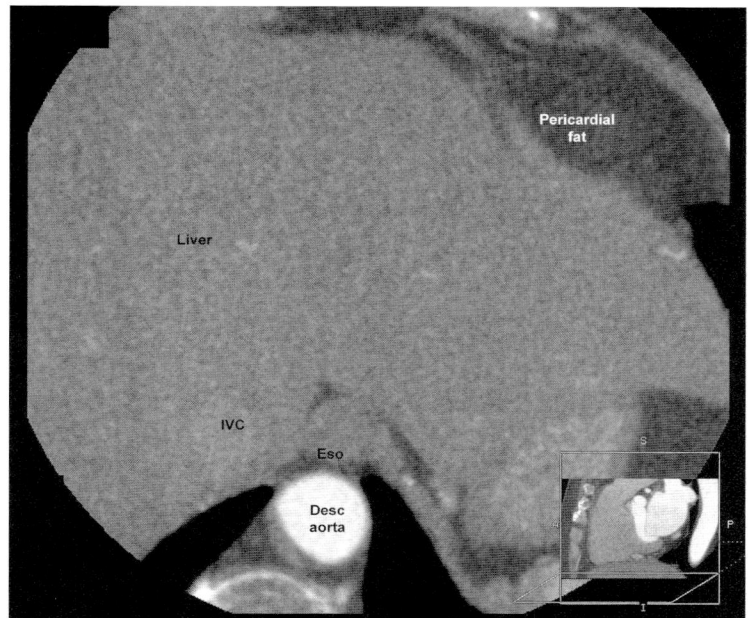

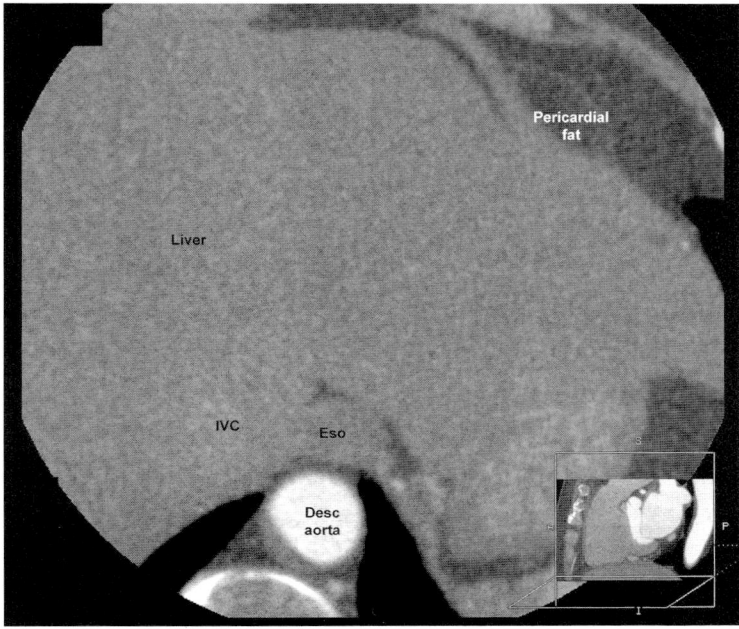

Index

Printed in the United States